TØ146112

Revitalization: Explorations in World Christian Movements
Pentecostal and Charismatic Studies
Series Editor—J. Steven O'Malley
Sub-Series Editor—D. William Faupel

1. *Who Healeth All Thy Diseases: Health, Healing, and
   Holiness in the Church of God Reformation Movement*, by
   Michael S. Stephens, 2008.

REVITALIZATION: EXPLORATIONS IN WORLD CHRISTIAN MOVEMENTS

This volume is published in collaboration with the Center for the Study of World Christian Revitalization Movements, a cooperative initiative of Asbury Theological Seminary faculty. Building on the work of the previous Wesleyan/Holiness Studies Center at the Seminary, the Center provides a focus for research in the Wesleyan holiness and other related Christian renewal movements, including Pietism and Pentecostal movements, which have had a world impact. The research seeks to develop analytical models of these movements, including their biblical and theological assessment. Using an interdisciplinary approach, the Center bridges relevant discourses in several areas in order to gain insights for effective Christian mission globally. It recognizes the need for conducting research that combines insights from the history of evangelical renewal and revival movements with anthropological and religious studies literature on revitalization movements. It also networks with similar or related research and study centers around the world, in addition to sponsoring its own research projects.

Michael Stephens's study of divine healing in the Church of God (Anderson) contributes to the knowledge of the proto-Pentecostal features of the holiness revival, with focus on one of the earliest and most influential radical holiness movements. It also offers important insights for understanding health reform in nineteenth century North America. For these reasons, it demonstrates congruence with the mission of the Center and serves to advance its research objectives.

J. Steven O'Malley, Director
Center for the Study of World Christian Revitalization Movements
Asbury Theological Seminary

WHO HEALETH ALL THY DISEASES

Health, Healing, and Holiness in the Church of God Reformation Movement

MICHAEL S. STEPHENS

*Revitalization: Explorations in World Christian Movements
Pentecostal and Charismatic Studes, No. 1*

The Scarecrow Press, Inc.
Lanham, Maryland • Toronto • Plymouth, UK
and
The Center for the Study of World Christian
Revitalization Movements
2008

SCARECROW PRESS, INC.

Published in the United States of America
by Scarecrow Press, Inc.
A wholly owned subsidary of
The Rowman & Littlefield Publishing Group, Inc.
4501 Forbes Boulevard, Suite 200, Lanham, Maryland 20706
www.scarecrowpress.com

Estover Road
Plymouth PL6 7PY
United Kingdom

British Library Cataloguing in Publication Information Available

Library of Congress Cataloging-in-Publication Data

Stephens, Michael S. (Michael Stanley)
  Who healeth all thy diseases : health, healing, and holiness in the Church of God
reformation movement / Michael S. Stephens.
    p. cm. — (Revitalization. Pentecostal and charismatic studies ; no. 1)
  Includes bibliographical references (p.   ) and index.
  ISBN-13: 978-0-8108-5840-4 (pbk. : alk. paper)
  ISBN-10: 0-8108-5840-1 (pbk. : alk. paper)
  eISBN-13: 978-0-8108-6270-8
  eISBN-10: 0-8108-6270-0
  1. Healing—Religious aspects—Christianity. 2. Spiritual healing. 3. Church of
God (Anderson, Ind.)—History. I. Title.
  BT732.2.S74 2008
  234'.1310882899—dc22   2008005097

♾™ The paper used in this publication meets the minimum requirements of
American National Standard for Information Sciences—Permanence of
Paper for Printed Library Materials, ANSI/NISO Z39.48-1992.
Manufactured in the United States of America.

For my parents
Stan and Christie Stephens

and my grandparents
B.R. and Pearl Smith
LaVerne and Jean Stephens

CONTENTS

THE PENTECOSTAL AND CHARISMATIC
SUB-SERIES

Of all the renewal traditions that have engaged the theological landscape, the Pentecostal Movement has undoubtedly made the most significant impact since it emerged at the turn of the twentieth century. Starting as a revival in a small African-American congregation on Azusa Street in Los Angeles, California, the movement soon swept the world, establishing itself in more than forty countries in the first three years. One hundred years later Pentecostalism has grown to an estimated 250 million global adherents or approximately twenty-five percent of all of Christendom. In the same manner that Wesleyanism burst beyond the bounds of Methodism to embrace an interdenominational holiness movement following the American Civil War in the nineteenth century, Pentecostalism transcended denominational lines in the form of the Charismatic Movement during the second half of the twentieth Century.

This sub-series is designed to explore the historical, theological, and intercultural dimensions of these twin twentieth-century Restorationist traditions from a global perspective. Included in the sub-series will be a few studies of proto-Pentecostal traditions that fall outside the exclusively Wesleyan/Holiness tradition. Michael Stephens's study of divine healing within the Church of God (Anderson) falls in this later category. As part of the Church of God Restorationists' tradition that began with Winebrenner's group founded in the early nineteenth century sweeping into the twentieth century with such Pentecostal bodies as the Church of God (Cleveland), Church of God of Prophecy, and the Church of God in Christ, the Church of God (Anderson) defined itself over against emerging Pentecostalism. Stephens's study shows that the movement's healing practices and measures of health reform were just as radical and all-embracing as that of early Pentecostalism. Yet, the Church of God (Anderson) abandoned the most controversial of those practices more quickly than did Pentecostalism, leading many to expunge them from its collective memory. Stephens's systematic, perceptive and sympathetic treatment of this dimension of early Church of God (Anderson) history helps to place both this church and Pentecostalism in their appropriate historical/theological contexts.

D. William Faupel
Sub-Series Editor

ACKNOWLEDGMENTS

I thank the Center for the Study of World Christian Revitalization Movements, Steven O'Malley, and Bill Faupel for producing such an interesting series and inviting me to be a part of it. Bill in particular has been a wise counselor through the editing process. I also thank Scarecrow Press. Their reference works about the Holiness and Pentecostal movements were a great help to my research, and now I am pleased to have my work join such a fine publishing house.

April Snider and Jayme Bartles, my editors at Scarecrow, have been everything I could want in editors: careful, patient, encouraging, and well versed in Microsoft Word formatting.

Many fine people have contributed to this project. I especially recognize Dale Johnson. He has been instrumental in every part of this study and has been a conversation partner, editor, and friend. Lewis V. Baldwin, Kathleen Flake, Darren Sherkat, Larry Griffin, and Anthea Butler have improved this study with creative and critical insights.

Friends and colleagues have helped with specific parts of this work, ranging from the theology of sanctification to modern discussions of medicine and religion to getting published. Chris Accornero, David Bundy, James P. Byrd, Barry Callen, Sandra Clark, Donald Dayton, Jack Fitzmier, Leonard Hummel, Charles Jones, Douglas Meeks, Sharon Pearson, Jana Riess, Rick Smith, Merle Strege, and Grant Wacker have given generously of their time and expertise. I also thank the Wesleyan Theological Society, the American Society of Church History, and the Church of God Historical Society for allowing me to present in preliminary form some of the ideas and findings in this book.

This study would not have been possible without the assistance of librarians and archivists. I thank Doug Welch, who granted me the run of the Church of God Archives, and Bill Kostlevy at the B. L. Fisher Library, Asbury Theological Seminary. My thanks also to Trish Janutolo at Nicholson Library, Anderson

University, who let me take a complete set of *Gospel Trumpet*s home to Nashville, albeit on microfilm.

Many family members and friends have supported me and my work through the years. I am grateful to each one of them. I especially thank my parents-in-law, Bill and Pat Harriss, for their love and support. I have dedicated this work to my parents, Stan and Christie Stephens, and my grandparents, Jean and LaVerne Stephens and B. R. and Pearl Smith. They have all been, in one way or another, ministers in the Church of God, although only B. R. has the ordination certificate to prove it. My love and gratitude to them are boundless. Credit for whatever is good about this work ultimately belongs to my family. I'll accept the blame for whatever is not, but I think we all know that the church bears some responsibility.

Most important are my love and thanks to Heather, Daniel, and Emma Anne.

INTRODUCTION

Willis M. Brown converted to Christianity in 1895 after witnessing the divine healing of a child. Brown soon began to feel a call to ministry and started to read the *Gospel Trumpet*, the newspaper of the Church of God Reformation Movement, also known as the Evening Light Reformation.[1] However, his life had been dissolute before his conversion, and years of drinking whiskey had so damaged his stomach that he continued to suffer physical debility even after his religious experience removed his taste for drink. An old remedy of soda and vinegar exacerbated his condition, but prayer brought a complete healing, and clean living kept him healthy and strong.[2] Brown and his eleven-year-old son Charles became evangelists in the autumn of 1895 and gained reputations for miraculous healing. According to a notice from the *Paducah News*, people from Kentucky, Tennessee, and Illinois converged on Paducah, Kentucky, for the Browns' revival: "Over 1,000 asked for prayers, above 800 freely declared themselves benefited, and half as many more left their crutches as a legacy of thanksgiving."[3]

In 1902, the Browns officially affiliated with the Church of God, and Willis attended the national camp meeting where over eighty ministers signed a statement asserting that divine healing was an essential part of the gospel that had to be preached and practiced by every minister. Despite his protests that he was new to the movement and was there to learn, the brethren convinced him to address the camp on the subject of divine healing.[4] Two years later, the Gospel Trumpet Company published Brown's autobiography, highlighting his healing ministry and showing how his radical change of life—from infidelity to Christianity—brought him health and happiness.[5]

In 1951, Willis's son Charles concluded his twenty-one-year tenure as the editor of the *Gospel Trumpet* by publishing the first history of the Church of God, *When the Trumpet Sounded*. Brown's own history with spiritual healing notwithstanding, his book barely mentioned health-promoting behavior or divine healing. Brown said the Church's traditional marks of a holy life (abstaining from medicine, sweets, alcohol, tobacco, coffee, and various other worldly behaviors) were "ascetic disciplines," and he gave no evidence that early Church of God advice books and *Gospel Trumpet* "Health Department" articles drew their material from health magazines and phrenological books, many of which were connected with the Seventh-day Adventists. Brown's neglect of the connection between holy behavior and the promise of physical health, intentionally or unintentionally, obscured the similarities between nineteenth-century health reform movements and the theology and practices of the Church of God.

Divine healing received even less historical attention than did health reform. The following disclaimer from the preface explained the omission:

> The records of the old days are full of miracles of healing and other remarkable happenings. I am an evangelical Christian. I believe these things with all my heart. I have personally participated as a leader in meetings where dozens and hundreds professed, and I believe received, healing. These things are very real to me and they mean much. Nevertheless there is a passage of Scripture which says, 'Cast not your pearls before swine.' I felt that if in this book I constantly emphasized the miraculous character of the ministry of the persons mentioned, I might not serve the cause I love; for constantly to emphasize these miracles without satisfactory corroborative testimony—which space did not allow— might actually stimulate the doubt I antagonize.[6]

Brown's statement was an unintentional call for a critical history of healing in the Church of God. It acknowledged that *When the Trumpet Sounded* omitted a highly significant part of the early ministry, and it suggested that the Church's opinion of healing had changed markedly over the years. The records of the old days were indeed full of healing.[7] Through the first two decades of the twentieth century, theological and biblical justifications of healing, healing testimonies, and advice for those seeking healing appeared in Church of God literature ranging from the children's magazine to the missionary paper. Physical healing was integral to the soteriology and ecclesiology—the life—of the Church of God. It functioned as evidence of the internal cleansing by the Holy Spirit, supported ministerial authority, and proved that God was using the movement to restore the New Testament church and its miracles. Healing was a visible sign of holiness that inspired faith and attracted converts. By the time Brown wrote his preface in 1951, however, healing was no longer essential for the Church's message. The old timers remembered and believed the miracles, but they also knew that claims about healing were more likely to inspire doubt than faith.

As of yet, no one has accepted the challenge to write a critical historical study of healing in the Church of God, a task that this study attempts to fulfill. A few works over the years have discussed the healing ministry of the early leaders. At most, they have described a few of the celebrated healings in the ministry of the Church's most influential healer, E. E. Byrum. In these accounts, healing appeared to be a particular emphasis of a few ministers but ancillary to the mission of the Church of God movement. In fact, in the early years of the Church, members believed that a ministry without physical healing was bereft of the gospel. The spiritual gifts of healing were prerequisites for ministers and evangelists, and the faith to trust God (rather than medicine) for healing was expected of all members, including children. No reader of these histories, however, would ever guess that healing was once a defining mark of the Church of God.[8]

Two mid-twentieth-century doctoral dissertations and one master's thesis included material useful for exploring healing in the Church of God. These differed from the previously-mentioned accounts because they showed that the Church's theology and practice of healing changed, but they still provided little analysis or context. Valorous Clear's sociological study mentioned the Church's changing opinions of both divine healing and distinctive behaviors as evidence of the movement's "social adaptation."[9] Aubrey Forrest's dissertation included a brief chapter about healing of the body that described the transformation from "extremism" to "the more evangelical Protestant teaching concerning the prayer of faith."[10] This chapter provided no context for the ideas and no explanation for the changes Forrest described; the implication was that the Church outgrew its youthful mistakes. Nonetheless, Forrest's was the most extensive description of divine healing in the Church of God for over forty years, but historical errors and the absence of citations hampered its usefulness. Dwight Dye's master's thesis adopted Brown's category of "ascetic disciplines" to connect otherwise independent chapters about fasting, diet, clothing, amusements, and life insurance. Dye produced a useful guide to articles about behavior and health in the literature of the early Church of God. Again, however, there was no historical context for this study. There was no discussion of similar behavior in the holiness movement, health reform initiatives, or Adventism. Further, Dye did not connect these behaviors with the theology of the Church.[11]

The best historical work on Church of God healing is by Merle Strege.[12] He has not only described the importance of healing for several of the early ministers, he also has begun the work of situating healing in the theology of the Church and explaining—rather than just describing—the doctrinal changes. Healing was not Strege's main interest in these books, however, so he did not show where the ideas came from or why they would have been appealing to the people of the nineteenth century. Still, *I Saw the Church* was an important beginning for establishing the theological and social importance of healing in the Church. It invited further study into the specifics of healing doctrine and practice.

Only recently has religious healing begun to gain widespread acceptance as a topic for serious history. Several pioneering studies about healing in the holiness movement, Pentecostalism, and Adventism appeared in the 1970s and 1980s, but they were received as minor miracles of judicious and empathetic scholarship that studied a quirky, nearly invisible set of practices and somehow managed to make them relevant to the study of religion.[13] A reviewer of David Harrell's 1975 study of the healing revivals of William Branham and Oral Roberts, *All Things Are Possible*, succinctly stated this opinion: "As if to illustrate that, indeed, all things *are* possible, David Edwin Harrell, Jr., has produced a book about healing revivalists that takes them seriously and treats them fairly."[14]

Religious healing remains an unusual topic for historians, but several trends have demonstrated its importance to historians. First is the growing connection between history and social scientific methods. Sociologists of religion, anthropologists, physicians, and medical historians have created a sub-field for studying the effect of religious beliefs on health and healing.[15] Second is the continuing influence of gender studies and the desire to understand religion as it is lived and experienced by adherents. Among the earliest groups with significant female leadership and intentional theological discussions of the physical body were Christian Scientists, Spiritualists, Adventists, and holiness groups. None of these makes sense, especially for scholars interested in religious experiences and the importance of the gendered body, apart from religious healing.[16] A third factor, related to the previous two, is the developing historical study of the Pentecostal movement. Healing has been a (some say *the*) defining emphasis of Pentecostalism, the most successful religious movement of the twentieth century.[17]

Once a person is sensitized to its presence, healing appears throughout religious history. As Amanda Porterfield argued in her 2002 presidential address to the American Society of Church History, "healing is a persistent and even defining characteristic of Christianity," and attention to it "can be extremely useful for historians."[18] Healing is not only a widely practiced aspect of Christianity with roots in the very beginning of the religion, it is also an enactment of belief where religion and culture intersect. First-century Christians and nineteenth-century Christians preached and practiced healing, but the practices and theological articulations were very different. One specific difference was that religious healing necessarily contrasted with contemporary medical care, and therefore nineteenth-century healers competed with antitoxins, X-rays, and other developments never dreamed of in the first century. Another difference was that nineteenth-century healers were trying to prove that they had the same power that the apostolic church did, so healing was freighted with meaning from the Bible and centuries of history. To quote Porterfield again, "Following the common thread of healing is one way of looking at the twists and turns that doctrine and practice had taken. Thus healing helps us think about change and diversity in Christian history, as well as continuity."[19]

Only two recent works on divine healing in America have included sections on the Church of God. Jonathan Baer's dissertation, "Perfectly Empowered Bodies: Divine Healing in Modernizing America," had a brief but very good account that identified divine healing with the Church of God's idea of the visible church. Baer correctly asserted that physical healing functioned to show the Church to the world and to give "concrete assurance" of holiness to believers.[20] Nancy Hardesty's account was much less helpful. It was less than a page long and relied on only two sources, one of which is *When the Trumpet Sounded.*[21] Nevertheless, these works show that scholars have begun to recognize that the Church of God movement was among the earliest and most radical of the groups that have taught divine healing. It belongs in the history of American religious healing, especially the history of holiness and Pentecostalism, but the Church's story has been inaccessible to scholars.

That is where this book fits. Using treatises, tracts, testimonies, and children's literature, it restores health and healing to the history of the Church of God and thereby inserts the Church of God into the history of religious healing. For the history of the Church itself this work makes several important contributions. It shows that healing was an essential aspect of Church of God soteriology and ecclesiology. Physical healing manifested and embodied the movement's claim that God was healing the universal church (the Body of Christ) by cleansing individuals from the corruption of inbred sin. Thus, healing was offered as visible evidence that God was doing something entirely new with the Church of God. Church members showed they were sanctified by repudiating medicine and self-destructive habits. Ministers showed that God had set them apart for ministry by performing healing. And God showed that a new age of Christianity had begun by giving health and healing to those with enough faith.

However, Church leaders adopted their descriptions of holy behavior and their doctrines of divine healing from contemporary healing movements. This study shows how culturally conditioned the Church of God movement's rejection of the world was. Church members were not rejecting all possible medical treatments (although they claimed to be); they were rejecting nineteenth-century medicine and were replacing it with nineteenth-century alternatives. This work will explore how the theology and practices of healing changed in the Church of God, and it will explain how healing first lost its power as evidence of holiness and then lost its place in the history of the Church.

From a wider perspective, this work will contribute to the study of religious healing by examining how ideas about divine healing were received, contested, and changed in a religious movement. Most studies of religious healing have focused on individuals who were primarily, if not exclusively, healing evangelists.[22] They preached salvation, living a good life, and turning away from sin, but the reason for their ministries was physical healing. They were for all practical purposes independent of their denominations or religious movements. The Church of God movement, in contrast, attempted—for a while—to integrate healing into every part of its ministry. Miraculous healings happened (or failed to happen) in communities of Church of God members. By studying a religious group that taught healing but was united by bonds of friendship, family, and belief, this work explores changes in the theology and practice of healing caused by persistent pain, unanswered prayers, legal prosecution, compulsory vaccination of schoolchildren, and medical advances.

The third contribution of this book is to the history of the American Pentecostal movement. The prevailing opinion of the Church of God among scholars of Pentecostalism is that it was the most strident, vitriolic, and mean critic of the tongues movement, which dismissed "Pentecostal converts as 'the very scum of sectism.'"[23] The other observation historians of Pentecostalism make about the Church of God is that, according to oral tradition, William Joseph Seymour, the founder of the Azusa Street revival, was ordained by the Church before he sought the gift of tongues.[24] How does one connect the former judgment with the fact that Seymour emerged as one of the most important Pentecostal leaders? Most accounts do not connect them at all and simply say that Seymour changed his mind or experienced a divine revelation.[25] This study does not complete the puzzle of Seymour's life, nor does it suggest that Pentecostalism began in 1881 with the Church of God. It does, however, show that the Church of God had several decades of experience debating, experimenting with, and praying for the spiritual gifts of Pentecost by the time the *Gospel Trumpet* began denouncing the "tongues heresy." This book is therefore preliminary work toward Augustus Cerillo's challenge to historians to "integrate into a coherent analysis or study the elements of continuity and discontinuity between a post-1901 Pentecostalism and the nineteenth-century holiness and evangelical movements."[26]

The study proceeds as follows. Chapter 1 sets the context for the rest of the work with an overview of health and healing in late nineteenth-century America. It briefly describes the state of orthodox medicine, health reform movements, and religious healing. The chapter concludes with a description of the Divine Healing movement and the post-Civil War holiness revival.

Chapter 2 tells the story of D. S. Warner's founding of the Church of God. It explores the links between health reform, divine healing, and Warner's holiness theology. Particular attention is given to Warner's soteriology, ecclesiology, and his idea of the "evening light" dispensation. The chapter concludes with a description of the institutional development of the Church of God from its founding in 1881 to the creation of the General Assembly in 1916.

Chapter 3 is a study of healing testimony. It shows how health and healing functioned in the creation and promotion of the early Church of God. It publicized the cause, provided physical evidence of spiritual sanctification, and functioned as a legitimization of leaders. This chapter shows that healing stories provided publicity that attracted outsiders and a divine stamp of approval that kept believers committed to the cause. Moreover, in the transition of leadership from D. S. Warner to E. E. Byrum in 1895, the doctrine of healing changed fundamentally from a sign of God's favor to *the* sign of God's favor.

Chapter 4 is a close examination of the development of the doctrine of divine healing from 1890 to 1905. The first half describes four overlapping but increasingly strict doctrines that culminated in the "divine healing in the atonement" doctrine. The second half explores how proponents of divine healing answered their critics and explained biblical texts that appeared to undermine divine healing doctrine. This chapter shows that the development of doctrine and practice in the Church of God paralleled that in the larger healing movement.

Chapter 5 studies health advice and health-promoting behavioral proscriptions the Church of God adopted from health reform and the holiness movement. The idea that the saints could obtain physical health by obeying the laws of nature existed throughout the history of the Church. At first this approach to health was presented as a blessing of sanctification, but in the 1890s it began to conflict with divine healing and was relegated to child-rearing literature. The didactic literature and the children's paper were full of articles about health and healing. By the early twentieth century, the concerns for cleanliness, sexual purity, and a happy home expanded beyond warnings to children and parents into lectures to adults about home, health, and success. This chapter shows that the increasing openness to medicine in the twentieth century was not as radical a departure as it might seem to those who listened only to the divine healing rhetoric of the Church. The use of material means to promote health existed in the Church from the very beginning.

Chapter 6 concludes the study with an examination of the decreasing importance of health and healing in the Church of God in the first quarter of the twentieth century. Court trials of parents who relied on divine healing for their children, the smallpox epidemic, compulsory inoculation of schoolchildren, improved medical treatments, and tragic deaths all forced a reassessment of healing in the Church. By 1926 the experiment was over. Radical healing sermons and testimonies were alienating potential converts and Church members alike. All of the radical statements about healing had been reversed. Church of God people continued to pray for healing, but they stopped using healing (or its absence) to prove anything. The Church's opinion of physical healing had changed from seeing it as the best possible evidence of God's redeeming power to believing that it was, as C. E. Brown suggested in his history of the movement, a pearl to be protected from swine.

Notes

1. This group was one of the first radical holiness churches. It began in 1881 with congregations in Indiana and Michigan united by Daniel Sidney Warner's newspaper, the *Gospel Trumpet*. Warner taught that a new age of the Christian church, the Evening Light (named for Zech. 14:7 "at evening time it shall be light"), was restoring the apostolic

church, or the "morning light." The group is now called the Church of God (Anderson).
Strongly opposed to denominations and denominational labels, the members favored the
biblical descriptor "Church of God" or "church of God." Since 1906, the publishing
house and the organizational center for the Church of God have been in Anderson, Indiana. The modifier "(Anderson)" is not officially part of the Church's name but distin-
guishes it from other "Church of God" groups. In 2004, statistics from the *Yearbook of
the Church of God* reported congregations in 91 countries and over 760,000 adherents
worldwide.

2. Willis M. Brown, *From Infidelity to Christianity: Life Sketches of Willis M.
Brown* (Moundsville, W.Va.: Gospel Trumpet Co., 1904). For Brown's conversion, see
133–35. For his healing and his call to preach, see 166–71.

3. Quoted in *From Infidelity to Christianity*, 261.

4. Charles E. Brown, *When the Trumpet Sounded: A History of the Church of God
Reformation Movement* (Anderson, Ind.: Gospel Trumpet Co., 1951), 169–70; Willis M.
Brown, *From Infidelity to Christianity*, 336–37. For the statement about divine healing at
camp meeting, see "Divine Healing in the Atonement," *Gospel Trumpet* [*GT*] 22:25 (June
19, 1902): 1–3.

5. The book was *From Infidelity to Christianity*. The first draft contained too much
infidelity; the assembly meeting at the 1904 camp meeting voted to suspend its publication because it contained objectionable material. Brown revised it for publication. ("Light
from the Lord," *GT* 24:24 [June 16, 1904]: 4.)

6. C. E. Brown, *When the Trumpet Sounded*, xi.

7. My purpose is not to adjudicate between "true" and "false" healings, as if that
were even possible. I am interested in the function of healing claims in religion: when
they were accepted, when they were rejected, and how they were used by ministers and
members of the laity. In this book, I say that a person who claimed to be healed was
"healed."

8. See Barry L. Callen, *The Wisdom of the Saints* (Anderson, Ind.: Anderson University Press and Warner Press, 2003), 29–33; John W. V. Smith, *The Quest for Holiness
and Unity: A Centennial History of the Church of God (Anderson, Indiana)* (Anderson,
Ind.: Warner Press, 1980), 69–71, 76, 134, 146; John W. V. Smith, *Heralds of a Brighter
Day: Biographical Sketches of Early Leaders in the Church of God Reformation Movement* (Anderson, Ind.: Gospel Trumpet Co., 1955), 68–75, 105; Harold L. Phillips, *Miracle of Survival* (Anderson, Ind.: Warner Press, 1979), 42, 256; and Robert H. Reardon,
The Early Morning Light (Anderson, Ind.: Warner Press, 1979), 34–37.

9. Valorous B. Clear, "The Church of God: A Study in Social Adaptation" (Ph.D.
diss,. University of Chicago Divinity School, 1953). Clear's revised dissertation was
published as *Where the Saints Have Trod: A Social History of the Church of God Reformation Movement* (Chesterfield, Ind.: Midwest Publications, 1977).

10. Aubrey Leland Forrest, "A Study in the Development of the Basic Doctrines and
Institutional Patterns in the Church of God (Anderson, Indiana)" (Ph.D. diss., University
of Southern California, 1948), 113–20.

11. Dwight Latimer Dye, "The Asceticism in the Church of God Reformation
Movement from 1880 to 1913" (Master of Religious Education thesis, University of
Tulsa, 1963).

12. See Merle D. Strege, *I Saw the Church: The Life of the Church of God Told
Theologically* (Anderson, Ind.: Warner Press, 2002), esp. 66–74 and 232–33; *Tell Me the
Tale: Historical Reflections on the Church of God* (Anderson, Ind.: Warner Press, 1991),

73–96; and *Tell Me Another Tale: Further Reflections on the Church of God* (Anderson, Ind.: Warner Press, 1993), 103–24.

13. Raymond J. Cunningham, "From Holiness to Healing: The Faith Cure in America, 1872–1892," *Church History* 43:4 (1974): 499–513; Ronald L. Numbers, *Prophetess of Health: A Study of Ellen G. White* (New York: Harper and Row, 1976); David Edwin Harrell, Jr., *All Things Are Possible: The Healing and Charismatic Revivals in Modern America* (Bloomington: Indiana University Press, 1975); Donald Dayton, "The Rise of the Evangelical Healing Movement in Nineteenth-Century America," *Pneuma* 4:1 (1982): 1–18; Donald Dayton, *Theological Roots of Pentecostalism* (Metuchen, N.J.: Scarecrow Press, 1987), chapter five.

14. William C. Martin, *Journal of Southern History* 42:4 (Nov. 1976), 603.

15. See Harold G. Koenig, Michael E. McCullough, and David B. Larson, eds., *Handbook of Religion and Health* (New York: Oxford University Press, 2001). See especially the preface, which describes how initial reactions from colleagues ranged from skeptical to dismissive, and the introduction, which provides an overview of current research.

16. See, for instance, Catherine Wessinger, ed. *Women's Leadership in Marginal Religions: Explorations Outside the Mainstream* (Urbana: University of Illinois Press, 1993). Five of the ten chapters are about religions that emphasized healing (Pentecostalism, Spiritualism, Christian Science, Theosophy, New Thought, and Unity). See especially Ann Braude's chapter, "The Perils of Passivity: Women's Leadership in Spiritualism and Christian Science," and pages 227–28 of Mary Farrell Bednarowski's conclusion, "Widening the Banks of the Mainstream: Women Constructing Theologies."

17. According to Donald Dayton, "perhaps even more characteristic of Pentecostalism than the doctrine of baptism of the Spirit is its celebration of miracles of divine healing as part of God's salvation and as evidence of the presence of divine power in the church" (*Theological Roots of Pentecostalism*, 115). See also Grant Wacker, "The Pentecostal Tradition," in *Caring and Curing: Health and Medicine in the Western Religious Traditions,* ed. Ronald L. Numbers and Darrell W. Amundsen (New York: Macmillan, 1986), 520–21. For the global expansion of Pentecostalism, see Harvey Cox, *Fire From Heaven: The Rise of Pentecostal Spirituality and the Reshaping of Religion in the Twenty-First Century* (Reading, Mass.: Addison-Wesley, 1995); and Vinson Synan, ed., *The Century of the Holy Spirit: 100 Years of Pentecostal and Charismatic Renewal, 1901–2001* (Nashville, Tenn.: Thomas Nelson, 2001).

18. Amanda Porterfield, "Healing in the History of Christianity," *Church History* 71:2 (June 2002), 227.

19. Porterfield, "Healing in the History of Christianity," 227.

20. Jonathan Baer, "Perfectly Empowered Bodies: Divine Healing in Modernizing America" (Ph.D. diss., Yale University, 2002), 175–84. The quote is from page 175.

21. Nancy A. Hardesty, *Faith Cure: Divine Healing in the Holiness and Pentecostal Movements* (Peabody, Mass.: Hendrickson, 2003), 46–47. The other source is Mary Cole's autobiography, *Trials and Triumphs of Faith* (Anderson, Ind.: Gospel Trumpet Co., 1914). Cole was an early evangelist in the Church and reported many experiences of divine healing.

22. An exception is William Boyd Bedford, Jr., "'A Larger Christian Life': A. B. Simpson and the Early Years of the Christian and Missionary Alliance" (Ph.D. diss., University of Virginia, 1992).

23. See Grant A. Wacker, "Travail of a Broken Family: Radical Evangelical Responses to the Emergence of Pentecostalism in America, 1906–16," in Edith L. Blumhofer, Russell P. Spittler, and Grant A. Wacker, eds., *Pentecostal Currents in American Protestantism* (Urbana: University of Illinois Press, 1999), 30 and 37. The quote is on page 30.

24. See, for instance, Douglas Jacobsen, *Thinking in the Spirit: Theologies of the Early Pentecostal Movement* (Bloomington: Indiana University Press, 2003), 61; Cecil M. Robeck, Jr., "William Joseph Seymour," in Stanley M. Burgess and Eduard M. Van Der Maas, eds., *New International Dictionary of Pentecostal and Charismatic Movements* (Grand Rapids, Mich.: Zondervan, 2002), 1054; David Bundy, "G.T. Haywood: Religion for Urbanites," in James R. Goff, Jr. and Grant Wacker, eds., *Portraits of a Generation: Early Pentecostal Leaders* (Fayetteville: University of Arkansas Press, 2002), 241.

25. For a work that claims that Seymour "maintained his Church of God orientation toward doctrine and Scripture" even after he began speaking in tongues, see Cheryl J. Sanders, *Saints in Exile: The Holiness-Pentecostal Experience in African American Religion and Culture* (New York: Oxford University Press, 1996), 32. Sanders identifies the Church of God movement's commitment to holiness, unity of the saints, and interracial community in Seymour's periodical *Apostolic Faith*.

26. Augustus Cerillo, "The Beginnings of American Pentecostalism: A Historiographical Overview," in Blumhofer and others, eds., *Pentecostal Currents*, 247. With respect to the Church of God and Pentecostalism, Charles Jones's work demands attention. Jones did not focus on healing, but he did identify the "Holiness independents" (Church of God [Anderson], Church of God [Holiness], and Holiness Church of California) as breeding grounds of Pentecostalism. According to Jones, "reliance on the guidance of the Holy Spirit occupied a prominent place in the thinking of Holiness independents and so opened the avenue to experience-centeredness and Spirit guidance so often revealed in later pentecostal thought. Future pentecostals in the Holiness ranks started in this direction intellectually very soon [after these groups began in the early 1880s]" ("Holiness Movement," in Burgess and Van Der Maas, eds., *New International Dictionary of Pentecostal and Charismatic Movement*, 726).

CHAPTER 1

HEALING IN THE LATE NINETEENTH CENTURY

Mary J. Sweeney and Dr. R. E. Sweeney of Chanute, Kansas, married in 1873. Mary was seventeen and had been a Christian for about a year. She felt it was her duty to conduct family worship but resisted because her husband was an unbeliever. Although the burden to follow the leading of the Holy Spirit grew heavier, she was timid and did not know how "to make a real consecration of all things to God." In February 1874, Mary became sick and was a "helpless invalid" for over nine years.[1]

Dr. Sweeney owned a large medical practice and devoted his considerable resources to curing his wife. He diagnosed her condition as "female trouble," specifically she had "antifluction and antiversion of the uterus, also mitritus, with ulcers at the os of the worst condition." He "perused some of the best works on Jinecology, such as West, Thomas, Monday and others, and consulted some of the best physicians" without success. For six years, Mary could not walk a step.[2]

Having exhausted all available medical options, Dr. Sweeney decided in the spring of 1881 to take Mary to the new healing resort in Eureka Springs, Arkansas. The mineral baths brought temporary relief, but Mary soon became blind and lost all but a whisper of her voice. All was not lost, however; at the springs she met people who taught the "holiness" doctrine of entire sanctification and showed her that it was her "privilege to be made whole both soul and body."

Mary testified that she had long felt that her spiritual life was deficient, but, until she heard the holiness message, she did not know what to ask for or how to obtain it. Her ministers at home had taught that "the day of miracles was past." Her new insight into holiness convinced her that Jesus would still heal just as he had in the New Testament, because he was "the same yesterday, today, and for-

1

ever." If, as her pastors had said, miracles ended with the apostolic church, then
it was true only because people no longer lived up to apostolic standards.

Mary was still an invalid when the Sweeneys returned to Kansas, but "a
sweet communion [with God] which words fail to explain" had replaced her
longings, doubts, and fears. She invited holiness people to her home to baptize
her and celebrate the Lord's Supper. Soon thereafter, on July 18, 1883, while
having grape juice and bread for breakfast, Mary felt the presence of Jesus and
his healing power. She claimed her healing, arose, and called her husband, saying, "Doctor, I am healed; will you believe it?" The evidence was irrefutable,
and Dr. Sweeney confessed that, though still an "unbeliever," he "was afraid to
deny the healing power of God." This began Mary's new life of preaching the
glory of God in family worship and in the world.

Mary Sweeney's experience was unusually dramatic but far from unique in
the late nineteenth century. Patent medicine advertisements, religious periodicals, and medical journals were replete with stories from people like her who
had suffered through various schemes and treatments before finally discovering
the secret of physical health. For some that secret was treatment by an orthodox
physician like Dr. Sweeney; for some it was in mineral baths, vegetarianism, or
fresh air; for others it was the touch of a divine healer or the power of prayer.
The simplest characterization is that there were options, each of which taught
that suffering was unnatural and avoidable—progress in science or spirituality
promised for the first time in history to overcome human frailty. One had only to
choose the correct regimen, commit to it, and healing would follow. The healing
was a tangible good, but more important it was proof that the individual had
discerned and joined the right group.

The unexamined factor in this story was healing. Everyone assumed that
physical healing was an objective truth that would serve as a common reference
point on which all reasonable people could agree. A healing was a healing was a
healing. A healed body was physical evidence that seemed to offer the best opportunity for an impartial and scientific comparison of religion and medicine.[3]
Divine healers expected physicians to confess the miraculous power of prayer,
and doctors believed devotees of healing ministries would acknowledge the
usefulness of drugs. All sides were arguing in essence that a tree shows its
goodness in its fruit. Years of interaction eventually demonstrated that different
beliefs and presuppositions affected the perception of supposedly objective
healing and thereby limited the usefulness of healing as evidence. In the late
nineteenth century, however, healing was still an objective truth with virtually
unlimited potential for promoting religion or medicine.

This does not mean that people evaluated medicine, prayer, or a health reform system with a simple calculus of success and failure. Adherents must have
derived some median benefits or they would have switched to another system,
but the benefit did not have to be a complete physical restoration. Among the
possible reasons for choosing a healing ideology were: a meaningful context for

suffering, integration into a community, a reduction in pain, or a persuasive promise of future benefits. Mary Sweeney, for example, embraced divine healing before she ever felt a physical change. Her spiritual suffering ended with her sanctification and communion with holiness people, well before her biological healing gave her the strength to preach and a compelling story to tell. Dr. Sweeney, in contrast, admitted that God had succeeded where years of doctoring had failed, but eight years later he was still a self-avowed unbeliever and a practicing physician.

Mary Sweeney's testimony was complex. For the purposes of this study, however, her story illustrates four points about healing in the nineteenth century. The first is obvious but so important that it bears emphasis: people who were suffering sought healing. In other words, people who experienced diseases and debilities were willing to reform, convert, and change their lives—depending on the sacrifice required—for the promise of a cure. Second, several groups competed to offer healing services. The most sophisticated of these—medicine, religious healing, and health reform—provided cosmologies and therapeutic techniques.[4] The cosmologies explained the existence of disease and showed that health was a possibility. The therapeutic techniques transformed the patient from sickness to health. Third, people seeking healing often took what they wanted from these groups and ignored the rest. Mary Sweeney, for example, tried dipping in the Eureka Springs but showed no interest in the larger hydropathic system of living harmoniously with nature through a vegetarian diet, careful chewing, loose clothing, fresh air, and deep breathing.[5] Similarly, divine healers frequently complained that notorious sinners asked for healing but not conversion, and doctors often failed to convince their patients to take their medicine. This tendency to experiment with remedies without fully committing to the corresponding cosmology diluted the influence of healing practitioners and led them to progressively more exclusive definitions of their respective systems. Divine healers began to preach that dabbling in medicine was a faithless act that invalidated prayers for healing, and doctors said that people needed protection from religious impulses and worked to outlaw divine healing. Despite these efforts, eclecticism remained common. Fourth, for those, like Mary and her husband, who did commit to a healing ideology, the changes could be profound. The healing itself was only the physical manifestation of a transformation that could alter one's relation to family, work, and the world. Choosing a path to healing could be deadly serious.

Medicine

The American Medical Association was founded in 1847 to promote the interests of regular physicians through lobbying for favorable legislation and controlling medical licensing and education.[6] That year the AMA's committee on

standards of medical education reported, "the profession of medicine has meas-
urably ceased to occupy the elevated position which it once did; no wonder the
merest pittance in the way of remuneration is scantily doled out even to the most
industrious of our ranks."[7] The professionalization of medicine was slow and
ultimately relied on therapeutic and educational advances that were not complete
until the middle of the twentieth century. By the end of the Civil War, the organization had begun to pay dividends in prestige and authority for its members.
The unmodified titles "physician" and "doctor" increasingly denoted a
practitioner recognized by the AMA, while Thomsonians, mesmerists, homeo-
paths, and eclectics became "irregular" physicians.[8] In the mid-twentieth century, educational reforms and regulation of physicians—though not without
controversy—frequently improved the medical care available to patients. In the
late nineteenth century, the practice of medicine was still primitive and American medical education was wholly inadequate.[9] The great success of the AMA
was in persuasively promoting its brand of medicine as the only scientific medicine, even when the practices of its physicians belied the claim.

Science was a magic word in the Gilded Age. Every group with an interest
in physical healing made at least a passing effort to claim scientific legitimacy.[10]
Technological advances in communication, transportation, and agriculture had
changed the lives of average Americans and had elevated science—profitably
applied—to new heights of cultural authority.[11] Medical advances were primarily in diagnosis and prevention of disease. Although great improvements came
from hygienic reform and city sanitation efforts, science had little positive effect
on medical therapeutics.[12] Nonetheless, the "success of science in revolutioniz-
ing other aspects of medicine and the growing recognition of the inadequacy of
the unaided and uneducated senses in understanding the world" improved the
confidence and authority of regular medicine.[13]

In the scientific—or better, "medicalized"—model, healing was entirely
material. The doctor was an expert who investigated and ultimately attempted to
remove or destroy a disease. The human being was a host for the condition but
was otherwise irrelevant to the diagnosis and treatment.[14] Without medical training, a patient could not possibly have helped the doctor with the examination;
therefore, physicians had no interest in listening to testimonies. The section
about the "Obligations of Patients to their Physicians" in the code of the AMA
said that the patient should not bother the doctor with "a tedious detail of events
on matters not appertaining to his disease" or with "the details of his business
nor the history of his family concerns."[15] The patients' experiences and feelings
were literally immaterial to the examination. True healing required the services
of a trained physician, which were "of such a character that no mere pecuniary
acknowledgement could repay or cancel them."[16]

Objectification of the patient continued beyond the examination. The same
AMA code also asserted, "obedience to the prescription of his physician should
be prompt and implicit. [The Patient] should never permit his own crude opin-

ions as to their fitness to influence his attention to them."[17] These demands for obedience and respect conflicted with the common experiences of nineteenth-century patients. For all the assertions of medical expertise, "until 1895, there were only three medicines capable of curing disease: quinine treated malaria, mercury treated syphilis and digitalis was often effective for heart disorders." In 1895, the discovery of the diphtheria antitoxin added a fourth and inspired "new faith in the potentially curative power of medicine."[18]

Many American physicians adopted these scientific advances unscientifically. That is, they simply added these medicines to their arsenal of drugs for attacking disease—any disease. The proven success of quinine as a treatment for malaria led doctors to prescribe it in such large doses that it caused heart failure. Calomel, a chloride of mercury, became the most common purgative because of mercury's success in treating syphilis. Many physicians adopted it as a panacea, even though extended use caused the teeth to fall out, the gums to become spongy, the upper and lower jawbones to loosen and rot, and finally parts of the tongue and palate to die.[19] Even the discovery of bacteria in the 1870s led to dangerous therapeutics. Researchers observed that whiskey in a Petri dish killed germs, so doctors inferred that alcohol would do the same to germs in the blood.[20] According to medical textbooks, the common dose for adults for the treatment of just about anything was one half to one ounce of whiskey every two or three hours. One half to two teaspoons every two to three hours was the dose for children and infants. By the end of the century, the American Pharmaceutical Association was publicly blaming physicians for the increase in opium addiction, and the Woman's Christian Temperance Union was accusing the medical community of creating a nation of alcoholics.[21]

Astonishing improvements in regular medicine occurred in the first decades of the twentieth century. The objective and materialistic understanding of the doctor/patient relationship continued, and this provided an opening for alternative medicines and religious healing which continues to today. However, the practical basis for the opposition to medicine decreased markedly. According to one medical historian, between 1910 and 1912 "a random patient, with a random disease, consulting a doctor at random had, for the first time in the history of mankind, a better than fifty-fifty chance of profiting from the encounter."[22] In the nineteenth century, before the odds improved, many alternatives proved appealing. A *Harper's Weekly* editorial from Christmas Day, 1897, said that Christian Science owed its success to the fact that medicine was in its "experimental stage, the doctors of which are in pretty constant disagreement with one another."[23] Less charitable critics saw the disagreements among doctors as proof that they were not scientific at all but rather ungodly materialists who were promoting themselves as the "saviors of the race."[24]

Health Reform

Living conditions were deplorable in the United States in the early nineteenth century. There was little if any public sanitation, and most people "rarely bathed, rarely opened a window, [and] rarely (in the case of town dwellers) took any regular exercise."[25] Alcoholism was rampant, and intemperate diets were at least as destructive as drink. Meals commonly included "gargantuan amounts of meat," food dripping with butter or made with lard, and starches for vegetables. Leafy vegetables and fruits were uncommon.[26] Gout and dyspepsia were nearly universal complaints, as were rashes, insect bites, and other preventable conditions. More acute health problems, such as cholera and yellow fever epidemics, reflected the poor state of hygiene and sanitation.[27]

In the 1830s, efforts to reform American hygiene and diets coalesced into a movement, complete with evangelists, zealous converts, and millennial predictions. Beginning as an attempt to reform specific behaviors, health reform caught the spirit of Jacksonian America, combined revivalism with a reverence for the laws of nature, and became a reformation of society based on the physical perfection of individuals.[28] Catherine Albanese has called health reform an example of "physical religion," and James Wharton has said that these reforms were "hygienic ideologies, idea systems that identify correct personal hygiene as the necessary foundation for most, even all, human progress."[29] Details varied from system to system, but all health reformers taught that obedience to a few simple laws of nature and nature's God would produce physical health. In contrast with patients of regular medicine, who depended on the expert opinions of physicians, adherents of health reform ideologies knew exactly what universal laws governed their health. Liberated from the priesthood of doctors, a person had a direct connection with healing power and could either earn health through "physiological rectitude" or lose it by sinning against nature.[30]

Health Reformers

Sylvester Graham—best known for his name's association with graham crackers—was the primary evangelist of the health reform movement. Trained as a Presbyterian minister but unable to secure a clerical appointment, Graham became a Temperance lecturer in Philadelphia in 1830. Within a year he converted to vegetarianism and added talks about the perils of meat-eating to those about the dangers of intoxicating drink.[31] By 1832, he had moved his ever-expanding lecture series on the "Science of Human Life" to New York City.[32] The arrival that year of Asiatic cholera stimulated interest in health and in Graham's lectures in particular. Cholera was a gastrointestinal disease, so it offered the perfect opportunity for promoting Graham's diet reform. Moreover, cholera had a reputation as a slum disease, God's judgment on the dissolute, filthy, drunken heathen.[33] Graham warned that people of all classes risked contracting cholera if they were not eating right; yet, his strict behavioral code—which prescribed frequent bathing and prohibited the consumption of alcohol, narcotics, meat, and spices—appealed to those who believed that cholera came to the United States because immigration and urbanization were eroding the Protestant roots of the nation. As with the Temperance movement, social control was as important for health reform as were the physical benefits.

In 1835 Graham began lecturing in Boston, the home of William Andrus Alcott, who was the other major health reformer of the Jacksonian period.[34] Due to the preparatory work by Alcott and to Graham's reputation from New York, these lectures were a huge success and made Graham into a national celebrity. Two years later, Alcott and Graham provided the health reform movement with a united front by founding the American Physiological Society, which promoted reforms involving "Air, Temperature, Clothing, Exercise, Sleep, Dress, Diet, and Drink." This society was home to major leaders of health reform in the early nineteenth century, such as Horace Mann, Dio Lewis, Larkin Coles, and David Cambell.[35]

Graham and Alcott developed their reform systems independently, but they relied on many of the same sources so their systems were essentially the same. They were popular applications of "vitalism, the belief that life transcends the simple inorganic sciences and can be understood only as a manifestation of unique physiological or vital forces."[36] These vital forces required careful regulation because every disease or debility resulted from an imbalance of vital forces created by unnatural "stimulation." Injurious stimulation or impediment of the life force resulted from the deranged appetites and self-destructive habits of modern life, such as sexual practices, restrictive clothing, lack of fresh air, poor hygiene, and countless other things.[37] Particularly dangerous was a diet that stimulated the gastrointestinal tract; hence, diet was usually the first recommended reform. A proper diet would produce an internal purification that reduced the desire to perform other physiological sins. By following a natural Graham diet, a person would easily adopt all of the other health reforms. The laws of health reform simply codified the instincts of a human being in a "pure state of nature," the "principles which, when strictly obeyed, will always secure [a person's] highest good and happiness."[38]

Health reform was no mere diet and exercise program. At the very least, it promised that every person could enjoy a life free from disease and debility.[39] Beyond the physical benefits, however, were promises of a moral reform of society. Men restructured by physiology and hygiene would naturally follow all of God's laws. They would not want to "own slaves, oppress women, or work their employees long hours in dirty factories for starvation wages." In short, they would be ideal republicans.[40] Sylvester Graham emphasized the millennial promise of health reform when he claimed that God was using him, "Not to teach men that they shall live by bread alone, but by every law of God in their nature and relations—by *every* law; physical, physiological, intellectual, moral, spiritual...that they may enjoy through true godliness 'the life that now is and that which is to come.'"[41] Health reform was the key to personal holiness and social harmony.

As an independent movement, health reform peaked in the antebellum period. Scores of periodicals and books advised about food, sex, childrearing, work, and play. Local health societies sponsored lectures in cities and towns, and traveling reformers (and salesmen) took the message to the frontier. In the 1840s, there were boarding houses governed by Graham's rules in most eastern cities. Existing institutions such as Bronson Alcott's Fruitlands, Brook Farm, and Oberlin College also enforced Graham diets and rules.[42]

After the Civil War, the health reform movement declined. Its grand claims for the perfection of society appeared naive when contrasted with the recent national tragedy, its reforms had become commonplace through repetition, and Sylvester Graham—the public face of the movement—had died.[43] That did not mean, however, that the message disappeared. It survived largely intact throughout the nineteenth century because religious and secular health reform movements incorporated it with little alteration. The millennial impulses, for instance, found a more comfortable home with the Seventh-day Adventists and the holiness movement, each of which expected the perfection and redemption of a holy remnant rather than of the whole society. Health reform's promises for individual health also persisted in alternative healing systems, especially practical phrenology and hydropathy.

Practical Phrenology

Franz Gall invented phrenology in Vienna around 1800. In the 1820s, J. K. Spurzheim brought the theory to Boston, but its significant influence in the United States began with George Combe's lecture tour of 1838–40, which produced several phrenological societies and the *American Phrenological Journal*.[44]

In simple terms, phrenology was the theory that the mind is composed of independent faculties localized in different organs of the brain. Because the development of these organs affected the size and contour of the cranium, a trained phrenologist could "read" a person's mental faculties by examining his or her head.[45] As a novelty and a party game, phrenological readings were very popular in the United States in the early 1840s. However, phrenology did not offer much beyond a diagnosis. What was one to do with an unsatisfactory reading? The determinism of phrenology limited its appeal and usefulness. The phrenological societies soon faltered due to declining interest.

That all changed when Orson and Lorenzo Fowler decided that the shape of the head reflected the current state of the mental organs but did not limit future development.[46] With proper exercise and care, a person could improve his or her mental faculties (such as "acquistiveness," "amativeness," "benevolence," "inhabitiveness," and "veneration"), even changing the shape of the head. The Fowlers called their system "practical phrenology" because it was useful. Head reading revealed the kind of work a person could do best, the kind of mate to choose to ensure a happy home and healthy children, the diseases one would likely contract, the religious feelings a person would be subject to, and just about anything else one could think of.[47]

Practical phrenology collapsed the distinction between the body and the spirit. A person's spiritual and mental conditions showed in the body. Phrenology itself was simply a tool for detecting how well a person followed the laws of nature. Graham's guide to health reform was relatively crude: either a person was sick or not. Phrenology offered a more precise diagnosis. Properly used, it promised perfect health and happiness to those who were willing to work toward harmony with nature.[48] As Orson Fowler wrote, "The plain fact is this, that we *need never be sick*. We have no *right* to be sick. We are *culpable* for being sick, for all of everything is caused. All sickness is caused, and caused directly by the violation of some physiological law."[49] Thus, practical phrenology offered hope to the suffering, but it also warned, "the show of their countenance testifies against them" (Isa. 3:9).

By connecting phrenological diagnoses with Graham's diets and Alcott's behavioral proscriptions, the Fowlers built a health reform empire that included the *American Phrenological Journal*, Fowlers and Wells Publishing Company, and the American Institute of Phrenology. The journal was on the brink of bankruptcy when the Fowlers bought it from George Combe, but it had 20,000 subscribers by 1852 and remained in publication into the twentieth century. The press operated throughout the nineteenth century, publishing a vast range of health-related books and tracts, including original works by the Fowlers and a reprint of Graham's *Science of Human Life*. Clinton Hall, the Fowlers and Wells headquarters at 121 Nassau Street, New York City, became a "lodestone for reformers and reform issues of the day." In 1850, it was the site of the opening meeting of the American Vegetarian Society. In attendance were the Fowlers, Sylvester Graham, William Alcott, and leaders of the water cure, Joel Shew and Russell Thatcher Trall.[50]

Hydropathy

Vincent Preissnitz developed hydropathy or "water cure" in Austria in the 1820s when he discovered the therapeutic virtues of drinking and bathing in pure water.[51] The water cure arrived in the United States in the 1830s, and, much like phrenology, it was transformed into an all-purpose "hygenic system." The five most influential American hydropaths were Joel Shew, Russell Thatcher Trall, Mary Gove Nichols, Thomas Low Nichols, and James C. Jackson. Each was a Grahamite with more than a passing familiarity with phrenology. According to

Richard Shyrock, what these hydropaths "really did was to superimpose Grahamism upon hydropathy, and later, in the most catholic spirit imaginable, to
add every other hygienic procedure available."[52] These various reforms integrated reasonably well into a system of human perfection. Phrenology provided
self-knowledge, health reform gave self-improvement, and the water cure introduced a substance with remedial power—pure water—that cured through im-
bibing, anointing, and washing. The quasi-religious nature of water cure benefited from the obvious association of hydrotherapy with Christian footwashing
and baptism, a connection water curists emphasized with the slogan, "Wash, and
be healed."[53]

    An important fact about hydropathy is that the treatments required pure
water, large bathtubs, and showers. These were not commonly available in
nineteenth-century houses. Those homes that did have the basic requirements
still could not compete with the pools, custom showers, and pure spring water of
hydropathic resorts, clinics, and boarding houses. There were over 200 such
institutions in the United States between 1840 and 1870.[54] They functioned as
gathering places for people interested in hydropathy and health reform. The
most successful added lecture series, publishing houses, and schools. Joel Shew
opened his water cure establishment in New York City in 1844 and began publishing the *Water-Cure Journal and Herald of Reform* in 1845. It had over
50,000 subscribers in 1851. When Shew died in 1855, R. T. Trall, another New
York City-based practitioner of the water cure, bought the *Journal*. Published
continuously—but under three different titles—for over fifty years, the *Water-
Cure Journal* was one of the most successful and influential health reform periodicals of the second half of the century. Trall also opened a hydropathic college
and published (through Fowlers and Wells) the *Hydropathic Encyclopedia* in
1857.[55] The school had the practical phrenologist Lorenzo Fowler as a faculty
member and the Seventh-day Adventist health reformer John Harvey Kellogg as
a student.[56] The encyclopedia was a convenient compendium of health reform
that preserved the tenets of the hydropathic system longer than periodicals,
tracts, and cheap books would have. As late as the early twentieth century, holiness periodicals quoted Trall's encyclopedia as a reliable source of science.[57]

    One final hydropathic resort requires attention because it was a physical
link between health reform and religious healing. James Caleb Jackson's "Our
Home on the Hillside" in Dansville, New York, was a popular retreat well into
the 1890s, long after most water cures had closed. Among the many visitors to
Our Home was Ellen G. White, prophetess of the Seventh-day Adventist movement.

    Several months after reading a tract by Jackson, White had a "vision on
June 5, 1863, which gave the divine seal of approval to health reform and hy-
dropathy" for Seventh-day Adventists.[58] In 1864, she spent three weeks in
Dansville, but found it unsuitable for Sabbath-keepers.[59] In 1866, in Battle
Creek, Michigan, White opened the "Western Health Reform Institute, a water

cure modeled after Our Home and the first link in what was to become a world-wide chain of Seventh-day Adventist medical institutions."[60] The Western Health Reform Institute, Ellen White, John Harvey Kellogg, and the Seventh-day Adventist publishing association effectively shifted the center of health reform to Battle Creek.

Holiness and Divine Healing

There was a wide variety of religious healing in the late nineteenth century. Seventh-day Adventism was the most obvious example of a movement that adopted health reform ideology, but several other groups (Mormons, holiness people, and Jehovah's Witnesses among them) also taught the spiritual benefits of clean living.[61] Christian Science, which began in the 1860s, drew from animal magnetism and mesmerism and taught a form of mind cure that denied the existence of disease.[62] The miraculous healing power of Lourdes water—first discovered in 1858—attracted the attention of American Catholics (and critics of Catholicism) throughout the century. Indeed, Lourdes is a pilgrimage site today.[63] Spiritualists not only bridged the chasm between the living and the dead, they also channeled healing power from beyond the grave.[64] Even the mainline Protestant denominations that traditionally separated the spiritual and the physical embraced "Muscular Christianity" and the YMCA.[65] Finally, the divine healing movement, which emerged from the holiness movement in the 1870s, taught that the age of miracles was not over and the prayer of faith would save the sick.

The Holiness Movement

The American holiness movement was an interdenominational network of people who were dedicated to promoting the doctrine and experience of "entire sanctification."[66] Very simply, this doctrine, which was attributed to John Wesley and the early Methodists, took seriously the injunction "be ye perfect as your Father in heaven is perfect" and asserted that a person can become "perfect in love or intention" in this life. It was a theory that should sound familiar after studying health reform: an experience of inner cleansing removed the desire to sin. A more common construction said that entire sanctification freed a person from sin. The holiness movement emerged from the perfectionist theology and the revivalism of the 1830s in which several important religious leaders—notably Charles Grandison Finney, Asa Mahan, and John Humphrey Noyes—preached "related but distinct bodies of perfectionism."[67] Phoebe Worrall Palmer, however, was the person who formulated and popularized the doctrine of entire sanctification that became the mainline of holiness.

Palmer and her sister Sarah Lankford were Methodists. Lankford experienced sanctification at a revival in 1835 and founded a weekly meeting for women interested in holiness, the Tuesday Meeting for the Promotion of Holiness. Lankford's example inspired Palmer to seek holiness, and she too experienced entire sanctification July 26, 1837.[68] Palmer soon became the leader of the Tuesday Meeting and began to expound her simplified theology of holiness, the "altar theology" or the "shorter way." According to Palmer, sanctification was neither mysterious nor elusive. Holiness was "the expected norm for Christian living rather than its culmination." Therefore, one could obtain sanctification by renouncing worldly desires and surrendering to God, trusting that God would honor his promise to sanctify those who (figuratively) laid themselves "upon the altar," and testifying to God's sanctifying grace. This altar theology reduced the importance of emotion in sanctification and empowered seekers to work for and claim holiness.[69]

Palmer's doctrinal reformulation was wildly successful. The Tuesday Meeting became so popular that she opened it to men, and several of them went home and started their own Tuesday Meetings. Palmer wrote popular books about holiness, became a famous revivalist at camp meetings, and in 1850 helped found the Five Points Mission in New York City. In 1864, she and her husband (a homeopathic physician) bought two periodicals and combined them as the *Guide to Holiness*. The circulation was up to 37,000 by 1870, and this periodical "tied the movement together."[70] From 1859 to 1863, Palmer and her husband led very successful holiness revivals in Great Britain, as did an evangelist named James Caughey. The reports of these revivals in the *Guide to Holiness* left a lasting impression on Americans who were in the middle of a war.[71]

If the Tuesday Meeting was the characteristic holiness gathering in the antebellum period, the camp meeting took over after the war. In 1867, Methodist holiness advocates in the United States founded the National Camp Meeting Association for the Promotion of Holiness.[72] Initially the National Association sponsored camp meetings at existing Methodist camps in the east, but soon they were nationwide. In the summer of 1871, for instance, it organized tabernacle meetings in Sacramento, San Francisco, Santa Clara, Salt Lake City, and Indianapolis.[73] The first president of the National Association was John Inskip, a Methodist minister from New York—in fact, all the presidents were ordained Methodists until 1942. This institutional connection seems to have helped with the organization, publicity, and recruitment to the meetings. The National Association was so successful that it began to look like a church within a church; this "created sharp tensions between the members of the National Committee and the Methodist Episcopal Church."[74] In the interests of preserving harmony and remaining ministers in good standing, the National Association ministers carefully policed their meetings to eliminate such divisive ideas as divine healing.[75]

Beginning in 1872 with the Western Holiness Association, regional associations were modeled on the national but were much less restrictive. Often the leaders were not Methodists, and the sermons covered topics related to sanctification, including healing, eschatology, and ecclesiology.[76] Yet, even these proved too restrictive for some proponents of holiness. Between 1879 and 1883—the same time as the flowering of the divine healing movement—the first of the radical holiness groups declared that holiness could not be contained or controlled by an association.

Divine Healing

The American Divine Healing Movement began in earnest with a homeopathic physician from Boston named Charles Cullis. Cullis experienced entire sanctification in 1862.[77] Two years later he opened a home For Indigent and Incurable Consumptives, which became the basis for Cullis's divine healing hospital. By 1870, he was convinced that the promise of divine healing in James 5:14–15 was still available to any who would pray the prayer of faith. As with the shorter way to sanctification, a faithful Christian could follow the instructions of the Bible to claim physical healing. In January 1870, Cullis prayed with and anointed Lucy Dake, and her tumor rapidly disappeared. Dake herself became a healing evangelist, and her testimony helped to spread Cullis's reputation as a healer. In 1869, he founded a periodical, *Times of Refreshing*, and a publishing house, the Willard Street Tract Repository. The press and the periodical were important vehicles for holiness, divine healing, and Cullis's healing organization. In 1879, Cullis published *Faith Cures,* a collection of testimonies to divine healing.

Through his hospital, press, and lectures at holiness camp meetings, Cullis attracted all of the national leaders of the divine healing movement. Directly associated with him were Sarah Mix, Carrie Judd Montgomery, A. B. Simpson, A. J. Gordon, William Boardman, R. Kelso Carter, and R. L. Stanton.[78] They were responsible for the most important divine healing books, periodicals, revivals, and conventions. Montgomery, Simpson, and Boardman followed Cullis's example and founded healing homes. Simpson also founded the Christian and Missionary Alliance, which had "healer"—along with "savior," "sanctifier," and "coming king"—as an essential part of the "fourfold gospel."[79]

The early theology of the divine healing movement simply asserted that the healings of the Bible were available in the present day. Cullis and his followers sought the benefit of physical healing they believed was promised by the Bible. Cullis maintained this position throughout his life, but, in the early 1880s, his followers created the "atonement doctrine of healing." This doctrinal formulation, a radicalization of holiness sanctification, used Isaiah 53 ("he was wounded for our transgressions, he was bruised for our iniquities: the chastisement of our peace was upon him; and with his stripes we are healed") to assert that Christ's atonement was for both sin and sickness. Therefore, divine healing was an essential aspect of the Gospel. God guaranteed healing to those with enough faith, so using medicine was evidence of a lack of faith.[80] After popularizing the atonement doctrine in 1882 in his *The Atonement for Sin and Sickness,* R. Kelso Carter publicly distanced himself from this radical doctrine in *Faith Healing Reconsidered,* returning to the moderate assertion that God does (sometimes) answer healing prayers.[81]

The atonement doctrine lived on in radical holiness movements and with the healing evangelists such as John Alexander Dowie.[82] These groups and healers further modified the doctrine of healing by exploring the possibility that healing power could reside in a human being as a spiritual gift. In the early twentieth century, divine healing (in the atonement and as a spiritual gift) was foundational for the Pentecostal movement, and it is in the Pentecostal churches that divine healing continues to find its most congenial home.[83]

Conclusion

Healing is about transformations, physical, mental, and spiritual. This chapter has described several of the options for healing in the late nineteenth century, along with the theological and metaphysical claims of each. It is important to recognize, however, that between the individual and the world were families, congregations, denominations, and communities. Successful and failed healings affected all of these associations, so healing also involved relational transformations. Before healing could save the world or the church, it had to save an individual, and then a family, and then a congregation. Around 1880, holiness people began to test (they would have said "trust") the power of divine healing and holy living to perfect the bodies of sanctified individuals and thereby heal the Body of Christ. The rest of this book will examine one such experiment and trace the role of health and healing in the gradual transformation of the Evening Light Reformation of 1880 into the Church of God (Anderson, Indiana) of 1925.

Notes

1. Mary J. Sweeney, "Nine Years an Invalid," July 29, 1891, in Enoch E. Byrum, *Divine Healing of Soul and Body* (Grand Junction, Mich.: Gospel Trumpet Co., 1892), 145–49.

2. Dr. R. E. Sweeney, "Corroborating Testimony," July 29, 1891, in Byrum, *Divine Healing of Soul and Body,* 149–51.

3. In 1872, John Tyndall added his support to an anonymous proposal designed to "confer quantitative precision on the action of the Supernatural in Nature." He believed that healing was the best test. The proposal was to choose two wings of a hospital offering the best in medical care. For the patients on one wing, Christians around the world

would regularly unite in prayer. The other wing would receive only medical care. Unfortunately, the original author believed this exact proposal was practically impossible, because "the unprayed-for ward would have attracted the prayers of believers as surely as the lofty tower attracts electric fluid." (John Tyndall, "The 'Prayer for the Sick:' Hints Towards a Serious Attempt to Estimate its Value," *Contemporary Review* 20 [1872]: 205–10.) See Robert Bruce Mullin, *Miracles and the Modern Religious Imagination* (New Haven: Yale University Press, 1996), 97–98; and Mullin, "Science, Miracles, and the Prayer-Gauge Debate," in David C. Lindberg and Ronald L. Numbers, eds., *When Science and Christianity Meet* (Chicago: University of Chicago Press, 2003), 203–24.

4. Remedies like patent medicines and commercial healing devices were also very popular in the late nineteenth century. This suggests that there was a large market for inexpensive products that made nearly incredible promises for health. It also shows that before the Pure Food and Drug Act of 1906 there was no regulation of medicine. However, these products were purely remedies, rather than healing systems. Typically, an advertisement for a patent medicine would assert that all the physical problems plaguing humanity stemmed from a deficiency of some substance or compound, 100 percent of which could be obtained from the medicine itself. All one had to do was buy and use the medicine. See Sarah Stage, *Female Complaints: Lydia Pinkham and the Business of Women's Medicine* (New York: Norton, 1979); Stewart H. Holbrook, *The Golden Age of Quackery* (New York: Macmillan, 1959); and James Harvey Young, "American Medical Quackery in the Age of the Common Man," *Mississippi Valley Historical Review* 47:4 (March 1961): 579–93.

5. See Susan E. Cayleff, *"Wash and Be Healed": The Water-Cure Movement and Women's Health* (Philadelphia: Temple University Press, 1987).

6. For the professionalization of medicine, see John Duffy, *From Humors to Medical Science: A History of American Medicine*, second ed. (Urbana: University of Illinois Press, 1993); John S. Haller, Jr., *American Medicine in Transition, 1840–1910* (Urbana: University of Illinois Press, 1981); Gerald E. Markowitz and David Karl Rosner, "Doctors in Crisis: A Study in the Use of Medical Education Reform to Establish Modern Professional Elitism in Medicine," *American Quarterly* 25:1 (March 1973): 83–107; Regina M. Morantz, "Feminism, Professionalism, and Germs: The Thought of Mary Putnam Jacobi and Elizabeth Blackwell," *American Quarterly* 34:5 (Winter 1982): 459–78; Charles E. Rosenberg, "The Therapeutic Revolution: Medicine, Meaning, and Social Change in Nineteenth-Century America," *Perspectives in Biology and Medicine* 20:4 (1977): 485–506; William G. Rothstein, *American Physicians in the Nineteenth Century: From Sects to Science* (Baltimore: Johns Hopkins University Press, 1972); Paul Starr, *The Social Transformation of American Medicine: The Rise of a Sovereign Profession and the Making of a Vast Industry* (New York: Basic Books, 1982).

7. Quoted in Rothstein, *American Physicians*, 108. For a description of the problems doctors had collecting fees, see Haller, *American Medicine in Transition*, 242–44.

8. For introductions to these medical systems, see Robert C. Fuller, *Alternative Medicine and American Religious Life* (New York: Oxford University Press, 1989); and Norman Gevitz, ed., *Other Healers: Unorthodox Medicine in America* (Baltimore: Johns Hopkins University Press, 1988).

9. See Abraham Flexner, *Medical Education in the United States and Canada: A Report to the Carnegie Foundation for the Advancement of Teaching* (New York: n.p., 1910). According to Duffy, reputable medical schools were only marginally better in the immediate postwar years than they had been in the early nineteenth century. The

proliferation of "diploma mills" at the end of the century likely made the state of medical education even worse than it had been at the beginning. (Duffy, *From Humors to Medical Science*, 165.)

10. The clearest example is Mary Baker Eddy's Christian Science, but other examples abound.

11. See James Rodger Fleming, "Science and Technology in the Second Half of the Nineteenth Century," in *The Gilded Age: Essays on the Origins of Modern America*, ed. Charles W. Calhoun (Wilmington, Del.: Scholarly Resources, 1996), 19–37.

12. Sand filtration of the water supply in the 1890s was very effective against typhoid, and regulation of the milk supply drastically cut infant mortality. (Starr, *Social Transformation of American Medicine*, 135.) For other successful hygienic reforms, see Nancy Tomes, *The Gospel of Germs* (Cambridge: Harvard University Press, 1998). According to Tomes, the therapeutic promise of germ theory eluded doctors until the twentieth century (46). Antiseptic surgery was possible after 1867. Lister introduced the techniques to the International Medical Congress in 1876, but the first antiseptic operation in the United States was in 1879. (Duffy, *From Humors to Medical Science*, 188–89; Starr, *Social Transformation of American Medicine*, 135.)

13. Starr, *Social Transformation of American Medicine*, 135.

14. For the idea of the "medical gaze," see Michel Foucault, *The Birth of the Clinic: An Archaeology of Medical Perception*, trans. A. M. Sheridan Smith (New York: Random House, Vintage Books, 1975). Catherine L. Albanese has contrasted the root metaphor of sight in medical healing with other dominant metaphors in various religious healing systems. See "The Poetics of Healing: Root Metaphors and Rituals in Nineteenth-Century America," *Soundings* 63:4 (Winter 1980): 381–406, esp. 394–400. A history of the body and the medical gaze is beyond the scope of this study. For more information, see James William Opp, "Religion, Medicine, and the Body: Protestant Faith Healing in Canada, 1880–1930" (Ph.D. diss., Carleton University, Ottawa, Canada, 2000), esp. 8–15.

15. *Code of Medical Ethics of the American Medical Association* (Chicago: American Medical Association Press, 1847), 96. See also Duffy, *From Humors to Medical Science*, 334; and Rothstein, *American Physicians,* 120.

16. *Code of Medical Ethics of 1847*, 97.

17. *Code of Medical Ethics of 1847*, 96.

18. Markowitz and Rosner, "Doctors in Crisis," 92,

19. Rothstein, *American Physicians*, 51; Haller, *American Medicine in Transition,* 77–90. According to Rothstein, the other common purgatives were nitre and jalap. Use of nitre reduced the force and frequency of the heartbeat, eventually causing it to stop. Jalap was so harsh that physicians mixed it with calomel "to make it more palatable."

20. Rothstein, *American Physicians,* 196.

21. Rothstein, *American Physicians,* 192–93.

22. Lawrence J. Henderson, quoted in Duffy, *From Humors to Medical Science*, 187.

23. Quoted in Paul Eli Ivey, *Prayers in Stone: Christian Science Architecture in the United States, 1894–1930* (Urbana: University of Illinois Press, 1999), 87.

24. E. E. Byrum, "A Medico-political Outrage," *GT* 31:33 (Aug. 31, 1911): 2.

25. Richard Shyrock, "Sylvester Graham and the Popular Health Movement, 1830–1870," *Mississippi Valley Historical Review* 18:2 (Sept. 1931), 174. See also Richard L.

Bushman and Claudia L. Bushman, "The Early History of Cleanliness in America," *Journal of American History* 74:4 (March 1988): 1213–38; and Tomes, *Gospel of Germs.*

26. Shyrock, "Sylvester Graham," 173; and Ronald L. Numbers, *Prophetess of Health: Ellen G. White and the Origins of Seventh-day Adventist Health Reform*, rev. and enl. ed. (Knoxville: University of Tennessee Press, 1992), 48–49.

27. Rothstein, *American Physicians*, 55. Yellow fever broke out in America every year between 1800 and 1879, with two exceptions. Cholera hit all the urban centers in 1832, 1849, and 1866. In 1853, between eight and nine thousand of the 150,000 inhabitants of New Orleans died from cholera.

28. Robert H. Abzug, *Cosmos Crumbling: American Reform and the Religious Imagination* (New York: Oxford University Press, 1994); Catherine L. Albanese, "Physical Religion: Natural Sin and Healing Grace in the Nineteenth Century," chapter four in *Nature Religion in America* (Chicago: University of Chicago Press, 1990); Albanese, "Physic and Metaphysic in Nineteenth-Century America: Medical Sectarians and Religious Healing," *Church History* 55:4 (1986): 489–502; Stephen Nissenbaum, *Sex, Diet, and Debility in Jacksonian America: Sylvester Graham and Health Reform* (Westport, Conn.: Greenwood Press, 1980); James C. Wharton, *Crusaders for Fitness: The History of American Health Reformers* (Princeton: Princeton University Press, 1982).

29. This is the title of chapter 4 in Albanese, *Nature Religion*. Wharton, *Crusaders for Fitness*, 4.

30. Wharton, *Crusaders for Fitness*, 5. Wharton describes this as "physical Arminianism." See also Ronald G. Walters, *Primers for Prudery: Sexual Advice to Victorian America* (Baltimore: Johns Hopkins University Press, 2000); and Guenter Risse, Ronald L. Numbers, and Judith Walzer Leavitt, eds., *Medicine Without Doctors: Home Health Care in American History* (New York: Science History Publications, 1977).

31. Wharton, *Crusaders for Fitness*, 45. See also Nissenbaum, *Sex, Diet, and Debility.*

32. First published in 1839, these lectures became a standard work in health reform.

33. A change in diet seemed a reasonable response to a disease that produced violent vomiting. One aspect of Graham's system was not so helpful, though. He taught that pure water was the only drink suitable for mankind. This was good in theory, but he had no idea about the microorganisms in the water that spread cholera and other diseases. As Wharton observed, for avoiding cholera, "cheap germicidal bourbon would have been a far safer drink" (*Crusaders for Fitness*, 46).

34. Alcott was a Yale-trained physician who worked as a teacher before becoming a health reformer. He was a more prolific author and had a greater range of interests than Graham. However, Graham's personality and self-promotion attracted more publicity. (Numbers, *Prophetess of Health*, 57.) For an introduction to Alcott, see Wharton, *Crusaders for Fitness*, 49–61.

35. Numbers, *Prophetess of Health*, 57–58.

36. Wharton, *Crusaders for Fitness*, 41. The immediate source of the theory of vitalism for both men appears to have been the French physician Francois Broussais. See Haller, *American Medicine in Transition*, 73–74; Nissenbaum, *Sex, Diet, and Debility*, 57–60; Wharton, *Crusaders for Fitness*, 41–43. Vitalism was common among physicians as well. See Charles E. Rosenberg, "The Therapeutic Revolution: Medicine, Meaning, and Social Change in Nineteenth-Century America," *Perspectives in Biology and Medicine* 20:4 (1977), 499.

37. Medical "stimulants" designed to produce violent physical reaction were obviously unacceptable. For a summary of Grahamism, see "The Graham System," *Graham Journal of Health and Longevity* (April 18, 1837): 17.

38. Sylvester Graham, *A Lecture to Young Men*, ed. Charles Rosenberg and Carroll Smith-Rosenberg (New York: Arno Press, 1974; original publication 1834), 11.

39. Graham, *Lecture to Young Men*, 11; Dio Lewis, *Our Girls* (New York: Harper and Brothers, 1871), 240–46. See also William Alcott's autobiography, *Forty Years in the Wilderness of Pills and Powders, or, The Cogitations and Confessions of an Aged Physician* (Boston: John P. Jewett, 1859). Note the biblical allusion in his title.

40. Wharton, *Crusaders for Fitness*, 117.

41. Quoted in Albanese, *Nature Religion in America*, 127. Emphasis in original.

42. Numbers, *Prophetess of Health*, 55; Robert Samuel Fletcher, *A History of Oberlin College: From Its Foundation Through the Civil War*, Vol. 1 (Oberlin, Ohio: Oberlin College, 1943), 318–31.

43. Wharton, *Crusaders for Fitness*, 132–33.

44. John D. Davies, *Phrenology Fad and Science: A 19th Century American Crusade* (New Haven: Yale University Press, 1955), 8–17; Robert E. Riegel, "The Introduction of Phrenology to the United States," *American Historical Review* 39:1 (Oct. 1933): 73–78; "Phrenology" in *Encyclopedia Britannica* 11th ed., vol. 21 (Cambridge: Cambridge University Press, 1910), 534–41.

45. Davies, *Phrenology Fad and Science,* 3–4.

46. See Madeleine B. Stern, *Heads and Headlines: The Phrenological Fowlers* (Norman: University of Oklahoma Press, 1971); Abzug, *Cosmos Crumbling*, chapter 7; Riegel, "The Introduction of Phrenology to the United States," 78; Wharton, *Crusaders for Fitness,* 124–25; Ruth Clifford Engs, *Clean Living Movements in America: Cycles of Health Reform* (Westport, Conn.: Praeger, 2000), 70–72.

47. See for instance George Sumner Weaver, *Lectures on Mental Science According to the Philosophy of Phrenology* (New York: Fowlers and Wells, 1852). According to Sumner, "By a critical self-exam, which every one should daily make, we can discover our weakest organs, and apply the only remedy" (60).

48. Orson Fowler, *Physiology Animal and Mental*, chapter 1, section 1 is "Happiness is the natural consequence of law obeyed; and suffering, of law violated."

49. Fowler, *Physiology Animal and Mental*, 109. Emphasis in the original.

50. Numbers, *Prophetess of Health*, 70; Stern, *Heads and Headlines.* See also Harriet P. Fowler, *Vegetarianism: The Radical Cure for Intemperance* (New York: Fowlers and Wells, 1886).

51. Susan Cayleff, "Gender, Ideology, and the Water-Cure Movement" in *Other Healers: Unorthodox Medicine in America*, ed. Norman Gevitz (Baltimore: Johns Hopkins University Press, 1988), 83–84; Cayleff, *Wash and Be Healed.*

52. Shyrock, "Sylvester Graham," 180. According to Wharton, Mary Gove Nichols was the first to connect the two. She owned a Graham boarding house when she began to experiment with the water cure. (*Crusaders for Fitness*, 137 and 154.) One of the more important related reforms was dress reform, inspired in part because long skirts interfered with the water cure treatment. See Gayle Veronica Fischer, "Who Wears the Pants? Women, Dress Reform, and Power in the Mid-Nineteenth Century United States" (Ph.D. diss., Indiana University, 1995).

53. This was the slogan of Joel Shew's *Water-Cure Journal* (Albanese, *Nature Religion*, 137).

54. Cayleff, "Gender, Ideology, and the Water-Cure Movement" in *Other Healers,* 83.

55. R. T. Trall, *The Hydropathic Encyclopedia: A System of Hydropathy and Hygiene, in Eight Parts, Designed as a Guide to Families and Students, and a Text-Book for Physicians* (New York: Fowlers and Wells, 1852).

56. Engs, *Clean Living Movements,* 96–97.

57. The importance of reference books should not be underestimated. Scientific knowledge changed very slowly among lay people and even with some doctors.

58. Ronald L. Numbers and David R. Larson, "The Adventist Tradition," in Ronald L. Numbers and Darrel W. Amundsen, eds., *Caring and Curing: Health and Medicine in the Western Religious Traditions* (Baltimore: Johns Hopkins University Press, 1998), 451.

59. Many other important Seventh-day Adventist leaders were associated with the water cure and with "Our Home on the Hillside." See Numbers, *Prophetess of Health,* 79. Jackson invented a cold cereal called "granula." Kellogg took the recipe and changed the name to "granola."

60. Numbers, *Prophetess of Health,* 101.

61. For introductions to health and healing in the Mormon and Jehovah's Witness traditions, see Numbers and Amundsen, eds., *Caring and Curing.* The relevant chapters are Lester E. Bush, Jr., "The Mormon Tradition," and William H. Cumberland, "The Jehovah's Witness Tradition." For holiness and health reform, see chapter five of this book.

62. Paul K. Conkin, *American Originals: Homemade Varieties of Christianity* (Chapel Hill: University of North Carolina Press, 1997), 226–75; Rennie B. Schepflin, "The Christian Science Tradition," in Numbers and Amundsen, eds., *Caring and Curing*; Sandra S. Sizer, "New Spirit, New Flesh: The Poetics of Nineteenth-Century Mind-Cures," *Soundings* 63:4 (1980): 407–22; Mary Baker Eddy, *Science and Health, with Key to the Scriptures,* 16th, rev. ed. (Boston: the author, 1886).

63. Sandra L. Zimdars-Swartz, *Encountering Mary: Visions of Mary from La Salette to Medjugorje* (New York: Avon Books, 1992), 43–67.

64. Ann Braude, *Radical Spirits: Spiritualism and Women's Rights in Nineteenth-Century America* (Boston: Beacon Press, 1989); Robert W. Delp, "Andrew Jackson Davis: Prophet of American Spiritualism," *The Journal of American History* 54:1 (1967): 43–56; and R. Laurence Moore, *In Search of White Crows: Spiritualism, Parapsychology, and American Culture* (New York: Oxford University Press, 1977).

65. See Clifford Putney, *Muscular Christianity: Manhood and Sports in Protestant America, 1880–1920* (Cambridge: Harvard University Press, 2001); and Donald E. Hall, *Muscular Christianity: Embodying the Victorian Age* (Cambridge: Cambridge University Press, 1994).

66. For narrative introductions to the holiness movement, see Melvin E. Dieter, *The Holiness Revival of the Nineteenth Century* (Lanham, Md.: Scarecrow Press, 1996); Paul M. Bassett and William M. Greathouse, *Exploring Christian Holiness: The Historical Development* (Kansas City, Mo.: Beacon Hill Press, 1985); Charles Edwin Jones, *Perfectionist Persuasion: The Holiness Movement and American Methodism, 1867–1936* (Metuchen, N.J.: Scarecrow Press, 1974); Timothy L. Smith, *Revivalism and Social Reform: American Protestantism on the Eve of the Civil War* (Baltimore: Johns Hopkins University Press, 1980, reprint). See also William C. Kostlevy, ed., *Historical Dictionary of the Holiness Movement* (Lanham, Md.: Scarecrow Press, 2001).

67. Kostlevy, ed., *Historical Dictionary of the Holiness Movement*, xi.

68. Susie C. Stanley, *Holy Boldness: Women Preachers' Autobiographies and the Sanctified Self* (Knoxville: University of Tennessee Press, 2002), 3–4; "Palmer, Phoebe Worrall," in Kostlevy, ed., *Historical Dictionary of the Holiness Movement*, 197.

69. Dieter, *Holiness Revival*, 24–28; Charles Edwin Jones, "The Inverted Shadow of Phoebe Palmer," *Wesleyan Theological Journal* 31:2 (1996):120–31; Kevin T. Lowery, "A Fork in the Wesleyan Road: Phoebe Palmer and the Appropriation of Christian Perfection," *Wesleyan Theological Journal* 36:2 (2001): 187–222; John Leland Peters, *Christian Perfection and American Methodism* (Nashville, Tenn.: Abingdon, 1956), chapter 4; Stanley, *Holy Boldness*, 71–73. See also Phoebe Palmer, *The Way of Holiness, with Notes by the Way; Being a Narrative of Religious Experience Resulting from a Determination to Be a Bible Christian*, second ed. (New York: Lane & Scott, 1849; reprint, Digital Edition 09/30/98 by Holiness Data Ministry).

70. Dieter, *Holiness Revival*, 42.

71. Dieter, *Holiness Revival*, 81.

72. In 1998 it became the Christian Holiness Partnership. See "Christian Holiness Partnership," in Kostlevy, ed., *Historical Dictionary of the Holiness Movement*, 48–50.

73. See Appendix II in Jones, *Perfectionist Persuasion*, for a list of all the meeting sites from 1867 to 1924. The National Association had very few meetings in the South, because of the division between the northern and southern branches of Methodism. The first southern meetings were in Knoxville, Tennessee, in 1872 and 1873. For regional tensions and the holiness movement, see Briane K. Turley, *A Wheel within a Wheel: Southern Methodism and the Georgia Holiness Association* (Macon, Ga.: Mercer University Press, 1999).

74. Dieter, *Holiness Revival*, 116.

75. Dieter, *Holiness Revival*, 252. However, many of the holiness evangelists in the National Association were in harmony with the divine healing movements. See also Kenneth O. Brown, *Inskip, McDonald, Fowler: "Wholly and Forever Thine," Early Leadership in the National Camp Meeting Association for the Promotion of Holiness* (Hazelton, Pa.: Holiness Archives, 1999), 109–10, 250–51. For an example of a member testifying that sufferings are "golden opportunities for the development of Christian character," see *Proceedings of Holiness Conferences, Cincinnati, November 26th, 1877 and New York, December 17th, 1877* (New York: Garland, 1985), 19–21.

76. Jones, *Perfectionist Persuasion*, 50; *Proceedings of the Western Union Holiness Convention Held at Jacksonville, Ill., Dec. 15th–19th, 1880* (Bloomington, Ill.: Western Holiness Association, L. Hawkins, agent, 1881).

77. W. E. Boardman, *Faith Work under Dr. Cullis, in Boston* (Beacon Hill Place, Boston: Willard Tract Repository, 1880), 23–24.

78. Baer, "Perfectly Empowered Bodies," 76–151; Raymond J. Cunningham, "From Holiness to Healing: The Faith Cure in America, 1872–1892," *Church History* 43:4 (1974): 499–513; Donald Dayton, "The Rise of the Evangelical Healing Movement in Nineteenth-Century America," *Pneuma* 4:1 (1982): 1–18; Nancy A. Hardesty, *Faith Cure: Divine Healing in the Holiness and Pentecostal Movements* (Peabody, Mass.: Hendrickson, 2003).

79. Hardesty, *Faith Cure*, 41–44; Bedford, Jr., "'A Larger Christian Life'".

80. For an in-depth discussion of healing doctrines, see chapter four.

81. Russell Kelso Carter, *"Faith Healing" Reviewed after Twenty Years* (Boston: Christian Witness Co., 1897).

82. Dowie was the most (in)famous faith healer in the United States at the turn of the century. See D. William Faupel, *The Everlasting Gospel: The Significance of Eschatology in the Development of Pentecostal Thought* (Sheffield, England: Sheffield Academic Press, 1996), 116–35; Grant Wacker, "Marching to Zion: Religion in a Modern Utopian Community," *Church History* 54 (1985): 496–511; Grant Wacker, Chris R. Armstrong, and Jay S. F. Blossom, "John Alexander Dowie: Harbinger of Pentecostal Power," in James R. Goff, Jr., and Grant Wacker, eds., *Portraits of a Generation: Early Pentecostal Leaders* (Fayetteville: University of Arkansas Press, 2002), 3–19.

83. Jonathan R. Baer, "Redeemed Bodies: The Functions of Divine Healing in Incipient Pentecostalism," *Church History* 70:4 (2001): 735–71; Dayton, *Theological Roots of Pentecostalism;* David Edwin Harrell, Jr., *All Things Are Possible: The Healing and Charismatic Revivals in Modern America* (Bloomington: Indiana University Press, 1975); David Edwin Harrell, Jr., *Oral Roberts: An American Life* (Bloomington: Indiana University Press, 1985); R. A. N. Kydd, "Healing in the Christian Church," in Stanley M. Burgess and Eduard M. Van Der Maas, eds., *New International Dictionary of Pentecostal and Charismatic Movements* (Grand Rapids, Mich.: Zondervan, 2002): 698–710.

CHAPTER 2

HEALING THE BODY OF CHRIST

> The light of eventide now shines the darkness to dispel,
> The glories of fair Zion's state ten thousand voices tell;
> For out of Babel God doth call His scattered saints in one,
> Together all one church compose, the body of His Son.
> (C. W. Naylor/A. L. Byers, "The Church's Jubilee")

The Church of God Reformation Movement traces its beginning to D. S. Warner's insight that entire sanctification of individuals is the biblical key to the unification of the one, holy, catholic, and apostolic church. The exact beginning date depends on whether one identifies the crucial event as Warner's initial discovery of that truth or his first public proclamation of it. In either case, the story asserts that a new and final age of the church—the "evening light" or the "final reformation"—began sometime between 1879 and 1881 with D. S. Warner. The Holy Spirit was cleansing individuals from the remnants of sin and calling them to separate from every worldly thing, thereby healing the body of Christ from the division of denominationalism.[1]

Thus, at the very center of Church of God theology was the idea that internal cleansing by the Holy Spirit produced a visible change in individual believers. Sanctified people exhibited holy behavior, and in turn they constituted the pure church, the recrudescence of the New Testament church. At first, this purification extended only to a spiritual cleansing and a moral perfection. Warner explicitly denied that sanctification would produce physical healing.[2] Before long, however, the implications for the health and healing of individual physical bodies proved impossible to ignore. The belief that entire sanctification purified the will and enabled a saint to follow God's laws perfectly suggested that the

23

sanctified might enjoy perfect health by eating right, exercising, and conforming to God's rules of health. The idea that entire sanctification immediately and supernaturally removed the effects of sin implied that divine healing might work similarly. Finally, the return of the organization of the New Testament church brought with it the hope that the gifts of healing exhibited in the early church would return as well.

This book will explore the various interpretations the Church of God gave to health and healing. Later chapters will explain specific doctrines of divine healing and the struggles the Church had over what health and healing (or the lack thereof) signified to individual believers and to the movement as a whole. The rest of this chapter will describe the connections among health reform, divine healing, sanctification, and ecclesiology in the Church of God. The first section is a brief biographical sketch of D. S. Warner's life up until the founding of the Church of God. It shows how he brought various broadly perfectionist ideas about health into the movement. The second section describes in detail the theology of the Church for the period covered in this work. The final section outlines the institutional developments of the Church from 1881 to the founding of the General Assembly in 1917.

D. S. Warner and the Beginning of the Church of God

Daniel Sidney Warner was born on June 25, 1842, in Bristol, Ohio, the fifth of six children of David and Leah (Dierdorf) Warner.[3] The Warners did not attend church, and Daniel remembered his father's hostility to religion. The antipathy may have stemmed from the fact that he was a tavernkeeper by trade. The year after Daniel was born, the Warners moved to the home they would live in until 1863 in New Washington, Ohio, and David became a farmer.

Little information exists about Warner's childhood other than the reminiscences he wrote much later in books and especially in his poem *Innocence*. Warner's first biographer, A. L. Byers, tried to reconstruct the story by interviewing Warner's relatives and descendants, but his work was strongly colored by Warner's own writings and by Byers's theological interest in showing the divine origin of the Church of God.[4] From Byers's account, we know that Warner was a talented public speaker and was employed to stump for Democratic candidates. He also appears to have been something of a class clown, but Warner himself described an unhappy childhood.[5] By the time Warner wrote his memories, his relationship with his father and his mother had become part of his personal testimony and are therefore suspect. Further, Warner had adopted such extreme views about alcohol and religion that it is not possible to say whether Warner's opinions colored his memories of his father or if his father's behavior led to Warner's opinions. That being said, Warner remembered an unhappy early life. He was sickly and weak and felt that his father despised him for his weakness.[6] He also remembered that his father was controlled by alcohol and his mother—though not formally religious—was a guiding spirit and a moral influence.[7]

According to Byers, Warner's initial conversion experience was fleeting and unexpected. Warner had displayed no interest in religion but did like to sing. One Sunday afternoon in 1864, he was singing gospel hymns at a neighbor's house and was "greatly affected." "God spoke to his conscience. His conviction was so strong as to cause him for several months to lose his love for the dance and to reflect seriously on his course of life." He had not, however, joined a church or any kind of community, and soon dancing replaced his religious convictions. Thus, at least in the way this story has been told in the Church of God, Warner's conversion—amorphous as it was—was to a faith that understood dancing and revelry to be incompatible with the Christian life. The crisis came when Warner went out dancing while his sister lay in bed gravely ill. His mother waited for his return, and at two o'clock in the morning she "expostulated with her boy regarding his sinful career." He fell to his knees and prayed for mercy. "From that time he was deeply convicted though to his companions he gave no evidence of a changed life, as he had not received the new birth." His friends believed he was planning mischief when he went to a revival at the local schoolhouse. However, Warner went to the altar and experienced the new birth that night in February 1865 at age 22.[8]

Less than a month after his conversion, Warner took his brother's place in the military draft and enlisted as a private in company C. of the 195th Ohio Volunteer Army. His tenure in the military was very brief. The war itself was quickly coming to an end, and Warner's poor health made him unfit for soldiering. Having served just over four months, he was honorably discharged in Wheeling, West Virginia, on July 21, 1865. He had contracted a "disease of the lungs" from marching and performing sentry duty. Warner never fully recovered from the disease and drew a disability pension of twelve dollars per month.[9]

Warner returned to northwestern Ohio intending to pursue a ministerial education. He had also fallen in love with a woman named Frances Stocking, and he proposed marriage. Stocking refused to wait for him while he went to college. Warner later wrote in his journal, "I took the matter to the Lord and was soon confirmed in the belief that our marriage was not ordained of God."[10] Stocking soon married someone else and moved to the West. Warner was confirmed in his decision when he later learned that she had left her husband and become a Spiritualist. This wrecked her "morally, mentally, and physically" and led her to an early grave.[11]

Instead of marrying, Warner enrolled in Oberlin College. His tenure there was very brief because he ran out of money after only two months. After teaching school for a brief period, he returned for the spring term and started again in the fall of 1866. He did not complete that semester either, because he decided that Oberlin was not helping to prepare him to preach the gospel. Unfortunately, we have no other information than the dates of his attendance, so it is impossible to document the college's influence on him.[12] Oberlin was a center of perfectionist theology and social reform. Charles G. Finney, one of the most influential revivalists and reformers in America, was president of the college and also professor of theology.[13] Oberlin was also a center of health reform. The cafeteria had experimented with planned vegetarian diets, and the school was one of the first to offer classes in hygiene and diet.[14] It is tempting to suggest that Warner chose Oberlin because he already had an interest in perfectionist theology, but his brief stay there and his apparent dissatisfaction with the course of study present problems for this argument. Further, Warner was extremely skeptical about perfectionist claims long after he left Oberlin.[15] Merle Strege has said, "it is interesting to note that late in life [Warner] adopted views on gender, race, and theology that closely resembled ideas in circulation at Oberlin during the middle of the nineteenth century."[16] I would add diet and hygiene to that list and say that it is almost certain that Warner was at least aware of these ideas. It is true that he was only briefly a student at Oberlin, but he was there preparing for ministry and presumably would have been interested in the theological and social ideas at the school. Moreover, Warner lived near Oberlin until he moved to Nebraska in 1873. He was working as a minister in northwest Ohio, a center of revivalism, perfectionist theology, and social reform. It would be surprising if he had not been aware of the holiness movement.

Warner did not affiliate with a denomination that emphasized the doctrine of entire sanctification. He gave his first sermon on Easter in 1876 at a Cogswell, Ohio, schoolhouse in a revival sponsored by the Methodist Episcopal Church, but he was licensed to preach by the West Ohio Eldership of the Church of God, a regional judicatory of the General Eldership of the Churches of God, in October 1867.[17] Evidently, the form of church governance was the most important issue for Warner when choosing a religious institution. He chose the Church of God because he believed it was the most compatible with what he understood to be the New Testament standards for the church. This denomination had German Pietist origins but had adopted Arminian theology. It was also the denomination of the minister who had conducted the revival in which Warner received the new birth.

Critics and supporters alike have charged Warner with taking his doctrine of the church from John Winebrenner.[18] There is no denying that Warner was strongly influenced by the ecclesiology of the Church of God (Winebrenner), including its assertion that the only biblically justifiable name for the church is the Church of God.[19] An outline from Warner's journal shows that he was already preaching anti-sect ideas by May of 1873.[20] Warner's mature doctrine of the church, however, differed from that of the Winebrennerian Church in that he came to determine that the basis of unity that held the anti-denominational church together was not an organization that called itself "the Church of God," granted ministerial licenses, and baptized converts into the Church. Rather, the

experience of entire sanctification was the basis of unity, and proof of membership was the holy life produced by the cleansing from all sin by the Holy Spirit.
A closer examination in the next section of Warner's theology will explain how
the Church of God movement combined the ecclesiology of the Winebrennarian
Church of God with the soteriology of entire sanctification from the holiness
movement. But Warner had not yet experienced sanctification or even accepted
it as a legitimate experience. He had rejected denominationalism and joined a
group that claimed to represent the church of the New Testament.

From the time he was licensed to preach until he resigned to become a holiness evangelist in 1877, Warner served ministerial appointments in the West
Ohio Eldership of the Church of God. His first circuits were in northwest Ohio,
but in June 1873 the Eldership appointed him to the Seward Mission in Nebraska.[21] He worked in Nebraska until the fall of 1875, when he returned to
assume the Ashland, Ohio, circuit.[22] Warner's experiences were the common
difficulties faced by homesteaders, circuit riders, and pioneer evangelists. His
work in building and leading congregations is well documented elsewhere and is
not relevant to this study, except to note that Warner achieved some prominence
in the Eldership. He served on numerous committees and was an invited speaker
at the annual ministerial assembly.[23] We will return to Warner's connection with
the West Ohio Eldership when we get to Warner's disciplining for unorthodox
theology (1877). The important point now, however, is that Warner's work with
the Eldership dramatically improved the historical record he left behind. He
began to write articles and reports for the denominational newspaper, *The
Church Advocate*. Warner also kept a daily journal from November 1872 to
December 1879.[24]

Warner's journal provides some insight into what he was reading and
thinking, and it is full of entries that relate to health and healing. The first thing
to note is that his interest in healing stemmed from his personal experiences with
pain, sickness, and loss. His chronically poor health has already been mentioned,
but his struggles continued throughout the period covered in the journal. The
most extreme incident was a coma-like blackout in 1878.[25] In addition to his
own health, Warner's immediate family suffered greatly in these years. Warner
married Tamzen Kerr on September 5, 1867. Their first child was born on December 29, 1868, and died soon after birth. Triplets were born in 1872 only to
die hours later. Soon thereafter, Warner's wife died as well.[26] On June 4, 1874,
he married Sarah Keller.[27] A healthy girl they named Levilla Modest was born to
them on March 18, 1875, but she died at age three from pneumonia.[28] Warner
also lost his mother and his father during this time. He had to leave his father's
body before the funeral so he could be with his daughter Levilla as she died.[29]
The infant mortality rate in the Midwest in the late nineteenth century was high,
and Warner's experience would not have been extraordinary. However, his journal entries indicate that these deaths affected him strongly and he continued to
reflect on them—and how to prevent that kind of loss—long afterward.[30]

Warner frequently prayed for divine healing and anointed the sick with oil following the instructions in James 5:14–15.[31] There is no evidence, however, that Warner understood prayers for divine healing to be anything more than a direct application of that passage from James. He was interested in divine healing early in his ministry and visited a "divine healing hospital" in 1873, but he did not conduct public healing services until after his sanctification.[32] He was disappointed when prayer did not bring an immediate healing, but healing was not so tightly integrated into his theology that failure would cause doubt about God's faithfulness or about Warner's ministry. Moreover, he used prayer as an *aid,* not an alternative, to medicine. His portrayal of doctors was generally positive.[33] The closest he came to expressing a negative opinion of doctors was really a condemnation of the poor dietary habits he observed among his congregants. He lamented that eating fried foods produced "families of living corps [sic] who sacrifice money, labor, health, and happiness to disease and doctors."[34] The only specific mention of a medical treatment was a surprisingly positive account of a doctor who used the yolk of an egg and salt to treat cancer.[35] Warner called a doctor to attend his wife when she had severe headaches.[36] He brought a doctor for his daughter Levilla at least four times. Once was merely for "counsel," but another time the doctor gave her medicine.[37] A third time Warner called the doctor after the saints had "bowed in prayer and anointed her bowels."[38] Warner himself saw a doctor for "bilious remittent fever and an attack of hemmorage [sic] of the lungs."[39] He maintained this practical approach to healing throughout his ministry. Indeed, one of the last articles he wrote challenged the exclusive dependence on faith and defended the use of natural remedies to help cure sickness.[40]

That is not to say that divine healing was without theological significance for him—around the time of his experience of sanctification in 1877, Warner began to focus more attention on divine healing, miracles, and explanations for unanswered prayers—but Warner was much more interested in the conglomeration of health-related theories and practices that were lumped together under the label "phrenology" than he was in divine healing or orthodox medicine. As early as February 1, 1873, he was studying phrenology, and just one month after that he was writing articles about it.[41] On occasion, he gave head readings, including a time when he concluded a revival service with phrenological analyses. He clearly saw no conflict between phrenology and religion. He visited a prison so he could study the heads of criminals, and he gave a phrenological interpretation of the Omaha tribe of Native Americans.[42]

The phrenological books mentioned by title in his journal were *Creative and Sexual Science* and *Physiology, Animal and Mental,* both by Orson S. Fowler, and George Weaver's *Mental Science.*[43] These books are particularly interesting for this study because they represented the progressive, hopeful, perfectionist strain of American phrenology.[44] They taught phrenology as a diagnostic tool that would unlock the power of self-improvement. Far from being fatalistic, they said that underdeveloped characteristics—as shown by the shape of the head—improve with exercise and work. The head would actually change shape to reflect mental and character development. Further, head reading would improve society by ensuring that people did work they were suited for, found compatible mates, and lived happy lives. Fowler was particularly expansive with his system. He insisted that he could prescribe a diet and lifestyle that would guarantee freedom from disease and debility.[45] Phrenology would also bring universal harmony and Christianity without division or creeds.[46] This last assertion had an interesting parallel in Warner's ecclesiology. On December 7, 1872, Warner wrote, "as Indians cause the heads of their children to develop into a peculiar shape by tying a board thereon, so human Creeds, bound upon unsuspecting converts mold them to their peculiar doctrine."[47] Warner never abandoned his early opposition to creeds.

It would stretch the evidence to say that D. S. Warner derived his holiness theology from health reform ideology, specifically the phrenology of Fowler and Weaver. Warner seldom mentioned phrenology after his sanctification, although he continued to recommend its practical teaching, and his library contained many phrenological books published after 1877. Yet the parallels are striking.[48] Phrenology was a key that unlocked the secrets of health, the Bible, and human progress. It claimed that perfect adherence to the laws of nature was possible. Fowler explicitly denounced creeds and denominations in favor of universal unity. Finally, phrenology, like holiness, asserted a correspondence between internal character and external appearance.

Warner most frequently used health-reform ideology in his ongoing struggle to combine his itinerant lifestyle with a healthful diet. He often complained that church socials were not only frivolous but also physically debilitating.[49] If people would have abandoned sweets, cakes, fried food, coffee, and tea, Warner argued, they would have been much healthier and more useful servants of God. Warner himself struggled with diet and his desire for sweets. His journal entry for Thanksgiving 1876 illustrates his evangelical commitment to diet reform:

> Read O. S. Fowler's Physiology, Animal and Mental. O God forgive me of the sin this book has convicted me of. By the grace of God, from this day forth I will reform in quantity, etc. of food as much as my irregular mode of life will allow. O how much I can improve the vigor of mind and the fervor of devotion.[50]

Warner wrote this journal entry five months before he began to seek entire sanctification. It indicates that he understood violation of the dietary recommendations of phrenology to be worse than physically harmful. Eating too much was a sin. That he continued to believe this after his own sanctification is clear from the "solemn covenant" he wrote on December 13, 1877, five months after his sanctification. In this covenant, Warner wrote, "*I bind myself to live,*

*act, speak, think, move, sit, stand up, lie down, eat [double underline], drink,
hear, see, feel, and whatsoever I do all the days and nights of my life to do all
continually and exclusively to the Glory of God.* I must henceforth *wear nothing*
but what *honors God.* I must have nothing in my *possession or under my control*
but such things as I can consistently write *upon 'holiness unto the Lord.'*"[51] An
even clearer connection between dietary rules and a sinless life is evident in the
rules Warner adopted for himself on the first of January, 1879. Many of these
came directly from Dio Lewis's book *Our Digestion, or, My Jolly Friend's
Secret.*[52]

By 1877, Warner had embraced phrenological perfectionism. He was
comfortable with the ideas that human beings could obey God's laws and that
obedience could be measured by examination of the physical body. There is a
correspondence between a person's internal state and his or her external
appearance. Moreover, phrenology taught that the fundamental means for
reforming society and the church was the perfection of individuals. Warner also
had strong opinions about the dangers of denominational Christianity, and
therefore it would seem that the theology of the holiness movement would have
been a natural fit for him.

Warner was more open to the secular perfectionism embodied in
phrenological reform than to the overtly religious perfectionism of the holiness
movement. Simply speaking, phrenology and holiness theology both promised
that individuals could progress to a higher state of existence in which they
would live "without sin." For phrenology, sin was a violation of the laws of
nature. In holiness theology, sin was more complex; however, the implications
of both movements for individuals looked very similar. Warner accepted the
idea of phrenological perfectionism before he embraced Wesleyan
sanctification. His opposition to holiness theology appears to have stemmed at
least in part from his experience with people who claimed to have been
sanctified. Early in his ministry, he attributed an acquaintance's suicide to the
man's recent profession of sanctification. Warner believed that the man
understood his new state of freedom from sin to be a deification, and reported
that the man had asserted that he could "lay down his life and take it back up
again" just before he killed himself with a pocketknife.[53] In addition to a fear of
fanaticism, Warner also faced institutional barriers in that many members of the
West Ohio Eldership considered holiness theology heterodox. Phrenology was
not a "religion" and therefore escaped the notice of the Eldership. When his in-
laws and his wife Sarah professed entire sanctification in April 1877, Warner
began to seek it as well.[54] He wrote in his journal for July 5, 1877, that he had
understood his conversion to be "a finished work" but had come to realize that
he had only asked God for pardon from past sin and relief from guilt. He went to
the altar again, feeling foolish for kneeling where he had invited so many
sinners, and God "directed" him to 1 Peter 5:10 and Eph. 3:14–20. The next day,

Warner experienced the second blessing. He wrote on July 8, 1877, "Thank God true holiness needs but to be tested to be proved genuine."

The testing of holiness took a number of forms in Warner's ministry. His commitment to the doctrine was tested, but the more important sense of testing is that he understood holiness to "prove" itself in a holy life and a visible church. Initially, the West Ohio Eldership tested Warner's commitment to sanctification. He had claimed the second blessing on July 7, 1877, and published his first two articles about holiness in the *Church Advocate* on July 28. On September 15, the annual assembly of the Eldership charged him with bringing "schism and division" to the Church of God by inviting "fanatics" into the assembly.[55] Warner denied the charges in his journal, but apparently not to the Eldership, and he quoted Joseph's words to his brothers, "Ye thought evil in your hearts, but God meant it all for good, for you see how much people he hath moved from death by the famine." Warner was unrepentant. He continued to study and preach holiness, but somehow managed to get his preaching license renewed.[56] On October 1, 1877, the ministerial credentials committee upheld the charges but "recommended me favorably to the body for license with this restriction, only that I do not bring holiness workers or any outside elements to hold a meeting anywhere in the churches of God without their [the Eldership's] consent." He agreed to the restrictions and received his license. That night he was the speaker at the Eldership's closing worship service and spoke about his sanctification. The meeting closed with the announcement of the new ministerial assignments, and Warner received a circuit that was supposed to be more hospitable to the message of holiness than was his old one. Even this proved too restrictive, and Warner resigned his appointment (but not his license) to become a holiness evangelist on November 23, 1877. On January 30, 1878, the standing committee of the Eldership found Warner guilty of "violating the rules of cooperation and dividing the church." He denied the charges but lost his license anyway. His opinion of the proceedings is clear from the title he gave the story in his journal: "Trial and Expulsion from the West Ohio Eldership of the Church of God for Preaching Full Salvation, for Following the Holy Spirit, and Helping to Save over 150 Souls in this Place."[57]

Warner's independence from the Eldership began as an intellectual separation and was completed by the official removal of his license. This independence appears to have contributed to his newly open preaching about divine healing. On the very day of his sanctification, Warner reported for the first time that the Holy Spirit had given him a message about divine healing and was leading him to pray for a specific individual.[58] He also began to seek miracles—as opposed to simply the grace—of healing and reported having prayed for a blind woman, a deaf boy, and a woman with severe spinal deformity.[59] Until Warner's expulsion from the West Ohio Eldership of the Church of God on January 30, 1878, all of Warner's divine healing activity appears to have been in private prayer services. Merle Strege has said that

Warner responded to his defrocking by adding services for divine healing with C. R. Dunbar.[60] Freedom from institutional restraint combined with an increased interest in divine healing led Warner to hold services specifically for healing. He conducted divine healing services in the Marion, Indiana, camp meeting and the camp meeting in Upper Sandusky, Ohio. In the latter, "special faith and gifts of healing were considered," and Warner miraculously obtained relief from a chronic cough that had plagued him since childhood.[61]

Several of the prayers for healing resulted in remarkable successes. A blind woman received both salvation and sight, "a poor colored sister on the verge of death by the consumption" was healed and strengthened, and Brother Kaufman's instantaneous healing astonished the medical doctor who had declared him to be beyond help.[62] Other prayers for healing had ambiguous results; however, the absence of immediate physical improvement did not seem to have caused Warner to question divine healing. Because he had no carefully developed theology of divine healing, his approach to healing prayers was experimental. Many were not healed, but there was no category for a "failure" of divine healing.

The attempts that failed to produce an immediate restoration to health revealed more about Warner's theology than the successes did. In several cases, Warner decided that the prayers had in fact helped. He anointed a young girl who then died several days later. Warner said that she had "got some better" and the healing had eased her death.[63] A boy received neither healing nor increased physical comfort but "felt at peace with God."[64] Thus, healing did not necessarily mean physical restoration. It could be a new sense of peace about the physical condition.

Another possibility was that conditions were not yet right for healing. A special meeting did not restore a deaf boy's hearing, but the saints were not discouraged. As Warner said, they would try repeatedly "just as we often have to do with those seeking pardon and sanctification."[65] Similarly, Warner and his wife confidently left a deformed woman "in the hands of Jesus," because they were "strongly impressed" that God would restore her in the future.[66] Warner's journal never returned to these cases, but he did describe a camp meeting in Marion, Indiana, where he and the saints prayed for God to heal two people. There was no immediate physical evidence of healing, and the two afflicted persons insisted that they were still sick. However, the group believed the healing had occurred and went to bed, leaving the sick people behind. In the night, their faith "joined on that of the party in the camp" and they received a complete healing. This success story notwithstanding, it is likely that Warner's itinerancy aided him in interpreting healing this way. He could leave the sick in the hands of Jesus.

The final explanation of "failed" healing prayers was that God was using the infirmity to communicate some message. The clearest example in Warner's journal was a time when his own "bilious remittent fever and an attack of hemmorage [sic] of the lungs" did not respond to prayer. It makes sense that Warner did not use the two previous explanations. He knew that he did not feel any better or enjoy any kind of spiritual advance, so the first explanation did not work. The second was not appropriate because it was from the perspective of an outsider, not of a sufferer. Therefore, he reasoned that the delay was a message from God:

> O Lord I thank thee for this affliction for I know it is all for the good of my soul. Thou hast shown me that I have boasted too much in my health and ascribed it too generally to my knowledge of and prudence in observing natural laws.[67]

Warner's own failed healing started to create the tension that the entire Church of God experienced in the 1900s. He identified a reason that God refused to grant healing, and thereby shifted the blame onto himself and protected the theory of divine healing from questioning. The problem he detected, however, was the first hint of a conflict between divine healing and the health reform ideology of willful adherence to the laws of nature. From here, it was a short step to saying that faith for healing required the abandonment of medical means and health remedies.

Some of Warner's influential followers did take that step, but Warner himself did not. His approach to health and healing was more practical than rigidly doctrinal. Divine healing had a place in his theology, but so did natural remedies and healthful diets. For instance, he ran a regular health column in his periodical years after claiming that God had told him he was taking too much credit for his own health. The most extensive phrenological analysis in Warner's journal appeared in the account of his only surviving child Levilla's death. Warner had rushed to her side when he heard that she was dying. When he arrived,

> [He] at once saw what was threatening the very life of the poor little sufferer. She was exquisitely fine in the texture of brain and her head measured 19 inches in circumference around the forehead—and had a very sensitive nervous temperament. Hence it was extremely important that the most perfect silence should be maintained in her presence, and with this strong nervous action with any sickness or weakness, much talk and noise would necessarily draw the disease to the brain.[68]

Warner removed her to a quiet room, but it was too late. Her obituary said that her parents had "imparted to her a good large physical structure" by carefully regulating her diet, but her mind "was of great nervous activity." The ladies of the church had not recognized the danger of her condition.

These examples show the importance of nurture and home life. The implication of the analysis of the crippled young man's mother was that she was responsible for his sin, which in turn prevented Warner's prayer of healing from working. With the man of "marked intellectuality," Warner was suggesting that the preachers (including Warner) should have recognized the way his mind worked and anticipated his questions. Finally, Levilla would likely have lived if her caretakers had given the proper treatment. "Scientific" techniques could produce health and belief.

Less than two months after Levilla's death, Warner and his wife attempted to create the perfect conditions for their next child. In preparation for procreation, "special attention was paid to diet and health, pleasure of mind, sociability, and practicable usefulness in order to endow the new contemplated immortal with the best physical, social, and holy executive abilities in our power to impart."[69]

After the West Ohio Eldership expelled him, Warner was an independent evangelist working with the loosely connected holiness camp meetings of Ohio and Indiana. In April, 1878, he traveled to Beaver Dam, Indiana, to meet with the Northern Indiana Eldership of the Church of God, a group formed "sometime in 1877" to protest the Winebrennerian Church's support of secret societies.[70] The Indiana Eldership was theologically similar to the West Ohio Eldership except that it explicitly denounced secret societies as contributing to the division of the church and it actively endorsed the doctrine of entire sanctification.[71] In July Warner approached the editor of the Indiana Eldership's newspaper, *The Herald of Gospel Freedom*, about adding a department on holiness. At the October meeting of the Indiana Eldership, Warner became a member, a resolution passed expanding the *Herald* and devoting it to holiness, and Warner was appointed associate editor.[72]

The paper consolidated in late 1880 with *The Pilgrim*, a holiness paper from Indianapolis, and Warner named the new publication *The Gospel Trumpet*. Although the *Trumpet* served as the official organ of the Indiana Eldership, the group does not appear to have contributed to it beyond the subscriptions of individual members. By the summer of 1881, Warner was its sole owner, publisher, and editor. With his acquisition of the *Gospel Trumpet*, Warner had the most important resource for his future ministry. The paper provided Warner with a forum for his ideas, means for organizing and promoting evangelistic meetings, and a position of authority. Moreover, "editor" and "publisher" were not ecclesiastical titles, so Warner was able to build a network of subscribers and adherents and still plausibly decry denominational organization. The *Gospel Trumpet* was so important to Warner's Church of God movement that a strong argument could be made for dating the beginning of the Church of God with the first issue, January 1, 1881. Years later, Warner provided support for this interpretation when he renumbered the volumes to erase the years of the *Herald of Gospel Freedom*.[73]

Two other events from this period also contributed to Warner's new religious movement, both having been identified as the beginning of the Church of God. First was Warner's insight into the nature of the church. His book *Bible Proofs of the Second Work of Grace* was published in 1880 by the Evangelical United Mennonite Press in Nappannee, Indiana. Most of the book was a collection of arguments common in the holiness movement showing the biblical foundations of the doctrine of entire sanctification. Chapters 24–26 were a departure from holiness theology in that they described "the great work of restoration in the latter times, when, through the preaching of holiness and the upholding of the full scriptural standards of the truth, God should bring his people into unity again."[74] In other words, Warner had come to believe that holiness was the means by which the Holy Spirit was going to restore the New Testament church. The anti-denominational beliefs of the Winebrennerian Church combined with Wesleyan holiness to create a new dispensation that Warner called "the Evening Light."[75] According to *Bible Proofs*, the "Holy Spirit in a special manner" gave him this new understanding of the church on the 30th of August 1879.[76] This insight, the intertwining of personal holiness and the restoration of the church as a visible unity of saints, became the central message of the Church of God.

Interpreters who have understood the Church of God as a Holy Spirit-directed reformation movement have tended to identify Warner's new "light on the church" as the pivotal event in the beginning of the movement.[77] This approach says that the Holy Spirit had begun to heal the body of Christ from division and impurity, and Warner was simply given the key to recognizing this divine initiative. Interpreting the Church of God in this way makes it much grander than the little association of people who read the *Gospel Trumpet*. The Holy Spirit was working everywhere. Warner and his band, therefore, were not creating or even organizing the church; instead, they were discovering it. The sign of the Church was the Holy Spirit working in individuals as it did in the apostolic period. Many signs existed, but one of the clearest proved to be divine healing.

Holiness and searching for the church did not lead to quietism. Warner was not only looking for evidence of the Holy Spirit, he also believed he was led to demonstrate with his life the visible Church of God. There was always the belief in the Church that while the Holy Spirit was doing its work around the world, it was also gathering the faithful to Warner and his followers. Thus, the beginning of the Church of God as a movement cannot be separated from the initial public testimonies made by Warner in 1881. That summer he withdrew his membership from the Western Holiness Association after attempting without success to abolish its constitutional requirement that all members of the Association also maintain membership in a Protestant denomination.[78] In October, at the annual meeting of the Indiana Eldership and just two years after his initial affiliation with that body, Warner withdrew because he believed that the Eldership's granting of ministerial credentials made it a denomination. Ministers should be known "by their fruits," that is by holiness and not by licenses. He claimed he "forever withdrew from all organisms that uphold and condone sects and denominations in the body of Christ."[79] He also managed to get five other members of the Eldership to withdraw with him. A few weeks later, Warner visited an Eldership in Michigan and made a similar speech that convinced several more people to separate from "sect Babylon."

The two groups that separated from the Indiana and Michigan Elderships formed the first two congregations in the Church of God. However, congregations were not the focus of the early movement. It was a publishing and evangelistic effort. Early Church of God people identified these acts of *separation* as significant steps in the founding of the Church of God. This interpretation identifies the importance of obedience to the leading of the Holy Spirit. For every statement that "the Shepherd has begun his long-divided flock again to gather into one," there was a balancing assertion that every saint must "*let* a holy life tell the gospel story."[80] Sanctification enabled perfect obedience to God's laws, and therefore the saints had a religious obligation to separate from all worldliness and live a pure life. No one had yet defined a "pure life," and this book will explore the options they eventually considered. For Warner, we have seen that the holy life included following the natural laws of health as described in phrenological diet reform literature.

By the end of 1881, all the pieces were in place for the Church of God movement. Warner had the beginnings of his soteriology and ecclesiology, he had the *Gospel Trumpet* to spread the message, and had convinced several people to follow him by severing their religious institutional connections. He had also convinced one of the "come-outers" from Michigan, J. C. Fisher, to join him as editor of the *Trumpet*. This proved to be an important decision because Fisher was a hymn-writer and an effective evangelist who contributed articles to the *Trumpet* and greatly increased the Church of God's presence in Michigan and northern Indiana.[81] Warner remained the central figure in the Church of God, but adding Fisher helped remove some of the focus from Warner.

The Church of God began as a publishing concern and a revivalist movement characterized by an overarching metaphor of the church as the pure and undivided body of Christ, a suspicion of human institutions, an interest in diet and health reform, and finally by a theology that invested every action with eternal consequences. The combination of such emphases can itself suggest how health and healing became central to the life and theology of the Church of God. A close examination of the soteriology and ecclesiology of the early movement will provide a context for interpreting the articles, testimonies, sermons, and advice literature that constitute the evidence for our study on health and healing in the Church of God.

Early Church of God Theology

The masthead of the earliest extant copy of the *Gospel Trumpet* declares the paper's object to be "The glory of God in the Salvation of men from all sin, and the union of all saints upon the Bible."[82] This preceded Warner's separation from the Eldership, and was less radical than the mottoes that followed his proclamation. Sometime between September 22, 1882, and August 15, 1883, the motto changed to the more militantly anti-denominational statement, "For the Purity and Unity of His Body, the defence [sic] of ALL His Truth, and the ABOMINATION of Sect Babylon."[83] This continued until the April 15 issue of 1884, at which point the motto became the statement that was used until 1892: "DEFINITE, RADICAL, ANTI-SECTARIAN. Sent Forth in the name of the Lord Jesus Christ. For the Purity and Unity of His Church, the Defence [sic] of ALL His Truth, And the Destruction of Sect Babylon." The motto grew increasingly definite and radical as the movement grew, defined its mission, and experienced conflicts with the holiness groups and the established denominations. However, the main ideas remained constant. Each motto says in effect that human beings can experience a work of grace that will save them "from all sin" and make them pure. The saints were those people who experienced this salvation, and they constituted the church. Both the doctrine of sanctification and the fact that God wanted a pure and unified church were believed to be "Bible doctrines" that the denominations and sects had deliberately obscured so that they could continue to lure people into their organizations, also known as "sect Babylon." The Church of God, therefore, was committed to preaching what they understood to be the plain sense of the Bible, or "ALL His Truth."[84]

Salvation

The early leaders of the Church of God brought the Wesleyan holiness doctrine of salvation—commonly known as "entire sanctification" or the "double cure"—with them into the new movement.[85] In essence, this doctrine asserted that the Bible promises every believer two distinct experiences of grace. The first forgives the guilt of sin, and the second perfects the moral nature, fills the heart with God's love, and frees from all sin.[86] The details and permutations of the theological expressions claiming to be "Wesleyan" perfectionism can be bewildering, and an extensive literature exists that attempts to untangle the development of holiness theology.[87] However, before exploring some of the specifics of Church of God soteriology, it is important to note that all of these movements—Wesley and his revivals, the nineteenth-century holiness revival, and the Church of God—were first and foremost evangelistic efforts. They were really only interested in making theological arguments that would lend biblical support to their descriptions of their experiences. Students of the nineteenth-century holiness movement and the early Church of God will search in vain for an academically consistent theology.[88] Instead, holiness theology was a general belief in the perfectibility of human beings that was supported by a set of shared stories, common interpretations of Bible passages, and technical terms.

The full title of D. S. Warner's first book, *Bible Proofs of the Second Work of Grace, or, Entire Sanctification as a Distinct Experience, Subsequent to Justification, Established by the United Testimony of Several Hundred Texts, Including a Description of the Great Holiness Crisis of the Present Age, by the Prophets*, illustrates many of the themes of holiness theology. It was a proof from "several hundred texts" in the Bible of two works of grace. It used the Bible to demonstrate that the prophets foretold the present holiness movement, and therefore the Church of God stood on biblical authority and was also part of salvation history. Finally, the focus was entirely on the second work. The book said almost nothing about justification, and, in fact, "justification" was an uncharacteristic term for the first work of grace, which was more commonly and accurately called "regeneration."[89]

The two works of grace corresponded to two types of sin. The first was "actual" sin, "willful acts of wrong which we commit by the consent of our own will after we reach the age when we have a knowledge of right and wrong."[90] This sin had eternal consequences. People were guilty of and damned for actual sin. The second type of sin was called "inherent," "inherited," or occasionally "original sin." It was a "sinful disposition which we receive through natural generation."[91] It was the failing that the flesh was heir to, and it produced the will to commit actual sins and violate God's laws. The second type of sin, it must be emphasized, was inherited corruption and not inherited guilt.[92]

The first work of grace removed the first type of sin and repaired the relationship between God and the human being. "Regeneration" was the favored term in both the Church of God and the larger holiness movement,[93] but other terms such as "justification," "conversion," and "the new birth" were common. In *What the Bible Teaches*, F. G. Smith, the third editor of the *Gospel Trumpet*, explained that each of these terms described an aspect of regeneration, but the exclusive use of any one of them would lead to misunderstanding.[94] Warner asserted that all holiness writers and teachers agreed that "regeneration includes the pardon of all past sins; the removal of guilt and condemnation; adoption into the family of God; the witness of the Spirit to pardon and sonship; spiritual life; and a new, moral nature including all the Christian graces."[95] In other words, regeneration did much more than absolve one of guilt. As far as sins were concerned, Christ gave himself as a ransom "so that we stand in the same relation to God as though we had never sinned."[96] The regenerated person was "born again" and returned to the state of childhood, before he or she committed any actual sins. The second birth was much better than the first, however, in that regeneration brought with it "the witness of the Spirit" and a "new, moral nature." Regeneration did not remove the corruption of inbred sin, but, by showing the converted person how inbred sin had led to actual sins that produced separation from God, it diminished its power. A child entering adulthood was without condemnation, just like an adult who was born again. The child, however, was completely at the mercy of inbred sin, because he had no idea that it was governing his thoughts and actions. The second birth brought an experience of love that enabled a struggle against sin and produced a growth in love toward God (1 John 4:19), toward enemies (Matt. 5:44–45), and God's people (1 John 3:14). This new experience of love both led and enabled a person to "go on unto perfection."[97]

Perfection came from the second work of grace, entire sanctification. This work completed salvation by destroying inbred sin, purifying the moral nature, and perfecting the believer in love.[98] Holiness people frequently omitted the modifier "entire" when talking with other believers. This was unfortunate for at least two reasons. First, there was an aspect of sanctification—not entire sanctification—in regeneration for which there was no name. In the Methodist Church two factions developed, each accurately claiming to represent Wesleyan sanctification but meaning very different things. The other problem was that members of Reformed and Lutheran traditions also believed in sanctification, but only as a gradual process not completed until after death. The modifier "entire" clarifies that, for the holiness movement and the Church of God, sanctification was an event, not a process, and it was "entire," not partial. "Sanctification—the second work of grace—includes the destruction of all the works of the devil; the restoration of man to the state of holiness from which he fell, by creating him anew in Christ Jesus, and restoring to him all that image and likeness of God which he lost in the fall of Adam."[99]

Regeneration and sanctification were works of God, and, technically speaking, human effort could not achieve them. However, this was a revivalist movement in which few people ever spoke with technical precision about theological questions. Moreover, entire sanctification depended on regeneration in such a way that it was difficult to separate human effort from divine initiative. God wanted a holy people, and regeneration produced in the believer a love for God and a desire to follow God's laws. Once a clear exposition of the Bible proved that God willed the sanctification of his chosen people, the believers would search for the second blessing.

The holiness preacher's job was to expound the scriptures to show that God demanded holiness. The role of the believer was more difficult to explain. At the most basic level, she would just follow the Holy Spirit to attain holiness with a "definite grasp of faith."[100] Regeneration produced a love for God that the Bible (and preaching) channeled into a desire for holiness. This in turn produced a searching after holiness that included prayer, "consecration," and a pursuit of holy living that would make the believer into a worthy recipient of the Holy Spirit.

Several questions that will be central to the rest of this book follow from the above description of sanctification. What were its limits? How did sanctification relate to human behavior and will? What function did sanctification play in the lives of believers and the life of the church?

Sanctification was a difficult doctrine to control. Warner himself was aware of at least some of the possible problems, and he initially opposed the doctrine because he feared that it would promote "fanaticism." Theologians and preachers tried to make clear that sanctification was only a perfection of the moral nature, and not a form of deification. As Warner wrote, "our moral nature alone is susceptible to perfection now, and that only in quality, leaving all the powers of the soul free to enlarge in magnitude." Human beings remained created beings, and were therefore subject to human limitations. The sanctified were still subject to mistakes, limited knowledge, and death.[101] Sanctification was not the end but rather the beginning of Christian development in holiness. However, the number and kind of limitations placed on the sanctified individual by the doctrine—as opposed to the limits that were discovered from the experience of living the sanctified life—were quite few, considering that the doctrine said that human beings were restored to the pre-Fall state. Ordinary believers as well as preachers reasoned that such a restoration would deliver a human being from such things as sickness and the condemnation of the law of God. Sickness came from sin, so sanctification should free one from sickness. Further, because inbred sin was the only impediment to fulfilling God's laws, the sanctified Christian should be able to follow God's will perfectly. Freedom from all the sins of the flesh became the practical focus of the teaching of sanctification. The perfect love for God—"serving God without fear in holiness and righteousness before him all the days of our life"—quickly gave way to the emphasis on pure living and the benefits that would redound to the believer.[102] That is to say, the experience of trying to live the implications of sanctification led to a contestation of the limits of sanctification.

The role of human effort in sanctification and the meaning of a holy life proved problematic. Sanctification always produced holy behavior, and preachers and *Gospel Trumpet* advice columnists frequently counseled addicts of all kinds to seek sanctification for a complete cure.[103] The *desire* to sin would disappear and would never return, unless sanctification was lost.[104] Holy living was therefore a testimony to sanctification. However, seeking sanctification involved abandoning the behavior that signified sin. "[E]verything which partakes of the spirit and nature of the world must be forsaken—worldly sentiments, worldly associations, worldly ambitions, worldly amusements, and worldly dress—everything that is not in strict accordance with the plain teachings of God's Word."[105] Forsaking such sins was supposed to be joyous, and regeneration provided the strength of faith necessary to forsake them. Hence, sinful behavior was a failure of will that had eternal consequences. To be sanctified and freed from sinful (and physically and mentally destructive) desires, one had to "be an overcomer" and work for the gift of the second blessing.[106]

Sanctification was a removal of inbred sin, a perfecting in holiness of the regenerated Christian. Several different dynamics described how sanctification affected the life of an individual. Frequently, preachers and writers described two or more of these dynamics without regard for potential conflicts among them. First, sanctification was an act of God. The Holy Spirit sanctified wholly, and the human being simply the received the blessing. All previously held sinful desires disappeared, leaving a holy life to "tell the gospel story" of sanctification. The second emphasis followed from the first but stressed the role of the individual. Sanctification enabled a human being to fulfill God's laws perfectly. The second blessing changed a person's will and perception and enabled her to read God's purposes in nature and in the scriptures. The final emphasis was on striving for holiness. One had to work for the "gift" by behaving as much as possible as if sanctification had already occurred. Each emphasis connected faith with behavior and proof of holiness. Each testified—to the redeemed, to God, and to the world—to the healing of the body of Christ.

Ecclesiology

The early mottoes of the *Gospel Trumpet* all emphasized the promotion of "Christian unity," which meant the gathering together of the sanctified.[107] The Church of God's concept of the church was of individuals separated from the world by God and perfected in holiness as a service to God and as a witness to the larger world. As in the book of Acts, the Holy Spirit guided the church.[108] Unlike the Lutheran and Reformed traditions, there was no "invisible church." Entire sanctification implied that the saved truly knew of their salvation and that their behavior would show their salvation to other saints, if not to the whole world. The Lutheran idea of "simultaneously justified and sinful" was accurate for those who had only experienced the first work of grace, and they might well be saved after death. However, in the opinion of the Church of God and the larger holiness movement, that teaching missed the emphasis on holiness that God demanded. That is, the classical Protestant doctrine of justification was technically correct but was incomplete and encouraged people to continue to sin. The justified sinners were not the church—the pure body of Christ. Unlike the Catholic Church, the Church of God rejected sacramental holiness, hierarchical church organization, and what they regarded as extra-biblical doctrine and church structures.[109] God added to the church those who were being saved (Acts 2:47). No one joined the church; sanctification joined them to the church.

Sanctification always included an experience of "light on the church" in that sanctification both created the church and enabled one to discern the church.[110] A characteristic statement from Church of God testimonies was "I saw the church," which meant that the person had experienced a fundamental change in perception and now understood that the body of Christ was not the same as any human institution.[111] Church of God ministers supported this vision of the church with various biblical passages. One of the most important was John 17:22–23, in which Jesus declares, "And the glory which thou gavest me I have given them; that they may be one, even as we are one: I in them, and thou in me, that they may be made perfect in one; and that the world may know that thou hast sent me and hast loved them as thou hast loved me." By interpreting the "giving of glory" in verse 22 as referring to sanctification, this passage connected holiness, unity of the saints, and God's will for the church. Warner used it to begin his discussion of ecclesiology in *Bible Proofs*.[112] Another important passage was Hebrews 12:25–29, because it formed the basis of Warner's understanding of how the Old Testament foretold the holiness movement's cleansing of the sects and denominations.[113] Church of God ecclesiology did not, however, come exclusively from a Holy Spirit directed reading of the Bible. Previous experiences with the denominations of the holiness movement also contributed to the doctrine of the church.[114] Warner recalled receiving his vision of the church the very next day after he lost his ministerial license: "On the 31st of January [1878], the Lord showed me that holiness could never prosper upon sectarian soil, encumbered by human creeds, and party names, and he gave me a new commission to join holiness and all truth together and build up the apostolical [sic] church of the living God."[115]

The first two congregations to follow Warner's vision for the apostolic church formed in Beaver Dam, Indiana, and Carson City, Michigan, in 1881, soon after the Indiana Eldership's October 1881 meeting.[116] The Michigan congregation was notable for the "Carson City Resolutions," a statement the saints in Carson City wrote to describe the basis of their union. This document warrants including because it describes the connection between sanctification and the church and because it shows the kind of language and arguments used in the early Church of God.

> **Whereas**, we recognize ourselves in the perilous times of the last days, the time in which Michael is standing up for the deliverance of God's true saints (Dan 12:1), the troublesome times in which the true house of God is being built again, therefore,
>
> **Resolved,** that we will endeavor by all the grace of God to live holy, righteous, and godly in Christ Jesus, 'looking for, and hastening unto the Coming of the Lord Jesus Christ,' who we believe is nigh, even at the door.
>
> **Resolved,** that we adhere to no body or organization but the church of God,[117] bought by the blood of Christ, organized by the Holy Spirit, and governed by the Bible. And if the Lord will, we will hold an annual assembly of all saints who in the providence of God shall be permitted to come together for the worship of God, the instruction and edification of one another, and the

transaction of such business as the Holy Spirit may lead us to see and direct in its performance.

Resolved, that we ignore and abandon the practice of preacher's license as without precept of example in the Word of God, and that we wish to be 'known by our fruits' instead of by papers.

Resolved, that we do not recognize or fellowship any who come unto us assuming the character of a minister whose life is not godly in Christ Jesus and whose doctrine is not the Word of God.

Resolved also, that we recognize and fellowship, as members with us in the body of Christ, all truly regenerated and sincere saints who worship God in all the light they possess, and that we urge all the dear children of God to forsake the snares and yokes of human parties and stand alone in the 'one fold' of Christ upon the Bible, and in the unity of the Spirit.[118]

The Church of God in Carson City carefully avoided calling its Resolutions a creed, and the members intended that affirming these principles would in no way be *sufficient* to ensure membership. The Resolutions were intended as a corporate description of the implications of their individual experiences of the Holy Spirit. It is worth noting, however, that from the beginning the Church of God created summaries and statements of belief that closely paralleled the creeds and doctrines they decried. The Church hailed the Bible as the only rule of faith, but, as with all restoration movements, church members emphasized some doctrines and ignored others.[119] The saints also believed that the Holy Spirit demanded that they regularly congregate. That required at least some planning.

It is tempting to suggest a fundamental conflict between early Church of God theology and practices. That is, if the Holy Spirit sanctified and showed the saints the church, why would they have needed a set of resolutions? Why would they have needed to *schedule* a meeting of the saints? If the Bible was the only rule of faith, what need was there for the Carson City Resolutions, *Bible Proofs of the Second Work of Grace*, or *What the Bible Teaches*? These questions, together with the assertion that the members of the Church of God were inconsistent, miss the context of the theological statements. When D. S. Warner withdrew from "sect Babylon," his language was absolute and phrased to imply that he was free from all the historical accretions that had developed since the New Testament church. In reality, he was participating in a specific debate over church organization and sanctification. The "sect Babylon" he intended at that time was the collection of denominations and holiness movements of late nineteenth-century America. When he wrote to show how holiness was the plain teaching of the Bible, he did so knowing that most of his audience had learned exactly the opposite in their home churches. Therefore, in Warner's opinion, the

doctrines and structures of Protestantism interfered with reliance on the Bible as
the sole rule of faith. Taking these statements out of context obscures their
function in the life of the church and in the competition for adherents.

Organs of the Church

Organization and doctrine always existed in the Church of God. In *What is the
Church and What is Not*, Warner wrote, "The Church is furnished with organs,
arranged in parts, and in due order; hence is an organic structure. But who is the
organizer of the same? Who furnished it with organs?" His answer was the Holy
Spirit, and his proof was 1 Cor. 12:8–11.[120] Warner's very statement—intended
as an authoritative interpretation of the Bible—was an example of church
organization and doctrine. There were also numerous unofficial church
structures. Most important was the *Gospel Trumpet* itself.[121] The paper held the
movement together, announced new congregations and camp meetings, and
provided doctrinal essays and opinions. The publishing house became the
organizational center of the Church. The camp ground nearest the publishing
house became the place of the annual national assembly. The publishing
building itself became a communal home for the press workers that also served
as a rest stop for missionaries. All of the early institutional developments of the
Church of God—evangelization teams, the publishing house, camp meetings,
missionary houses, the Children's Home, the Old People's Home, the
missionary board, and the General Assembly—grew from the publishing effort,
either as a direct aid to publishing itself or as an aid to distribution of gospel
literature.

   In 1881, "publishing house" was too grand a description for the hand press
Warner used to print a four-page semi-monthly paper from a kitchen in
Indianapolis. Warner's press moved six times in the first seven years searching
for adequate facilities and gradually building a subscription base.[122] After an
insecure start, the publishing effort grew impressively. In 1882, Warner reported
runs of 2,000 papers on a hand-operated press.[123] By 1902, the number of regular
subscribers to the *Trumpet* was between 8,000 and 10,000, and the company had
just completed a ten-cent subscription drive that netted an additional 45,000
subscriptions. The Gospel Trumpet Company also published a newspaper for
children, a German-language version of the *Trumpet*, books, hymnals, and
tracts. The year-end report of the work for 1902 said that the "Trumpet Family"
(workers who lived at the publishing house) was "now at 116 persons, including
children. About three tons of papers are mailed each week. About 300 letters are
received each day. Over twenty-eight thousand orders for books and tracts were
filled and sent out through the mails, besides several tons sent by express and
freight during the year 1902."[124]

A parallel to the publishing work and the growth of the *Gospel Trumpet* were the evangelistic teams known as the "flying messengers." These were small groups of people, usually consisting of a preacher and singers, who traveled around the country staging revivals, preaching the doctrines of the Church of God, and distributing Gospel Trumpet Co. literature. Warner organized his "company" early in 1885. It consisted of him, "Mother" Sarah Smith, Nannie Kigar, Frances (Frankie) Miller, and Barney Warren.[125] Warner was the primary preacher and Warren was the main songwriter. However, all testified publicly and Mother Smith frequently preached.[126] Other ministers copied Warner's group, and it was the standard form of ministerial organization at least until the turn of the century. These teams were particularly well suited to spreading the message of the final reformation and did not create a settled, denominational structure. However, the resulting congregations eventually wanted full-time ministers. Warner resisted the congregational system, and in 1892 he wrote, "Beware how you through selfish motives of having frequent preaching lay a snare to entangle God's flying messengers. ... This is the time of the end, and God's messengers must run to and fro."[127] A warning from Warner was a strong deterrent, but even Warner could not prevent settled pastorates forever. By 1919, 925 of the 1,097 congregations had resident pastors.[128]

Literature campaigns and traveling evangelists tended to produce isolated or very small groups of converts. The Church of God did not provide resident pastors or even regular preaching circuits, so adherents who wanted to congregate with other Church of God people often had to travel. Regional camp meetings became extremely important for the Church of God.[129] The saints could count on meeting with like-minded people and hearing a Church of God minister. Evangelists knew that camp meetings would likely supply a receptive crowd and opportunities for additional meetings in the area. Reports of the meetings, complete with the number of conversions, sanctifications, and healings, printed in the *Trumpet* attracted people to meetings, increased the drawing-power of evangelists, and showed readers that the Church of God reformation was progressing and growing. Camp meetings retained an important place in the life of the Church of God long after congregational ministry became the standard organizational form.

Of all the camp meetings, the June meeting nearest the publishing house was the most important. Warner first called it the "general assembly of the saints" in 1883, and this annual meeting functioned as a General Assembly long before the official incorporation of the General Ministerial Assembly in 1917.[130] It was the closest thing the Church had to a governing board for the first thirty-seven years and the meeting served as an opportunity for united action. The ideal of Holy Spirit-leadership in the Church of God led to an opposition to all forms of voting. The saints relied instead on the "spirit of unanimity," and therefore overt acts of legislation do not exist from the early years of the camp meeting. Persuasion was extremely important, and this was the opportunity for the most persuasive speakers in the movement to address all of the evangelists. The governmental function of the camp meeting is clear from a number of cases. The vast majority of decisions like this were declarations that someone was not in harmony with the Church of God and should be avoided.[131] However, the saints issued at least one statement of belief. At the 1902 camp meeting, the ministers "arrived at a uniform understanding of [healing in the atonement]" and submitted it in writing to "the ministers and saints scattered abroad."[132]

The publishing house was also important because it served as a base of operations for many of the evangelists in the Midwest. They would visit to replenish their supply of literature and would stay a while to rest.[133] On occasion, evangelists would leave their children at the Home while they went on a preaching tour. To help care for the children, the Church opened a children's home sometime in the late 1880s.[134] This was the first institution other than the publishing house in the Church of God, and its construction produced strong opposition and concern. An article explaining that the home needed reorganization based on sound business principles said, "Do not get the idea that this is a human church organization. It is nothing of the kind."[135] The children's home eventually separated from the publishing house and became a mission to orphans rather than a service to the children of evangelists. The changing pattern of ministry along with improved transportation and a growing network of established places for evangelists to stay enabled evangelists to take their children with them. The new problem became housing for "retired" evangelists. The man who ran the children's home opened an Old People's Home in South Haven, Michigan. This institution was even more problematic than the children's home because of the fear that some ministers would be lured into the work by the promise of future security.[136] However, it proved to be an important service to the Church that prefigured the Church's pension plans of the twentieth century.

The Trumpet Home was an actual home with additions for children and the elderly. This model served as a justification for building missionary homes that would be bases of operation for evangelists on the coasts and in big cities.[137] The first homes were built in the early 1890s as rest stops for ministers and as literature distribution sites. Their purpose expanded markedly as the turn of the century approached. Some of the homes, such as the one in Oakland run by J. W. Byers, became divine healing homes.[138] Byers's Gospel Healing Home had regular divine healing services and produced its own periodical, *Tidings of Healing*.[139] Others, such as the Open Door Mission in Chicago and the Church of God Missionary Home in New York City, became rescue missions and urban evangelization centers. The Chicago and New York homes in particular were large operations that regularly provided shelter for the homeless, ran soup kitchens, and conducted religious services.[140]

In addition to providing services to the poor and to traveling ministers, the missionary homes also attracted young converts who wanted to learn how to be ministers. The Church of God had no official system for educating those who felt a call to ministry. Some aspiring evangelists attached themselves to an evangelistic company to serve an informal apprenticeship. However, the missionary/healing/rescue missions were very attractive for young ministers. They provided opportunities for preaching without the burden of attracting a congregation or staging a meeting. Perhaps the most important function of the homes was providing a place where the new minister could meet the leaders of the Church. Thus, "the training of young people became a standard feature of almost all of" the homes. Those in New York City, Spokane, Washington, and Kansas City, Missouri, developed into schools for training ministers, complete with regular and correspondence classes.[141] A school also grew from classes offered in the Trumpet Home itself. In 1917, the Anderson Bible Training School opened. It eventually became Anderson University and the Church of God School of Theology. The school was centrally located, relatively well organized, and more prestigious than the other schools in the movement and led to their closure.[142]

Missionary homes facilitated the spread of the Church of God's message, and training schools helped to ensure that the Church would have well-prepared women and men working as evangelists. Neither the homes nor the schools, however, provided any central planning for evangelization. For home missions, the informal direction of the *Gospel Trumpet*-aided network of pastors appears to have worked well enough. Ministers went where they were called, stayed with subscribers to the *Trumpet*, visited the missionary homes, and hoped to support themselves on offerings. Foreign missions were a much greater undertaking, and "traveling by faith" (relying on donations from those who hear the message) to places without missionary homes or even converts made by the *Trumpet* was risky. Missionaries went anyway, but a better system was needed if the Church wanted to continue foreign missions.[143] The *Trumpet* for October 1898 announced the establishment of a "Missionary Fund" to help provide a centrally managed distribution to missionaries of funds solicited from the entire Church of God. In 1909, the Church of God formed its second organized ministry, the Missionary Committee, to help rectify the "overlapping work, differing mission philosophies, poor communication, improper preparation for cross cultural-ministry, and financial inefficiency" the Church's informal approach to missions had permitted.[144] In 1917, the Church incorporated the Missionary Board of the Church of God under the laws of the State of Indiana and made the Board wholly responsible to the newly formed General Ministerial Assembly.[145]

From a beginning as D. S. Warner's publishing effort, the Church of God had grown by 1917 into a Church with a General Assembly, a school for ministers, a missionary board, numerous missionary and rescue homes, settled congregations, and a full-service press. The Church of God gradually grew to look like a denomination. The organs of the Church resembled the organs of other religious movements more than the body of Christ. The point is not that the early Church of God people were inconsistent or self-deluded. Rather, it is that early Church of God theology and ecclesiology *put them in danger* of the charge of inconsistency and self-delusion. There was a great fear of "man rule," which meant overstepping the leading of the Holy Spirit and organizing the church based on human desires. The only guarantees against this were the Bible's description of the apostolic church and the witness of the Holy Spirit. Thus, the Church of God was always looking for evidence of God's favor and for a correspondence between the movement and the church of the apostles.

Notes

1. For the church as the "body of Christ," see 1 Cor. 12:12–31.

2. D. S. Warner, *Bible Proofs of the Second Work of Grace* (Goshen, Ind.: Evangelical United Mennonite Press, 1880), 10.

3. There are two modern biographies of D. S. Warner, but neither is a full, critical treatment of his life. Thomas A. Fudge's *Daniel Warner and the Paradox of Religious Democracy in Nineteenth-Century America* (Lewiston, N.Y.: Edwin Mellen Press, 1998) is an important contribution to the literature on the Church of God, especially since this is the only book on Warner written by someone outside the Church of God. However, Fudge's interest in Warner was as an example of "spiritual dictatorship" in the context of the democratization of American Christianity, and therefore his focus was quite narrow. Barry L. Callen's *It's God's Church! The Life and Legacy of Daniel S. Warner* (Anderson, Ind.: Warner Press, 1995) ranges over Warner's entire life and is a great source of information about Warner, but it was not intended to be a scholarly work. The best academic works on Warner are the first two chapters in Merle Strege's *I Saw the Church: The Life of the Church of God Told Theologically* (Anderson, Ind.: Warner Press, 2002). See "D. S. Warner and the Early Church of God" and "The Theology of D. S. Warner." The most complete—but completely uncritical—biography of Warner is A. L. Byers, *Birth of a Reformation, or The Life and Labors of Daniel S. Warner* (Anderson, Ind.: Gospel Trumpet Co., 1921). It cannot be ignored, however, because much of the later works have had to rely on Byers as the only source for much of Warner's early life. Works with significant sections about Warner include Dieter, *Holiness Revival*, 208–17; John W. V. Smith, *The Quest for Holiness and Unity: A Centennial History of the Church of God (Anderson, Indiana)* (Anderson, Ind.: Warner Press, 1980); idem, *Heralds of a Brighter Day* (Anderson, Ind.: Warner Press, 1955); Harold L. Phillips, *Miracle of Survival* (Anderson, Ind.: Warner Press, 1979); and Brown, *When the Trumpet Sounded.*

4. Byers, *Birth of a Reformation.* The title itself suggests its theological purpose. For Byers's explicit statement of the importance of the Church of God Reformation and Warner's role as a reformer, see pages 25–29. For a description of his sources used, see pages 4 and 5 of the Preface.

5. Byers, *Birth of a Reformation,* 35–37. In *When the Trumpet Sounded,* Brown wrote, "D. S. Warner enjoyed pioneer life to the utmost." However, his father's drunkenness seemed to have caused Daniel to take "a middle way between fanaticism and vice." See p. 46.

6. Warner's poem *Innocence* (Grand Junction, Mich.: Gospel Trumpet Co., 1896) was written for a recitation on the last day of school at the Church of God's Children's Home, May 31, 1895. That institution was a home and school for the children of missionaries and evangelists, and the setting likely explains the poem's theme of a terrible childhood leading to an adulthood of full salvation and happiness. A few of the relevant stanzas that biographers have used are as follows. His sickness is shown by: "But life held on its tender thread/Days, unexpected grew/To weeks: and still he lived./Why, Heaven only knew." His father's cruelty: "It seemed the special pleasure of/Another certain one,/To quite demolish everything/His heart was set upon." His father's alcoholism: "He never knew that "Father" was/A sweet endearing name./Its very mention was a dread,/His life's most deadly bane./The demon of intemp'rance there,/Infused the wrath of hell./And most upon this sickly head/The storm of fury fell."

7. Warner dedicated his first book "To the sacred memory of my sainted mother, whose tender affections were the only solace in my suffering childhood, and whose never-failing love, and whose pure and innocent life, were the only stars of hope that shone in the darkness of my youth." Warner, *Bible Proofs*, dedication page.

8. Byers, *Birth of a Reformation*, 38–40.

9. This information is from a report to the Commissioner of Pensions by the Assistant Secretary of Pensions for the Army (name illegible). Warner's third wife applied for his pension after he died, but her claim was rejected "on the ground that she had no title under said act, not having been married to soldier until after the passage of said act." The report said that Warner applied for his pension in 1890, less than three months after the passage of the Pension Act of June 27, 1890. This was well after his sanctification and numerous experiences with divine healing. See "Report on Warner's Pension," Church of God Archives, W656, 1994A, Box 1, "Warner, Daniel Sidney Papers," Legal Pensions.

10. Warner, journal, June 11, 1874. Callen, *It's God's Church*, 40.

11. On Spiritualism, see Moore, *In Search of White Crows,* and Braude, *Radical Spirits.* For the opposition to Spiritualism in the Church of God, see for example, John E. Roberts, *Spiritualism or, Bible Salvation vs. Modern Spiritualism, The Doctrine of the Bible arrayed against the Doctrine of Devils* (Grand Junction, Mich.: Gospel Trumpet Co., n.d.).

12. Byers, *Birth of a Reformation,* 40–42.

13. Finney retired from the presidency in 1866 but remained a professor of theology until 1875. See the article on Finney in Henry Warner Bowden, *Dictionary of American Religious Biography* (Westport, Conn.: Greenwood Press, 1977). There are no sources connecting Warner and Finney, other than the fact that they were both at Oberlin at the same time. For discussions of the similarities between the two men, see Fudge, *Daniel Warner*, 185, and Harold L. Phillips, "Warner and Charles Finney," *Vital Christianity* (Oct. 6, 1974): 7–8.

14. Fletcher, *A History of Oberlin College*, chapter XXII.

15. Warner continued to oppose perfectionist theology even after he embraced such kindred movements as phrenology and diet reform. He did not accept the idea of entire sanctification until 1877. Warner thought that perfectionist claims led to "fanaticism" and "delusions." Warner's journal entry for Nov. 11, 1872 reported on a perfectionist meeting he attended. "Heard a great noise, but to the congregation it appeared as a tinkling cymbal and sounding brass, evidently having no effect. Nearly all blew loudly the horn of sanctification but manifested little of its fruits, such as travail of soul for the sinner and sympathy for the one soul at the altar, to whom none gave a word of encouragement, but

each in turn arose and boasted of his holiness. Oh, the delusions of Satan! How manifold they are!" C. E. Brown quoted this passage in *When the Trumpet Sounded,* 56.

16. Strege, *I Saw the Church,* 2.

17. Report of the 11th Annual Eldership of West Ohio, Oct. 16, 1867, *Church Advocate* 32, no. 27, 214. The General Eldership of the Churches of God is now formally known as the Churches of God, General Conference. It is informally known as the Winebrennerian Church or the Church of God (Winebrennerian) for its founder, John Winebrenner. "Arminian in theology, these churches consider the Bible the sole rule of faith and practice. They believe in justification by faith; repentance and regeneration; the Triune God; the office and work of the Holy Spirit; practical piety; observance of the Lord's Day; and the resurrection of the just and unjust at the final judgment." There are to be no creeds, and "sectarianism is held to be antiscriptural." See Frank S. Mead and Sam Hill, *Handbook of Denominations in the United States* (Nashville, Tenn.: Abingdon Press, 1995), 119–20. For information about John Winebrenner, see Richard Kern, *John Winebrenner: Nineteenth Century Reformer* (Harrisburg, Penn.: Central Publishing House, 1974). There are numerous accounts of Warner's connection with the Winebrennarian church in books about the history of the Church of God (Anderson). See, for example, Strege, *I Saw the Church,* 3–4; Brown, *When the Trumpet Sounded,* 40–41; Barry L. Callen, *Radical Christianity: The Believers Church Tradition in Christianity's History and Future* (Nappanee, Ind.: Evangel Publishing House, 1999).

18. In the early years of the Church, it was unacceptable to suggest that Warner's ecclesiology came from Winebrenner. William G. Schell, the man who preached Warner's funeral sermon, was disfellowshipped in 1903. One of the charges was that Schell had implied that "this work has been shaded more or less with Winebrennerianism." See the report in D. O. Teasley, "Departed from the Faith," *Gospel Trumpet* 23:25 (June 18, 1903): 5. In the 1940s, Charles Wesley Naylor made a similar but broader and more constructive charge in his privately published pamphlet *The Teaching of D. S. Warner and His Associates.* Naylor had been a leader in the Church for many years when he wrote this analysis, but the Gospel Trumpet Co. was not willing to publish it. Excerpts of this pamphlet have been reprinted in Barry L. Callen, ed., *Following the Light: Teachings, Testimonies, Trials and Triumphs of the Church of God Movement, Anderson* (Anderson, Ind.: Warner Press, 2000), 148–51. In 1954, the Gospel Trumpet Co. published *When Souls Awaken: An Interpretation of Radical Christianity* in which C. E. Brown challenged the idea that the Church of God was the "Last Reformation" and instead attempted to place it in the context of radical reform movements. Brown said that Warner had adopted the ideas of Winebrenner, Thomas and Alexander Campbell, and J. N. Darby into his understanding of the church. See pages 19–41 in particular.

19. John Winebrenner, *A Brief Scriptural View of the Church of God,* revised edition (Harrisburg, Penn.: Board of Publication of the Church of God, 1878). See also, F. D. Rayle, J. A. Parthemore, Jr., and J. Harvey Gossard, *The Church—Nature and Organization* (Harrisburg, Penn.: Central Publishing House of the Churches of God, General Conference, 1975).

20. Warner's journal entry for May 28, 1873, reports that he preached "in La Rue on the Church of God. Text. Eph. 1:10." The text is "That in the dispensation of the fulness of times he might gather together in one all things in Christ, both which are in heaven, and which are on earth; even in him." Warner wrote his outline in his journal, and it shows clearly that the church must be one and visible, and its name must be "Church of

God." For the outline, see Strege, *I Saw the Church,* 12, note 11, or Byers, *Birth of a Reformation,* 72.

21. *Church Advocate* 38, no. 7, 3. Callen, *It's God's Church,* 51–52.

22. *Church Advocate,* 40, no. 30, 2.

23. Callen, *It's God's Church,* 47–66. An example of Warner's committee work is that on the same day he was ordained, he was appointed to the committees on Rules and Order, on Religion, and on Obituaries, and was elected to the Stationing Committee (*Church Advocate* 33, no. 28, 211).

24. The Church of God archives in Anderson, Indiana, has the original handwritten journal. Typescript copies are housed at the archives and in the libraries of Anderson University and Warner Pacific University. I have used a photocopy of the typescript version. Warner does not say why he began to write the journal or why he stopped. One possible explanation is that the journal would have helped him to prepare his annual reports to the Eldership and to avoid repetition on his preaching circuits. He carefully noted where he preached and what texts he used. He also kept a tally of converts. By the time he stopped writing in the journal, Warner no longer had a preaching circuit and was settling into his position as an editor.

25. For examples of serious illness, see the journal entries for Feb. 23, 1877, when an "acute pleurisy of the side" prevented him from preaching, and Oct. 2, 1878, when a "bilious remittent fever" left him unconscious for three days. Aubrey Forrest also traces Warner's interest in healing to his poor health. See Forrest, "A Study of the Development of the Basic Doctrines and Institutional Patterns in the Church of God," 117.

26. Byers, *Birth of a Reformation,* 49. Byers used the Warner family Bible for the dates. Warner's journal notes that May 28, 1873 was the first anniversary of his wife's death, but Byers claims she died on May 26. There is no available death date for the first child.

27. See Warner's journal for Jan. 4, 1874. See also Callen, *It's God's Church,* 59–60.

28. Warner, journal, March 18, 1875, and June 24, 1878.

29. Warner, journal, June 18, 1878.

30. On April 4, 1874, Warner wrote in his journal about visiting the graves of his triplets.

31. Warner, journal, Dec. 4, 1872, and May 29, 1873. This passage from James says, "Is any sick among you? let him call for the elders of the church; and let them pray over him, anointing him with oil in the name of the Lord: And the prayer of faith shall save the sick, and the Lord shall raise him up; and if he shall have committed sins, they shall be forgiven him." This was the classic text for proving that divine healing was a permanent gift to the church.

32. Warner, journal, July 2, 1873.

33. I am following Warner's use of the labels "Doctor" and "medicine." It is impossible to say what kind of medicine they practiced. For information about the variety of treatments, theories, and professional organizations that existed and competed under the umbrella term "medicine" in the nineteenth century, see chapter one.

34. Warner, journal, Dec. 1, 1877.

35. Warner, journal, May 12, 1874. According to Warner, "it is said to be a highly successful treatment in taking them out."

36. Warner, journal, Dec. 30, 1876.

37. Warner, journal, Jan. 24, 1876, and Jan. 20, 1878.

38. Warner, journal, Sept. 28, 1877.

39. Warner, journal, Oct. 2, 1878.

40. Warner, "Question," *Gospel Trumpet* 15:42 (Oct. 24, 1895): 2. In this article Warner answers a reader's request that he "Please explain I Tim. 5:23." Warner says this passage in which Paul advised Timothy to "take a little wine for your stomach's sake," was a biblical warrant for the use of natural remedies. The article appears in its entirety in Warren Roark, ed., *Divine Healing* (Anderson, Ind.: Warner Press, 1945), 114–19. We will explore this article in greater depth in chapter three.

41. References to phrenology appear throughout Warner's journal, ranging from reports on head readings to the use of its technical language. The earliest such reference says simply, "studied frenology [sic]" and is from Feb. 1, 1873. On March 24, 1873, he reported writing an article but did not indicate his audience or intended publication. He had learned to spell "phrenology." See also June 25 and 26, 1873, where Warner reported that he attended a lecture on phrenology by "Bro. Everitt," who examined Warner and gave him a "chart of charter and instruction." On Feb. 22, 1875, Warner "examined Bro. Mitchell and gave him a phrenological chart," and on June 1, 1877, he spoke to the Excelsior Society about "the interrelation between mind and body and their mutual dependence."

42. Warner reported studying prisoners on July 29, 1876, and the Omahas on Feb. 12, 1875. He was serving a church in Nebraska at the time.

43. Orson S. Fowler, *Creative and Sexual Science: Or Manhood, Womanhood, and Their Mutual Interrelations; Love, Its Laws, Power, Etc; Selection or Mutual Adaptation* (New York: Fowlers & Wells, 1875); Orson S. Fowler, *Physiology, Animal and Mental: Applied to the Preservation and Restoration of Health of Body, and Power of Mind* (New York: Fowlers & Wells, 1851); George S. Weaver, *Lectures on Mental Science According to the Philosophy of Phrenology: Delivered to the Anthropological Society of the Western Liberal Institute of Marietta, Ohio, in the Autumn of 1851* (New York: Fowlers and Wells, 1852). The reference to "Sexual Science by O.S. Fowler" in the journal appeared on Jan. 15, 1875. Warner read "O. S. Fowler's Physiology, Animal and Mental" on Nov. 30, 1876. And the journal reference to "Weaver's Mental Science" is from the entry for Nov. 19, 1877.

44. Stern, *Heads and Headlines*; Davies, *Phrenology Fad and Science*; Riegel, "The Introduction of Phrenology to the United States," 73–78.

45. According to Fowler, "if we obey all the laws of our being, we shall become as PERFECTLY Happy as it is possible for human nature to become or endure." Further, "all diseases taken in season, can be warded off by a correct physiological regimen, ALL can therefore preserve health and escape disease." The emphases are in the originals and the quotes are from *Physiology, Animal and Mental*, 26 and 49.

46. Fowler was not a Christian theologian and did not care to be. His real interest was in phrenology, which he believed was a gift from God that explained God's will for all people. He said that if phrenology and the Bible were to prove incompatible, then he would have to abandon the Bible. However, he was convinced that such a conflict could never happen, because both phrenology and the Bible were examples of God's self-revelation. He was "Christian" only in the sense that for him all true religion was "Christian." The atonement was of no interest to him; Jesus was a phrenologist who came to bring the message of moral development. Fowler believed that denominational Christianity had lost the original message of Jesus and had created creeds and divisions that both appealed to and promoted different intellectual faculties. Calvinists, for instance, had a "large rev-

erence." Through phrenology, Christians could progress beyond divisive doctrines. See
O. S. Fowler, *Religion; Natural and Revealed, or, The Natural Theology and Moral
Bearings of Phrenology and Physiology,* 10th ed. (New York: Fowlers and Wells, 1847),
41–62. In no sense am I suggesting that Warner shared the details of Fowler's religious
beliefs, only the desire to reform the church through the perfection of individuals.

47. Warner, journal, Dec. 7, 1872.

48. Barry Callen has called Warner's interest in phrenology one of his "faulty judg-
ments" and said it was "a passing curiosity" (*It's God's Church,* 157). It is true that Warner seldom mentioned phrenology explicitly after he founded the *Trumpet,* but I believe
that it was much more than a passing interest and that phrenology continued to influence
Warner's thinking throughout his life. I am arguing that phrenology and holiness reinforced each other in Warner's worldview, each connecting behavior and belief, internal
transformation and external evidence. Historians have underestimated the importance of
phrenology in the Church of God and in the wider holiness movement for at least two
reasons. First, orthodox medicine in the twentieth century has so thoroughly discredited
phrenology that it is very difficult for historians who have not studied the history of
American medicine to understand the pervasiveness of phrenology in the nineteenth
century. The tendency is to assume that a rational person could not possibly have chosen
phrenology over medicine, and therefore reading heads must have been a hobby or a di-
version. In fact, phrenology was a well-developed system founded on a theory that was at
least as coherent (although we now know that it was based on a mistaken assumption) as
the theories underlying homeopathy, osteopathy, etc. The language, periodicals, and
leaders of phrenology are no longer familiar and are easily overlooked or discounted.
Second, much of the history of the Church of God and the holiness movement is apolo-
getic. If not actually written to demonstrate the legitimacy of holiness, this history at least
assumes that the historical interpretation of the Church or the movement is fundamentally
the same as the religious interpretation. The leaders said they were rejecting the world,
and therefore there is little point in looking for cultural influences other than to see what
the Church rejected. They certainly would not have adopted some discredited portion of
nineteenth-century culture. Even if they did, this misstep did not reflect the true message
or beliefs of the Church. Numerous articles in the *Trumpet* indicate that Warner's interest
in phrenology continued into the 1890s. However, none of the articles mentions "phrenology" explicitly. For example, in 1892 Warner recommended that readers of the *Trumpet* buy Fowler's *Physiology, Animal and Mental,* the first page of which was a picture of
a head with a chart showing the "numbering and definition of the organs." Warner provided his readers with an address for ordering the book. *GT* 12:18 (Feb. 18, 1892): 4. It is
also worth noting that a traveling phrenologist examined Warner's head and the heads of
several other members of the Gospel Trumpet Co. on July 23 and 24, 1889 (Diary for
1889, Noah Henry Byrum papers in the Church of God archives).

49. Warner, journal, Sept. 16, 1876; June 17, 1877; Oct. 28, 1877; and Dec. 1, 1877.
See also Wallace Thornton, *Radical Righteousness: Personal Ethics and the Development of the Holiness Movement* (Salem, Ohio: Schmul Publishing Co., 1998) for the
larger holiness opposition to church socials.

50. Warner, journal, Nov. 30, 1876.

51. Warner, journal, Dec. 13, 1877. Emphasis in original.

52. Warner's rules were as follows: "1. Sleep no longer than eight hours out of 24.
When at home retire at 9 and arise before 5. 2. Each morning after a towel bath devote at
least one hour to reading the Bible and worship. 3. Frequent closet devotion during the

day. 4. Breakfast at 7 to 8 A. M. 5. Dinner at 2 to 3 P.M. 6. Eat absolutely nothing between these two meals. 7. Eat slow and as little as will supply natural wants. 8. Since
eating fruit unnecessarily has been my strongest temptation to intemperance, God helping
me I will henceforth entirely abstain between meals and will indulge in no more than two
small apples or one medium or large apple immediately after meals, and that only when
the meal was without fruit and when conscience does not remonstrate on the ground of
having already eaten all the stomach will welcome." The schedule is from Lewis, and the
1872 imprint of *Our Digestion* is in Warner's library at the Church of God archives. His
library also includes T. L. Nichols, *Diet Cure* (1881); A. J. Bellows, *How Not to be Sick,
a Sequel to "Philosophy of Eating"* (1869); and M. L. Holbrook, *Eating for Strength; or,
Food and Diet in their Relation to Health and Work, together with Several Hundred
Recipes for Wholesome Food and Drinks* (1888).

53. Warner, journal, June 1, 1874.

54. Callen, *It's God's Church*, 49.

55. Warner, journal, Sept. 16, 1877.

56. On Sept. 26, 1877, Warner wrote that he was reading *Purity and Maturity* by J.
A. Wood. This book by one of the founders of the National Holiness Association was an
extended defense of the place of the doctrine of holiness in the Methodist Church. Wood
collected hundreds of quotes from authorities ranging from John Fletcher and Daniel
Steele to Charles Spurgeon and Charles Hodge to show that Christianity is meant to save
from sin not save while in sin. Immediate sanctification and its relationship to growth in
holiness are the particular concerns. The 1882 self-published edition is available as
Digital Edition 07/26/95 from Holiness Data Ministry.

57. Warner, journal, Jan. 30, 1878. Opinions about entire sanctification varied
widely in the Church of God (Winebrennerian). According to a history of the General
Conference, "Beginning in 1865, and continuing for over 20 years in an intensive
fashion, the Church was in continual debate over the meaning of 'Sanctification.' The
question revolved around whether it were a "second definite work of grace" or not. The
result was the unfortunate loss to the Churches of God of one of its best pastors, Dan
Warner, and some of his close followers. ... He left the church, possibly more because of
some less-than-laudatory attitudes on the part of his fellow Ohio pastors than because of
his attitude toward sanctification." Richard Kern, Jack Parthemore, and Richard E.
Wilkin, *Time for Review: Facts about the Founding of the Churches of God, General
Conference* (Harrisburg, Penn.: Central Publishing House, 1975), 7. It does not appear,
however, that this acceptance of entire sanctification extended to the editorial board.
Warner's final article for the *Church Advocate* was an "Answer to Questions on
Sanctification," *Church Advocate* 42 (April 10, 1878): 2–3. At the end of the article, the
editor appended the following note: "Brother Warner's connection with the Eldership
having ceased, we grant him this privilege of replying to questions that had been
previously asked. Hereafter, unless he is restored, we cannot permit our columns to be
used by him to advocate a doctrine that we think is radically wrong, and which to our
mind has always done more harm than good. We believe that Christians should be pure
and clean from sin, but this sanctification doctrine is a complete perversion of Bible
sanctification."

58. For journal entries that report the Holy Spirit's guidance, see July 7, 1877, Aug.
11, 1877, and Feb. 14, 1878.

59. The grace of healing was for removing illness and disease. It cleansed the body
and returned it to a state it previously had enjoyed. The idea was that the illness just had

to be removed so the body could function normally. In contrast, miracles restored damaged body parts. Say a person was deaf because he had a very high fever as a child. The removal of the disease and the fever would not repair the ears, so a simple healing would not either. A miracle was needed to repair or regenerate the eardrum.

60. Strege, *I Saw the Church*, 7.

61. Warner, journal, Sept. 12, 1878, and Sept. 10, 1879.

62. Warner, journal, Nov. 19, 1879, Feb. 14, 1878, and Feb. 22, 1876.

63. Warner, journal, May 6 and 12, 1876.

64. Warner, journal, Feb. 6, 1877.

65. Warner, journal, Nov. 18, 1879.

66. Warner, journal, Aug. 11, 1877.

67. Warner, journal, Oct. 2, 1878.

68. Warner, journal, June 18, 1878.

69. Warner, journal, Aug. 6, 1878. William Alcott's *The Physiology of Marriage* (1855) said that the time and conditions of conception were essential for the future health of the child. See Wharton, *Crusaders for Fitness*, 97.

70. See the chapter on the Indiana Eldership in C. H. Forney, *History of the Churches of God in the United States* (Harrisburg, Penn.: Board of Directors of the Publishing House and Book Rooms of the Churches of God, 1914). "Support" of secret societies is not exactly accurate, but that is how the Indiana Eldership understood it. A resolution denouncing secret societies failed to pass in the national meeting.

71. Brown, *When the Trumpet Sounded*, 75.

72. Brown, *When the Trumpet Sounded*, 75. Brown has reprinted the Prospectus for the *Herald* on pages 76–77. Among the more interesting paragraphs are the following: "Viewed from a human standpoint, the *Herald* may appear to possess two separate features; namely that of an organ of the Church of God and an advocate of holiness. But viewed from a pure Bible standpoint these distinct features naturally blend into one effort and propagate the pure religion of the Bible. Church signifies 'called out.' The divinely given title, Church of God, therefore denotes the called out of God or separated unto God. Holiness means the same thing; that is to be separated from all sin and wholly given to God."

73. See D. S. Warner, "Explanation" *GT* 9:15 (Aug. 1, 1889). Warner provided an extensive and confusing explanation of the renumbering. The *Herald* ran for almost three years before Warner changed the name to the *Gospel Trumpet*; however, the renumbering reduced the volume number only by two, because the beginning issue changed as well. The main point is as follows: "But since that *Herald* was started back in the fogs of babylon, and died before it saw the evening light clearly, we have desired to drop off its three years and cast it back to the burning city where it belonged, and have our volume indicate the actual number of years that the TRUMPET has been sounding."

74. Byers, *Birth of a Reformation*, 196. Byers reprinted these three chapters in his book.

75. "In the evening it shall be light" (Zech. 14:7). Warner used this passage as a label for the new dispensation of holiness that would return the church of the apostolic age, also known as "the morning light." Useful introductions to the use of apocalyptic literature in the Church of God are John Stanley, "Unity Among Diversity: Interpreting the Book of Revelation in the Church of God (Anderson)" *Wesleyan Theological Journal* 25:2 (Fall, 1990): 64–98, and Steven L. Ware, "Restoring the New Testament Church: Varieties of Restorationism in the Radical Holiness Movement of the Late Nineteenth

and Early Twentieth Centuries" *Pneuma* 21:2 (Fall, 1999): 233–50. For a full statement, see D. S. Warner and H. M. Riggle, *The Cleansing of the Sanctuary; or, The Church of God in Type and Antitype, and in Prophecy and Revelation* (Moundsville, W.Va.: Gospel Trumpet Co., 1903).

76. Byers, *Birth of a Reformation*, 200–209, and Strege, *I Saw the Church*, 17–22. Specifically, the Holy Spirit directed him to Hebrews 12:25–29 and showed him "the key to the prophetic description of the great work of holiness." The two "shakings" in the passage from Hebrews do not relate, as many had supposed, to the last day. Rather, "'earth' here means the unconverted world, and 'heaven' the church." Thus, there is a "purification" of the church that will come out of the holiness movement. Warner, *Bible Proofs*, 114.

77. See F. G. Smith, *The Revelation Explained* (Anderson, Ind.: Gospel Trumpet Co., 1907), 206. In *A Brief History of the Church of God Reformation Movement* (Anderson, Ind.: Warner Press, 1976), John W. V. Smith wrote, "It is customary to speak of 1880 as the year in which the movement started. From available information it would be much easier to designate 1877 or 1878 as the crucial turning points in the lives of the early leaders" (11).

78. This was a regional organization existing under the umbrella of the National Camp Meeting Association for the Promotion of Holiness. Warner was one of the invited speakers at the regional meeting in 1880. See *Proceedings of the Western Union Holiness Convention held at Jacksonville, Ill., Dec. 15th-19th, 1880* (Bloomington, Ill.: Western Holiness Association, L. Hawkins, agent) for Warner's sermon, "The Kind of Power Needed to Carry the Holiness Work." Selections from the sermon appear as Appendix C in Callen, *It's God's Church.*

79. John W. V. Smith, *Heralds of a Brighter Day*, 42. This quote is from the June 1, 1881, issue of Warner's newspaper, *The Gospel Trumpet.* Warner was not the only one to use the language of disease and the body, according to page 185 of C. H. Forney, *History of the Churches of God in the United States* (Harrisburg, Penn.: Board of Directors of the Publishing House and Book Rooms of the Churches of God, 1914), "During several of these years the Eldership was contending against the inroads of heresies advocated by D. S. Warner. It had finally to resort to the old remedy of excision in order to prevent the spread of the disease and restore the body to good health."

80. These quotes are from two important Church of God hymns. First is "The Church's Jubilee," by C. W. Naylor and A. L. Byers, first published as no. 62 in *Reformation Glory*, ed. A. L. Byers and B. E. Warren (Anderson, Ind.: Gospel Trumpet Co., 1925). The second is "A Child of God," by B. E. Warren, first published as no. 205 in *Truth in Song*, ed. B. E. Warren and others (Anderson, Ind.: Gospel Trumpet Co., 1907).

81. Gale Hetrick, *Laughter among the Trumpets: A History of the Church of God in Michigan* (n.p.: General Assembly of the Church of God in Michigan, 1980).

82. *GT* 4:13 (July 1, 1881): 2. For a brief discussion of the mottos, see Harold L. Phillips, *Miracle of Survival* (Anderson, Ind.: Warner Press, 1979), 21–22.

83. The issues of the *Gospel Trumpet* between 5:11 (Sept. 22, 1882) and *GT* 5:22 (Aug. 15, 1883) are missing. Between these issues, Warner moved the press from Indianapolis to Cardington, Ohio. The issue numbers indicate that Warner did print papers in between these two. See Smith, *Quest for Holiness and Unity*, 62–63.

84. Clear, *Where the Saints Have Trod*, 41–42. Clear highlights the "anti" language, in contrast to the more common "nondenominational."

85. Warner's library included Phoebe Palmer's *Pioneer Experiences*, George D. Watson's *Secrets of Spiritual Power*, and Daniel Steele's *Milestone Papers*. On pages 82–83, Warner included a long quote from *Milestone Papers* in *Bible Proofs of a Second Work of Grace*. In his journal, Warner reported reading J. A. Wood's *Perfect Love* (July 15, 1877) and *Purity and Maturity* (Sept. 26, 1877). Wood was the man who had the initial idea for the National Camp Meeting Association for the Promotion of Holiness, and he formulated the definition of sanctification adopted by that body in 1885. *Purity and Maturity* was a collection of statements supporting holiness theology by important Methodists ranging from John and Charles Wesley to contemporary leaders. He read Dr. Steele's *Love Enthroned* on Sept. 30, 1877. Warner also attended a lecture by Steele. His journal said that, "Dr. Steele from New York was reading his interesting Bible lessons, giving the benefit of the Greek" (Aug. 3, 1877). Warner also reprinted holiness articles in the *Gospel Trumpet*, including a selection from *Wesley's Sermons* (*GT* 6:1) and one from *Finney's Lectures to Professing Christians* (*GT* 6:1).

86. For a brief description of holiness doctrine, see Susie C. Stanley, *Holy Boldness: Women Preachers' Autobiographies and the Sanctified Self* (Knoxville: University of Tennessee Press, 2002), 1–5. For a lengthy study, see Leslie D. Wilcox, *Be Ye Holy: A Study of the Teaching of Scripture Relative to Entire Sanctification with A Sketch of History and the Literature of the Holiness Movement* (Salem, Ohio: Schmul Publishing Co., 1994).

87. The history of the development of holiness theology is the story of changing emphases in the doctrine of sanctification. No one denies that John Wesley preached about sanctification and the importance of the recovery of that doctrine for Christianity. All of the key terms and scriptural passages appeared in Wesley's sermons and essays. However, most interpreters see a significant difference between the way Wesley described sanctification as a possibility in this life, and the later holiness movement's assertion that sanctification is the pentecostal experience of Baptism with the Holy Spirit and is an absolutely necessary preparation for salvation. Unfortunately for the historian, those who taught the latter interpretation insisted that they were merely preaching the pure Wesleyan gospel, so a clear delineation of the changes in the doctrine is very difficult. Useful introductions to the study of the holiness movement are: David Bundy, "The Historiography of the Wesleyan/Holiness Tradition," *Wesleyan Theological Journal* 30 (Spring, 1995): 55–77; William Kostlevy, "Historiography of the Holiness Movement" in *Holiness Manuscripts* (Metuchen, N.J.: Scarecrow Press, 1994), 1–40; and Donald Dayton, "The American Holiness Movement: A Bibliographic Introduction" in Donald Dayton, William Faupel, and David Bundy, eds., *"The Higher Christian Life": A Bibliographic Overview* (New York: Garland Publishing, 1985).The current state of the field of Wesleyan holiness studies is best explored in the *Wesleyan Theological Journal*, *Methodist History*, and *Pneuma*.

88. Modern descendents of these movements have attempted to provide their traditions with systematic explanations, but typically they are commentaries on holiness texts rather than fully developed systematic theologies. The Exploring Christian Holiness series by Beacon Hill Press is the most comprehensive such attempt. Its first volume presents the "biblical foundations" of holiness. The second volume is a historical study of the doctrine of sanctification, both before and after Wesley. The final volume is "the theological formulation" of holiness. The first attempted systematic theology in one of the holiness churches that developed from the holiness revival was Russell R. Byrum's *Christian Theology* (Anderson, Ind.: Gospel Trumpet, 1925).

89. "Justification" accurately described the legal aspects of the first work of grace, and Wesleyans continued to use the term. However, it often proved problematic because the term "justification" served as shorthand for "justification by faith alone" for members of the Reformed and Lutheran traditions. This doctrine brought with it an understanding of sin that was not compatible with the soteriology of the holiness movement.

90. F. G. Smith, *What the Bible Teaches: A Systematic Presentation of the Fundamental Principles of the Truth Contained in the Holy Scriptures* (Anderson, Ind.: Gospel Trumpet Co., 1914), 165. See also D. S. Warner, *Salvation: Present, Perfect Now or Never* (Grand Junction, Mich.: Gospel Trumpet Co., n.d.), 30. A characteristic Bible passage for this interpretation was Rom. 3:23: "all have sinned and fall short of the glory of God."

91. Smith, *What the Bible Teaches*, 165. See also C. E. Brown, *The Meaning of Sanctification* (Anderson, Ind.: Gospel Trumpet Co., 1945), 84–103; Warner, *Salvation*, 31. Biblical texts included Psalms 58:3; 51:5; Eph. 2:3.

92. According to Peters, Wesley believed that "original sin, despite its non-volitional character is not only sin but the very essence of sin. It is the inherent force, the root stock, from which sins as 'voluntary transgressions' spring. It is distinguished as sin without specific guilt—for Wesley held that 'by means of Christ, all men are cleansed from the guilt of Adam's actual sin'—yet with universal consequence—which needs and requires the grace of God in no less measure, though in differing relationship, than 'deliberately violating a known law of God'" (*Christian Perfection and American Methodism*, 42).

93. In the Church of God, see Henry C. Wickersham, *Holiness Bible Subjects* (Grand Junction, Mich.: Gospel Trumpet Co., 1890), 63. See also Strege, *I Saw the Church*, 5. For the larger holiness movement, see the definition of sanctification the General Holiness Assembly adopted in 1885: "Entire sanctification is a second definite work of grace wrought by the Baptism with the Holy Spirit in the heart of the believer subsequent to regeneration, received instantaneously by faith by which the heart is cleansed from all corruption and filled with the perfect love of God." This quotation is from page 23 of George Failing, "Developments in Holiness Theology after Wesley," *Insights into Holiness*, ed. Kenneth Geiger (Kansas City, Mo.: Beacon Hill Press, 1962), 11–32.

94. Smith, *What the Bible Teaches*, 127.

95. Warner, *Bible Proofs*, 16.

96. Smith, *What the Bible Teaches*, 127. Smith's reference is to Romans 3:2–28.

97. The quote is from Hebrews 6:1; it was frequently used in the Church of God and also the wider holiness movement. This description of regeneration borrows heavily from the chapter on "Salvation" in Smith's *What the Bible Teaches*, 123–38. Smith divides regeneration into "justification," "conversion," "the new birth," and "knowledge of salvation." This last section provided the explanation of how growth in love leads to the desire for entire sanctification. See also Strege, *I Saw the Church*, 13–22, and D. S. Warner, *Salvation*, 12–16.

98. Warner, *Bible Proofs*, 10. See also Wilcox, *Be Ye Holy*, 59–78. This doctrine reflected an understanding of sin as corruption or disease that could be cured. According to Harald Lindström, "[Wesley] is fond of describing sin as a injury, as corruption, as disease. . . . As sin is thus regarded as an illness, it follows that salvation will be seen primarily from a subjective-medical rather than an objective-judicial angle. Salvation is called a healing: man is cured of his inherent sinfulness as of a disease" (*Wesley and Sanctification* [Grand Rapids, Mich.: Francis Asbury Press, 1980], 41).

99. Wickersham, *Holiness Bible Subjects*, 63. According to Peters, "Wesley's tendency to use 'sanctification' where he meant 'entire sanctification' is another instance of terminological carelessness. The uncritical interchange of terms became especially characteristic of Wesley's later years. It was an unfortunate practice rather generally adopted by many of his followers. The result was that there arose in Methodism two groups using the same term, 'sanctification,' but with crucially different meanings." *Christian Perfection and American Methodism*, 63.

100. Warner, *Bible Proofs*, 6.

101. Warner, *Bible Proofs*, 10.

102. The quote is from Smith, *What the Bible Teaches*, 160, and is a reference to Luke 1:75. For more information about the importance of behavior in the Church of God and also in the larger holiness movement, see Charles Jones, "Tongues-Speaking and the Wesleyan-Holiness Quest for Assurance of Salvation," *Wesleyan Theological Journal* 22:2 (1987): 117–24, and Thornton, *Radical Righteousness*. According to Thornton, "Warner and his colleagues were contributing to yet another shift in the motivation of behavioral standards." The first shift was when Phoebe Palmer used behavior to show "surrender"; the second was when "Warner saw [standards of behavior] as indicating separation" (75).

103. The following are examples of articles that recommended sanctification as a cure for addiction to tobacco and alcohol: Charles Ford, "Tobacco" *GT* 16:9 (May 7, 1896): 3; J. E. Forrest, "Tobacco an Enemy to Good Health" *GT* 24:24 (June 16, 1904): 2; Robert Rothman, "Talks on Healthful Living. Article XIV—The Cure of Drunkenness" *GT* 28:12 (March 19, 1908): 4–5; P. Casteel, "The Tobacco Sin" *GT* 28:32 (Aug. 13, 1908): 4.

104. Both sanctification and salvation could be lost and regained. See Wickersham, *Holiness Bible Subjects*, for the article "Backslidden in Heart," 278. Wickersham bases his article on Proverbs 14:14, "The backslider in heart shall be filled with his own ways."

105. Smith, *What the Bible Teaches*, 154. For support Smith quotes 1 John 2:15–17, which says, "Love not the world, neither the things that are in the world. If any man love the world, the love of the Father is not in him. For all that is in the world, the lust of the flesh, and the lust of the eyes, and the pride of life, *is not of the Father, but is of the world.* And the world passeth away, and the lust thereof; but he that doeth the will of God abideth forever." The italics were in Smith's quotation.

106. See the hymn "Be an Overcomer" by C. W. Naylor and A. L. Byers, first published as no. 174 in *Truth in Song*, ed. B. E. Warren and others. The final verse declared, "Be an overcomer, forward boldly go/You are strong enough if you count it so/Strong enough to conquer through sustaining grace/And to overcome every foe you face/Never yield a step in the hottest fight/God will send you help from the realms of light/In Jehovah's might put the foe to flight/And the victor's crown you shall wear at last."

107. See mottoes on page 37.

108. See Acts 2:37–47. Church of God authors frequently used verse 47: "And the Lord added daily to the church those who were being saved."

109. This does not mean that the Church of God avoided these things; that would be a theological judgment for another kind of study. We will see that they did have doctrine, hierarchy, and extra-biblical sources of authority, but they rejected these *ideas.*

110. Warner, *Bible Proofs*, 8.

111. Merle Strege, the official Historian of the Church of God, titled his most recent book *I Saw the Church: The Life of the Church of God Told Theologically.*

112. Warner, *Bible Proofs*, 6.

113. See Dieter, *The Holiness Revival of the Nineteenth Century*, 211–12.

114. In addition to his membership in various Elderships of the Church of God, Warner had some connections with the Evangelical United Mennonites in Indiana. From April 1881 to February 1882, he was an Adjutant-General in the Salvation Army.

115. Dieter, *The Holiness Revival of the Nineteenth Century*, 209. The quote is from Warner's journal, March 7, 1878. See also Brown, *When the Trumpet Sounded*, 71–72. Warner recorded this insight in 1878, three and a half years before he announced his breaks with the holiness movement and the Indiana Eldership of the Church of God.

116. Immediately after the Indiana meeting, Warner visited some like-minded members of the Michigan Eldership. The most important were J. C. and Allie Fisher. J. C. became an editor and co-owner of the *Gospel Trumpet*, and he and Allie founded the work in Michigan. Strege, *I Saw the Church*, 11; Smith, *Quest for Holiness and Unity*, 43–48.

117. At this time, "church of God" was more common than "Church of God."

118. The saints in Carson City adopted their Resolutions in 1881. The Church of God Archives had an original copy of the Carson City Resolutions. For reprints, see Callen, *Following the Light*, 71, and Smith, *Quest for Holiness and Unity*, 46–47.

119. For Primitivism in American religious history, see Richard T. Hughes, ed., *The American Quest for the Primitive Church* (Urbana: University of Illinois Press, 1988), and Richard T. Hughes and C. Leonard Allen, eds., *Illusions of Innocence: Protestant Primitivism in America, 1630–1875* (Chicago: University of Chicago Press, 1988). For the holiness movement in particular, see Melvin Dieter, "Primitivism in the American Holiness Tradition," *Wesleyan Theological Journal* 30:1 (1995): 78–91.

120. D. S. Warner, *What is the Church and What is Not* (Grand Junction, Mich.: Gospel Trumpet Co., n.d.), 13–14.

121. The history of the Gospel Trumpet Company is a fascinating story but is well beyond the scope of this book. See Phillips, *Miracle of Survival*, for the basic story and detailed explanations of changes in editorial policies, the legal status of the company, personnel, and connections with the Church of God. Another interesting history is N. H. Byrum, *Familiar Names and Faces; a Collection of Cuts from Photographs of Ministers, Gospel Workers, Writers, and others, whose Names are Mostly Familiar to the Readers of the Gospel Trumpet...also a History of the Gospel Trumpet Publishing Work, with Cuts representing the same and other things of interest* (Moundsville, W.Va.: Gospel Trumpet Co., 1902). According to Strege, the centrality of the *Gospel Trumpet* for the Church of God conferred on the editor the role of "primary theological educator of the new movement" (*I Saw the Church*, 11).

122. From 1881 to September, 1882, it was in Indianapolis, first at 70 North Illinois Street and then at 625 West Vermont Street. From Indianapolis Warner moved to Cardington, Ohio, but by June of 1883 he had moved the twenty miles to Bucyrus, Ohio. In April 1884, he moved to Williamston, Michigan, where for the first time he "had sufficient space to house several persons and by January 1885 there were eight people assisting Warner in the publishing work." The operation quickly outgrew the plant in Williamston and moved to Grand Junction, Michigan in 1886. The next move, in 1898, was to Moundsville, West Virginia. This was the base of operations until the final move in 1906 to Anderson, Indiana. See Smith, *Quest for Holiness and Unity*, 59–67.

123. Smith, *Quest for Holiness and Unity,* 62. Smith cites his source as the Feb. 8, 1882 volume of the *Gospel Trumpet.*

124. "The Office Work," *GT* 23:3 (Jan. 15, 1903): 4. Further evidence of the growth of the publishing effort comes from a report on the office work from March that gave the places the Trumpet Family workers came from. It said that the present workers were from: Indiana: 22; Ohio: 16; Michigan: 13; Penn.: 11; W.Va.: 10; Ill.: 7; MO: 5; Kans.: 3; Iowa: 3; Tenn.: 2; Arizona: 2; Wisc.: 2; NY: 2; Neb.: 2; KY:2; Cal.: 2; Minn.: 2; Maine: 1; Colo.: 1; Maryland: 1; Ala.: 1; Canada: 1; Sweden: 1; Germany: 1; Scotland: 1; Italy: 1. See "Office Items," *GT* 23:12 (March 19, 1903): 4.

125. Smith, *Quest for Holiness and Unity,* 124; Callen, *It's God's Church,* 107–29.

126. Women frequently preached and led congregations in the holiness churches. Many of the early leaders in the Church of God were women. In 1925, 32 percent of the congregational pastors in the Church of God were women, as were many of the well-known evangelists. Women's leadership in the Church of God is a more contentious issue now than ever before. An increasing openness to ecumenical dialogue with the broader evangelical culture has led to a more male-dominated pastorate. For women's leadership in the holiness movement, see Stanley, *Holy Boldness*; Donald Dayton, "Yet Another Layer of the Onion; Or Opening the Ecumenical Door to Let the Riffraff In," *Ecumenical Review* 40:1 (1988): 87–110; and Lucille Sider Dayton and Donald Dayton, "Your Daughters Shall Prophesy: Feminism in the Holiness Movement," *Methodist History* 14 (1976): 67–92. *Holy Boldness* includes a section about Sarah Smith's autobiography. For an early defense of women's preaching, see Warner, "Woman's Freedom in Christ, to pray and prophesy in public worship" *GT* 10:7 (April 1, 1890): 1, 4. There are many autobiographies and biographical sketches of women who served as leaders in the early Church of God. See for example Sarah Smith, *Life Sketches of Mother Sarah Smith: "A Mother in Israel"* (Moundsville, W.Va: Gospel Trumpet Co., 1902) and Mary Cole, *Trials and Triumphs of Faith.*

127. Quoted in Smith, *Quest for Holiness and Unity,* 124.

128. Smith, *Brief History of the Church of God,* 73.

129. See Gale Hetrick, *Laughter Among the Trumpets,* for how the legal requirements for owning and administering the Michigan state campground led to the growth of the Michigan ministerial assembly.

130. "First General Assembly in Ohio," *GT* 6:2 (Oct. 15, 1883): 3.

131. The disfellowshipping of William Schell in 1903 is a notable case, because Schell had been an extremely influential evangelist and writer. Many of the saints expected him to take Warner's place as the de facto leader of the movement. See D. O. Teasley, "Departed from the Faith," *GT* 23:25 (June 18, 1903): 5. An earlier case was that of T. H. Low, who was disciplined in 1885 for "ridiculing the idea of divine healing." Byers, *Birth of a Reformation,* 328–29.

132. "Divine Healing in the Atonement," *GT* 22:25 (June 19, 1902): 1–3.

133. The Trumpet Family workers did not always appreciate the presence of the evangelists. Rhoda Keagy was one of the printers and office workers in the late 1880s. Her diary entry for Tuesday, May 29, 1888, said, "It does 'beat every thing I ever heard tell of' to see how people will string in here & settle down for a season as though it was their home." Rhoda Keagy diary, Church of God Archives.

134. Smith, *Quest for Holiness and Unity,* 76.

135. A. B. Palmer, *GT* 16:25 (June 25, 1896): 2.

136. Smith, *Quest for Holiness and Unity,* 76.

137. The justification was not entirely successful, and in 1908 the debate entered the *Trumpet*. H. M. Riggle admitted that the New York and Chicago homes were "successful in every way," but he thought the others were a waste of resources and were distracting the Church from the more productive rural fields of evangelism. See Riggle's articles, on "Faith Homes" in *GT* 28:50 and 51 (Dec. 17 and 24, 1908). Both articles are on page 10. J. W. Byers, the man who started the Oakland home, responded that Riggle was right about the limited resources of the Church, but said that *every* home should be a missionary home. The problem was not with the homes but rather with the lack of support from the Church. "Missionary Homes," *GT* 29:3 (Jan. 21, 1909): 11–12. The debate in the *Trumpet* concluded with an article from Claudine Heald, one of the superintendents of the home in Kansas City. Heald detailed the amount of work they do in the city and urged the saints to send support and workers. "What We Do in the City," *GT* 29:3 (Jan. 21, 1909): 14.

138. In the late 1880s, there were more than thirty divine healing homes in the United States. They resembled boarding houses, but were intended for people who were seeking divine healing. The more influential homes included Charles Cullis's faith home in Boston, Carrie Judd Montgomery's Home of Peace in Oakland, and A. B. Simpson's Berachah in New York. In the late 1890s, John Alexander Dowie's home in Chicago became the most important. See R. Kelso Carter, "Divine Healing or 'Faith Cure,'" *Century Magazine*, March 1887, 777–80. See Hardesty, *Faith Cure*, 56–71, and Paul Gale Chappell, "Healing Movements," in Stanley M. Burgess and Gary B. McGee, eds., *Dictionary of Pentecostal and Charismatic Movements* (Grand Rapids, Mich.: Regency Reference Library, 1988), 353–74.

139. The operation of the periodical eventually became burdensome and in 1898 the *Tidings of Healing* merged into the *Gospel Trumpet* and Byers became a contributing editor for the *Trumpet*. See the notice in *GT* 18:18 (May 5, 1898): 4.

140. The superintendent of the Chicago mission reported having fed 10,172 men between Jan. 1 and March 10, 1896, in the March 19, 1896 *Trumpet* (quoted in Brown, *When the Trumpet Sounded*, 199). See also Smith, *Quest for Holiness and Unity*, 239–42. Smith includes a list of the forty-five known Church of God homes. Urban rescue work in the holiness movement is most closely associated with the Salvation Army; however, all of the holiness churches conducted social ministries in the big cities. See Norris Magnuson, *Salvation in the Slums: Evangelical Social Work, 1865–1920* (Metuchen, N.J.: Scarecrow Press, 1977). For a contemporary account, see Seth Cook Rees, *Miracles in the Slums* (New York: Garland, 1985; originally self-published in 1905).

141. Smith, *Quest for Holiness and Unity*, 236–37; Strege, *I Saw the Church*, 81. See especially Robert H. Reardon, *The Early Morning Light* (Anderson, Ind.: Warner Press, 1979), 5–8. Dr. Reardon was the President of Anderson University and one of the most influential leaders in the Church of God. He was also the son of an extremely influential minister, E. A. Reardon. In the Foreword, he relates that his family's first contact with the Church of God came because his grandmother and her two sisters were interested in the divine healing literature published by some of the workers in the Open Door Mission in Chicago. They visited the mission and were converted. When Reardon's father felt the call to ministry in 1899, he went to the Chicago home for training.

142. Strege, *I Saw the Church*, 77–82. See also Barry L. Callen, *Guide of Soul and Mind: The Story of Anderson University* (Anderson, Ind.: Anderson University and Warner Press, 1992).

143. The first missionary work outside of the United States appears to have been D. S. Warner's meetings in Ontario in 1888 (Brown, *When the Trumpet Sounded*, 327). The Canadian border was porous and the holiness movement was well established in Canada, so this trip did not create any particular difficulties for the evangelistic company. The first foreign missionary trip appears to have been B. F. Elliott's trip to Mexico in 1892. See Douglas E. Welch, *Ahead of His Times: A Life of George P. Tasker* (Anderson, Ind.: Anderson University Press, 2001), 46–47.

144. Callen, *Following the Light*, 121–22. The first organized ministry was, of course, the Gospel Trumpet Company. The Missionary Committee was the first ministry of the whole Church—as opposed to the missionary houses that were owned and operated by individuals in behalf of the Church—that was not completely controlled by the Board of Directors of the Gospel Trumpet Co. See also Strege, *I Saw the Church*, 82–87, and Lester Crose, *Passport for a Reformation* (Anderson, Ind.: Warner Press, 1981). For an early explanation of the changes in the Church relating to missions see, J. W. Phelps, *Our Ministerial Letter*, Nov. 1912. It is worth noting that at the first meeting of the Missionary Committee, twenty-seven missionaries already in the field were recognized. "British Isles, four; China, two; Japan, four; British West Indies, two; Germany, four; and India, eleven." Callen, *Following the Light*, 123.

145. Smith, *Brief History of the Church of God*, 74. See also Strege, *I Saw the Church*, 134–64.

CHAPTER 3

TESTIMONY

Let the redeemed of the Lord say so,
Whom he hath redeemed from the hand of the enemy.
(Psalm 107:2)

While at the mercy seat I knelt,
My Lord I did behold.
No tongue can tell the joy I felt,
'Tis better felt than told.
(H. R. Jeffrey, "'Tis Better Felt than Told")

The saints took seriously the biblical injunction to testify to God's redeeming power, and the literature of the Church of God is full of these stories.[1] Sources include the pages of the *Gospel Trumpet* devoted to testimony and reports of divine healing, camp meeting reports that showed that people were giving oral testimonies in the meetings, and full-length autobiographies that told of a journey "from infidelity to Christianity."[2] Hundreds of these testimonies reported on health or divine healing. More important, the stories were often specific where doctrinal articles were general. Instead of merely asserting God's desire to heal all diseases, testimonies told how, when, and where God had healed a broken leg, a blind eye, or a serpent's bite. Occasionally, a testimony declared that healing had not yet come. These personal stories indicated how the readers of the *Gospel Trumpet* applied the doctrine of divine healing to their own diseases and how they integrated ideas of healing into their religious beliefs.

The hymn verse at the head of this chapter is in the form of a testimony but is unusually explicit about the disjunction between the religious experience and the report of that experience.[3] As such, it is a good introduction to our study of the relation between testimony and divine healing. The first part of the verse, "While at the mercy seat I knelt, My Lord I did behold," introduces the point that these are reports of supernatural power. For readers of the *Trumpet* who were sympathetic to the message of the Church of God, testimonies (first to sanctification and later to healing) showed the spread of the movement and the dawning of the evening light dispensation. The saints saw them as dispatches from the front lines of the movement, confirming their belief that God was starting a new age of sanctification and unity, and leading them to look for "greater things than these."[4] Testimony from all points of the compass reinforced the sense of wonder and the hope for the return of spiritual gifts and miracles—such as healing of diseases and the physical restoration of damaged bodies—which existed in the apostolic church. Therefore, stories of sanctification and healing fueled a desire for even clearer signs and amazing stories.

Yet even the most sympathetic audiences in the Church of God demanded some evidence before they believed a testimony. The second part of the hymn verse, "No tongue can tell the joy I felt, 'Tis better felt than told," suggests a reason for skepticism. These stories were attempts to convey an ultimately incommunicable feeling, and that feeling came from an experience that forever changed the person's status with God. If accepted by the saints as legitimate, it also changed one's status in the Church of God movement. The power of the stories combined with the gap in communication introduced the possibility for error or even fraud. The *Trumpet* reported numerous warnings about preachers who intentionally counterfeited testimonies for personal gain. Whole congregations went astray by listening to deceiving spirits or by misinterpreting the signs of God. Testimony could be extremely powerful. If accepted as true, it could change the whole worldview of a convert. It could reshape the entire movement by introducing new beliefs and practices, and it had the potential to alter the authority structure of the Church by increasing one person's reputation for holiness.[5] Thus, testimony had to present evidence appropriate for the chosen audience. In the Church of God, the two main audiences were the saints and the sinners, those who already proclaimed sanctification and those who had not.

The task of testifying to the saints involved conveying that the experience in question fell within the vaguely defined boundaries that marked legitimate experiences of God's grace. The theological commitment to unity restricted adversarial relations to only the extreme cases—those "handed over to Satan"—and obscured the evaluation of testimony.[6] Not all testimonies were equal. Those that introduced no new doctrine were innocuous enough. If no evidence to the contrary existed (such as riotous living or flashy attire), the saints would accept the testimony even if it were not particularly convincing. If the testimony contradicted or challenged the beliefs of the saints, however, the only real chance it had of succeeding was if the person testifying had a long and respected reputation for holiness and discernment of God's will. Testimony had to conform to

the expectations of how God interacted with human beings. The saints already
believed in sanctification, so the task was to demonstrate the legitimacy of this
particular instance of sanctification. A model sanctification narrative developed,
complete with standard vocabulary and characteristic passages from scripture.
The testimony hymns helped further standardize the stories by putting the words
of testimony into the mouths of the congregation. However, as useful as mor-
phology of sanctification was, the saints wanted more tangible and affective
evidence of God's work. Divine healing eventually met this need. It gained acceptance through doctrinal arguments connecting it to the benefits of sanctification and biblical proof of God's desire to heal people. Further, divine healing
proved useful in spreading the message of sanctification to the unconverted.

Testifying to the unconverted differed from testifying to the saints because
the goal was not to gain acceptance in an established group but rather to attract
someone to this group. Divine healing and affective testimony were very useful
for this purpose. Secular newspapers frequently reported on notable healings or
large divine healing meetings. In addition to the publicity, healing was a tangible
good. Potential converts could hear a testimony and not quite understand why
they needed sanctification, or even what sanctification was. Nevertheless, they
knew about illness and suffering and could easily see the benefits of free and
immediate healing through prayer. The members of the Church of God believed
that God was using divine healing to attract new members to the Church, just as
Jesus used healing to attract people to the gospel.[7]

Healing did more than attract converts, however. It provided metaphors for
thinking and talking about holiness and the unity of the saints.[8] Sanctification
was difficult to explain and even harder to demonstrate. The doctrine said that
sanctification was a deliverance from inbred sin; the external evidence of it was
a "holy life." That may have worked well in small congregations of Wesleyans
where the members were all convinced of the truth of sanctification and were
intimately involved in one another's lives. It did not translate to testimonies in a
periodical or an evangelistic meeting, where the audience had no personal connection with the testator. Divine healing stories proved much more accessible
and effective than sanctification stories. The testimony of the Church of God
gradually changed from testimony to sanctification to testimony to the "divine
healing of soul and body."[9]

The change from sanctification as a cleansing to sanctification as divine
healing of the soul was easy for the Church. The description of sanctification the
Church of God adopted from the holiness movement explained that inbred sin
was a corruption of the soul. It was a disease that sanctification would heal. In
fact, the language of healing the soul preceded widespread testimony to physical
healing in the Church. An early Church of God hymn, "The Great Physician,"
illustrates this well. Its title referred to a classic divine healing proof text. However, the verses clearly show that the hymn is about sanctification, not physical
healing.[10] The development of testimony in the Church of God was not linear.

The descriptions of sanctification as a healing led to increased interest in miraculous physical healing, and experiences with divine healing of the body inspired models of sanctification based on healing of the soul. They were mutually reinforcing. Once the Church embraced divine healing, however, it proved extremely useful as a visible parallel to the invisible grace of sanctification.

Published testimonies provide much of the extant information about divine healing in the Church of God. In addition to the stories, the centrality of testimony in the life of the Church became important for the emphasis on divine healing. Testimonies—especially those describing sanctification—created difficulties in communication that divine healing helped to solve. Healing served as evidence for the members of the Church that God was restoring the apostolic church. Moreover, divine healing attracted potential converts and introduced them to the theology of the Church. This chapter explores how testimonies promoted divine healing. The final chapter will return to this topic to explore how testimonies to failed healings eventually undermined the significance of divine healing for the Church.

Healing Testimonies

In 1911, Herbert M. Riggle, the erstwhile "Boy Preacher of the Reformation" and the Church's reigning expert on eschatology, contributed his assessment of divine healing in the Church of God to *200 Genuine Instances of Divine Healing*. According to Riggle, "It would take a larger book than Webster's Unabridged Dictionary to contain all the testimonies of the multitudes who have been healing in this blessed light, and it would include all the diseases mentioned in the New Testament that were healed and as many wonderful miracles."[11] Excepting a few diaries and some personal correspondence, this study explores only published healing testimonies. Even with that limitation, reprinting all the healing testimonies published by the Church from its beginning to the year Riggle's quote appeared in print (1911) would indeed require a large book and would include a wide range of healings.[12]

According to the testimonies, faith cured diseases ranging from cancer to consumption to the common cold.[13] God instantly healed broken bones and restored eyesight to the blind and hearing to the deaf.[14] The Church resolutely rejected taking up serpents in worship, so testimony about poison had to be carefully stated. However, numerous testimonies proved that the prayer of faith protected against accidental poisonings from snakes, toadstools, and strychnine.[15] Divine healing repaired damage from minor or major accidents. Jennie M. Byers wrote a six-page testimony about the insight she gained into God's power from the instantaneous healing of her cut finger.[16] Charley Halstead reported that God had healed a cut he received from a rotary saw that exposed his spine.[17] A Gospel Trumpet Co. worker fell through the floor of the Trumpet

Home and was impaled on a sharp board that stuck under his arm. Remarkably, he was able to return to work after three days.[18] A few testimonies even reported resurrections from the dead.[19]

Most of the published testimonies followed a standard form. It is impossible to determine the extent to which this form reflected editorial policy because rejected testimonies have not survived. The editors may have changed the stories for publication, or they may have only accepted accounts that followed a common pattern.[20] The shaping of testimonies likely was subtler than mere editorial imposition. Testimonies were offered as evidence of God's interaction with humans in the Church. They served as models by which people interpreted their own experiences, and they guided their expectations and shaped their explanations. This alone could account for the similarities. Further, the *Trumpet* and testators both had an interest in telling compelling stories. Testimonies were dramatic narratives intended to capture attention and impress an audience with a feeling of the healing.

Whether due to authors or editors or some combination, the majority of the testimonies had the following structure:[21]

1. The person had lived a sinful life. Shorter testimonies or those written by people who became sick while already sanctified often omitted this point.

2. The statement of the affliction.

3. If the person was not a member of the Church of God, this part frequently stated that he or she heard from a non-Church of God preacher that the age of miracles was over. If in the Church of God, he or she had not heard divine healing preached as effectively as it should be.

4. The testator sought medical help. This functioned as apparently independent, professional verification of the affliction. The physician either proclaimed the case incurable or prescribed medicine. The medicine in turn exacerbated the condition, or the person refused to take it because it was a religiously forbidden substance such as alcohol or opium.

5. The person heard the Church of God's message of divine healing and decided to investigate further.

6. After searching the Scriptures, divine healing and sanctification were found to be "Bible promises."

7. Prayer was offered. The details of this step depended on how the person was connected to the Church of God. If he or she was near a congregation or was attending a camp meeting, then the elders would have laid on hands and anointed for healing. If the only contact was the *Gospel Trumpet*, the person could have simply followed John 15:7 ("If ye abide in me, and my words abide in you, ye shall ask what ye will, and it shall be done unto you").[22] Many wrote to the *Trumpet* to request that

prayer be offered at a specific time. After 1895, the person could have requested an anointed handkerchief.[23]

8. Any of the following that needed to be done, in this order: regeneration, sanctification, healing.

9. The symptoms returned. Doubt caused the person to lose healing and possibly sanctification.

10. Recommitment brought back sanctification and healing, and strengthened the person's faith so that the person would never doubt God's healing power again.

11. New health enabled the person to work for the Lord.

12. The example has led others to salvation and healing.

Testimonies fitting the above outline came from the leaders of the movement as well as from otherwise unknown Church members. By 1891, even young children submitted healing testimonies, a fact that suggests that both the belief in divine healing and the culture of testifying were pervasive.[24] The significance of most of the testimonies is simply the evidence that Church members were practicing divine healing for a wide variety of illnesses. However, some particular testimonies affected the movement as a whole. The following examination of one of the best-documented healing testimonies in the history of the Church will give some indication of the impact of stories of miraculous healings.

"God's Wonderful Dealings with Sister Emma Miller"

Emma Miller's healing testimony was the first to capture the imagination of the Church of God movement.[25] Four other healing testimonies had already appeared in the *Trumpet*, but Miller's account was exceptional for at least two reasons. First, she was healed of total blindness. The other stories were remarkable in their own right; most notable were a healed broken bone and a restoration of hearing. However, nothing could compete with the restoration of sight as a sign of God's healing power. Everyone knew that Jesus had healed the blind and physicians could not. It was the gold standard of healing and, as one Church of God writer asserted, it was evidence that the time in which "the eyes of the blind shall be opened" was now here.[26] Moreover, the miraculous transformation from blindness to sight resonated with the movement's emphasis on "seeing" the evidence of holiness and, ultimately, seeing the Church. Ideally, testimony itself would open the eyes of the spiritually blind. The second reason for the effect of Miller's testimony was more mundane. It was the first public healing accompanied by corroborating evidence.

According to her testimony,[27] Miller had grown up in the Methodist Episcopal Church, but had only received "defective religion."[28] In 1880 or 1881, she
lost her eyesight but did not say how. She was "converted to God" on August 2,
1882, and sanctified the next day. Apparently, she knew of the Church of God
but did not yet accept the Church's ecclesiology. She remained a member of the
Methodist Church until a year after her healing. Sanctification did not heal
Miller's eyes, but she began to have "visions" of Jesus in which he told her of
things printed in the *Trumpet*. In his second appearance, Jesus told her that she
would be healed sometime in the future. In June 1883, a member of the Church
of God who had been healed of some undisclosed affliction at a camp meeting
invited Miller to the Bangor, Michigan camp. A "brilliant light, like a flame of
fire" enveloped Miller, and the Lord assured her that she would be healed at the
meeting. She was so confident that she took paper and pens with her to Bangor
so she could write letters to her friends reporting that her sight had returned. On
the fourth morning of the camp meeting, Jesus told Miller that she would be
healed that day, and so she sat on the platform to give everyone a good view. J.
C. Fisher prayed and laid hands on her, and at about five in the afternoon Miller
was healed. There was great shouting and rejoicing, and "many believed unto
salvation when they saw the miracle."[29] Miller gained spiritual sight as well as
physical so that she was "wholly absorbed in divine things." Or rather, she saw
that the mundane was also divine. Her follow-up testimony reported that after
her healing Jesus would whisper "wipe them for me my child" to her while she
did the dishes. Yet, she still had not withdrawn from the Methodist Church. At
the Williamston camp meeting, she told God that if it was his desire for her to
align with the saints forever, to lead her to baptism and give her a sign. Before
the baptism, a red glory enveloped her so that she could barely move, forcing
Warner to wait for her to come into the water. That was the sign, and she sent a
letter to her pastor resigning from the rolls.[30] One year after her healing, the
symptoms returned but a sister showed her that it was a temptation of the devil.
She recommitted for healing. The symptoms disappeared, and Miller gained new
strength. Several other afflictions beset her, but she always relied on divine healing and "found [God] faithful to his word."[31]

Miller's first healing happened quite literally in front of the saints at the
Bangor camp meeting. The initial publication of her testimony included a con-
firmation by the minister, J. C. Fisher, and an eyewitness testimony by Brother
Benjamin Bell, who happened to be in the office when Fisher was preparing the
story for the *Trumpet*. Fisher noted that "there were men base enough to insinu-
ate that it was a case of feigned blindness; but when the powers of God came
upon the camp, and the Lord touched the sister's eyes, conviction struck their
hearts and their mouths were stopped."[32] The editor of one of the secular papers
obtained a copy of Fisher's account and published it under the caption "Tougher
than a Snake Story." Fisher dismissed this as "latter day scoffing at the work of
the Almighty" and warned that "men who treat with contempt all divine interpo-

sitions that exceed their credulity usually pride in their reason [sic], but what is more reasonable that that the God who formed the universe should be able to 'heal all manner of diseases.'"

Miller's healing attracted the attention of the saints and the secular press. The members of the Church of God who attended the camp meeting saw the miracle for themselves, and the readers of the *Trumpet* had testimonies from Miller, Fisher, and Bell. As added proof, however, the account of the "Third General Assembly of the Saints in Michigan" in the October 15, 1883 issue reported that Emma Miller had attended, that she was still healed, and that someone had brought written statements from her father and her physician corroborating the healing.[33]

Published testimonies provide information about the structure of the Church and the theology of the editors of the *Trumpet*. Evidence also supports the conclusion that the presence of healing testimonies in the periodical and at Church of God camp meetings attracted converts to the Church. However, the information from most testimonies stops right where they might appear to be the most useful: the local situation of the person giving the testimony. Did the members of the local congregation rejoice at the healing, or did they reject it as the ranting of a lunatic? Were testimonies that were published in the *Trumpet* or witnessed at a camp meeting easier to accept than testimonies from members of a local congregation? Did the influence of testimonies change over time as miraculous stories became familiar or even expected? There are no definite answers to these questions. Yet, it is important to consider the power a healing testimony could have had in a family or a congregation.

The Emma Miller healing is attractive for historical study because it left a published trail of influence. Testimonies commonly asserted—as did Miller's—that the healing had led many witnesses to "believe unto salvation" or to pray for their own healing. Often stories reported a chain of healing in a family or a congregation. In the vast majority of these cases, however, internal evidence is the only source available for determining its influence. Either the *Trumpet* did not publish any follow-up reports, or the evidence is so fragmentary that it is impossible to determine the connections between two stories. These familial and congregational connections may have been common knowledge among Church members at the time of publication, but they are now lost.

"The Eyes of the Blind Opened": Josephine (Miller) Courtney

The Emma Miller testimony was admittedly unusual. It was the first major healing, it was a public event, and the Church was still very small and interconnected. The influence of this testimony on the development of divine healing in the Church was important in and of itself. It also suggests how divine healing testimonies attracted converts and increased the personal authority of those who testified.

As has already been stated, Emma Miller was healed of blindness at the Bangor, Michigan camp meeting in June 1883, and her testimony appeared in the September 15 issue of the *Trumpet*. In the October 15 issue, J. C. Fisher reported that Emma Miller's sister, Josephine (Miller) Courtney, had heard about Emma's healing and, being similarly afflicted with blindness and also "mental difficulties," came to the camp on the last day of the meeting. Fisher judged that she was sanctified and had faith to get healed, so he scheduled a special healing service for the following day. After praying and laying-on hands, the Lord healed her blindness.[34]

Courtney's follow-up to Fisher's report appeared May 1, 1884, under the heading "Made Every Whit Whole." Courtney confirmed that her eyes were healed at the Bangor meeting, but when she arrived at home, she realized that she should have asked God for a "complete healing." Having spent December 31st fasting and praying for God to reveal what was lacking, she took up the *Gospel Trumpet* and her eyes first rested on an article by Sister Willard headed "Faith before Sight." Courtney understood the title to be a message that she had to trust God's promise before the symptoms would disappear. She fell on her knees with the *Trumpet* and asked God to make her "every whit whole" (John 13:10). Then she arose and declared that she was healed, although she had no other evidence than her faith in God's word.[35] Two months later, Courtney reported that her healing was a complete success, and she had begun a Bible study in Petoskey, Michigan. This Bible study was the foundation of the first Church of God congregation in Petoskey. Courtney had submitted her testimony to the *Petoskey Record* and the *Battle Creek Weekly*. Another letter from Courtney to the *Trumpet* said that the Petoskey paper had published her story, and it had attracted three new women to her Bible class. Two of them had already been healed, and the third was confidently seeking healing.[36] In addition to its physical benefits, Courtney's divine healing gave her the personal authority and the publicity to start a new congregation.

Courtney's preaching and personal influence—as opposed to her written testimony—led to at least two additional healing testimonies. The first was from Rhoda Keagy, one of the first members of the Trumpet Family. Keagy testified that D. S. Warner and Josephine Courtney prayed and laid hands on her in Battle Creek in 1885. She was healed, and Jesus showed her that she should leave school and go to work for the Trumpet office. Keagy's diary shows that her decision was extraordinarily important for the success of the fledgling Church of God movement. Keagy and her coworker Celia Kilpatrick worked as editors, writers, printers, mechanics, cooks, and janitors for the Trumpet Home. When Warner was absent conducting evangelistic tours, they produced the *Trumpet* and ran the house. They were the only experienced workers left to keep the presses running in the leadership transition from J. C. Fisher to the second office manager, E. E. Byrum.[37] Further, they both married E. E. Byrum. Kilpatrick and he wed on March 4, 1888, but she became ill and died on December 11. The next year, Byrum and Keagy were married.[38]

The second healing testimony that mentioned Josephine Courtney belonged to her eight-year-old daughter Belle. In the "Little Letters" column of the January 1, 1892 issue of *The Shining Light*, Belle Courtney reported that she was not yet saved, but her mother had promised her that God would give her a "new heart." She had been healed of the catarrh in her head. Belle had believed that God would heal her and was anointed. Then "Mama and two sisters who had faith laid hands on my head and prayed, and God did heal me."[39] A follow-up report in 1893 brought the sad news that Belle had died, "but she lived long enough to receive the desire of her heart, and to know that her mother's word and the promise of God were fulfilled. She gave herself to the Lord and he truly gave her a new heart, and filled her soul with his love and glory." She had "gone to be with Jesus."[40] This story shows that the saints had faith enough in divine healing to trust it with their children's health. Moreover, their understanding of divine healing was not so rigid that a death—even the death of a child—could undermine it. The editor of the *Shining Light* regretted that Belle did not receive physical healing but exulted in the much more important healing of her soul. There is no way to know how Belle's death affected Josephine; however, an article she wrote for the *Trumpet* two years later reaffirmed her belief that prayer was the only divinely warranted treatment for the sick.[41]

In addition to her preaching and personal influence, at least one testimony in the *Trumpet* credited Josephine Courtney's published testimony with producing a healing. An extended version of Courtney's testimony from the *Trumpet* appeared first in *Divine Healing of Soul and Body* (1892) and later in *Familiar Names and Faces* (1902). Emma J. Billig wrote to the *Trumpet* in June 1902 that "Sister Courtney's testimony" in the latter book answered her prayer. Billig had been healed nine years earlier, but the disease had returned the previous winter. Courtney's testimony showed her that the symptoms were merely a test. She rebuked "the enemy" and claimed divine healing. She was now every whit whole. This is an example of the influence of a written testimony on a reader who, as far as can be determined, had no other connection with the writer. Billig was a member of the Church of God, but not a minister or a leader. This testimony was her only contribution to the *Trumpet*.[42]

"Healed by the Power of God": Frankie Miller

A year after Emma Miller's healing and several months after Josephine Courtney's, another member of the extended Miller family, Sister Frankie Miller, was healed of "partial blindness" at the Bangor camp meeting.[43] She attended the 1884 Bangor camp meeting "with a sin sick soul and a body wrecked with disease, and praise God! I returned home saved and sound."[44] Her eyes had troubled her for ten years, and had become increasingly worse in the past two. She had been a dressmaker, but her vision had deteriorated such that she could no longer work. One of the "prominent physicians of Battle Creek, Michigan" treated her. She did not specify what kind of medical attention she received, but after the third treatment she could no longer walk. While in this condition, she heard that her cousin Emma Miller had been healed. Later that fall, Frankie also heard about her other cousin, Josephine Courtney. Frankie decided to attend the next Bangor meeting, even though her condition made the trip extremely difficult. She arrived safely but was too weak to sit up, so "the dear saints made a bed for [her] beside the pulpit." During the meeting, God pardoned her sins and gave her "a clear witness that [she] was accepted." The next day she "presented [her] body a living sacrifice, and died the death unto sin." Only then did she feel that she could ask God for healing. Following the instructions in James 5:14–15, D. S. Warner, J. C. Fisher, and Jeremiah Cole laid hands on her and anointed her in the name of Jesus. She was enduring many trials from the devil and was unable to testify to God's healing power at the meeting. She wrote in the *Trumpet* that this cheated God of the glory that was rightfully his; the written account was intended to fulfill her obligation.[45]

Two months after the meeting, Frankie Miller had a relapse, as had her cousins. Josephine Courtney counseled her to "trust God over all the bad feelings" and claim the healing. It worked and Frankie decided to enter the ministry of the Church of God. She traveled all over the country singing and testifying as a member of D. S. Warner's evangelistic company. After his second wife died, D. S. Warner married Frankie Miller.

This brief account of the chain of influence of testimony from the Miller family suggests the networks that operated in the Church of God. Conversion to the healing doctrine spread through families, camp meetings, and print. People turned to testimonies for evidence of how God worked and—as in the case of recurring symptoms—for information about what to do to regain health. The testimonies themselves were dramatic stories of extended suffering, failed doctoring, struggles with temptations, and finally victory over sin and sickness. Sanctification was a prerequisite for healing, but received little attention when compared with healing the body. Further, in these three stories (Emma Miller, Josephine Courtney, and Frankie Miller), there is the suggestion that divine healing completes the sanctification. Each of these women had a relapse that required a special exercise of faith. This brought about a new understanding of faith and a deeper level of trust in God's plan. For Josephine and Frankie, it was the second experience of healing—not sanctification—that propelled them into the ministry.

Enoch E. Byrum: Miracles and Healing

Testimonies from the Miller family initiated the first phase of divine healing in the Church of God movement. These were testimonies by laywomen. The form of the testimonies fit perfectly the early theology of the Church—the Holy Spirit led them to camp meetings where they obeyed the scripture and received healing. The stories pay remarkably little attention to the role of the minister in the healing. In fact, all three regained their healing without benefit of the clergy.[46] Healing came thorough grace, and the relevant biblical passages emphasized that Jesus was still healing through the Church.[47] The Church merely followed God's commands and discovered the return of divine healing.

Ministers began the second phase, most notably Enoch E. Byrum. He was D. S. Warner's successor as the editor of the *Trumpet* and became the Church's divine healing specialist. This phase was marked by a new intentionality in promoting divine healing. Chapter four will show how this new focus culminated in the belief that physical healing was an integral part of the gospel, and therefore one could not preach the "whole gospel" without preaching divine healing for soul *and* body. The increased importance of the minister's role was evident in the new emphasis on the "gifts" of divine healing that God imparted to individuals. Further, the expectation of healing in the Church increased to the point where using medicine became a sign of a sinful lack of faith and continuing afflictions aroused suspicion.

In June 1887, immediately after completing his second year at Otterbein University, Enoch E. Byrum met D. S. Warner at the Bangor camp meeting. Warner asked Byrum to replace J. C. Fisher as the publisher and business manager of the Gospel Trumpet Co. Fisher was no longer in harmony with the saints, because he had filed for divorce and taken up with another woman.[48] Byrum had no experience in publishing or business, and his only qualifications seem to have been that he had saved a small amount of money and was relatively well educated. He initially protested that he was unprepared for the work, but then he remembered a vow he made to God several years before. While plowing a field, Byrum had promised that if God would enable him to go to college, he would answer God's call to work, whatever it might be.[49] Two weeks later, Byrum assumed the most influential position in the Church of God movement.

D. S. Warner and E. E. Byrum had radically different styles. Warner was a charismatic leader, a skilled preacher, a poet, and a songwriter. He was able to persuade people to seek sanctification and to accept his vision of the Church beyond the division of denominationalism.[50] However, he was a poor organizer by temperament and by theological conviction. Under his leadership, the Gospel Trumpet Co. barely broke even. E. E. Byrum was by his own admission a poor preacher. After his first camp meeting sermon, he heard one of the congregants remark, "Brother Byrum can not talk at all."[51] He was rigid, deductive, and careful with details. His were the qualities that enabled the Gospel Trumpet Co. to grow in twenty years from a single-press operation worth a few hundred dollars into a publishing house that required twenty-six railroad cars to move the machinery and inventory from Moundsville, West Virginia, to Anderson, Indiana.[52] It has been observed that when Warner died "the Church lost a leader but gained a manager."[53]

As much as the Church benefited from Byrum's managerial ability and editorial precision, organization remained a dirty word in the Church. It was simply unthinkable for the editor of the *Gospel Trumpet* to be more of an editor than a minister.[54] Byrum was acutely aware that he needed ministerial authority from his first days at the company. He found it in the ministry of divine healing, substituting the charism of healing for the charismatic personality necessary to preach sanctification. Displays of the power of divine healing helped to dispel concern that Byrum's authority derived from his position in the Church's informal hierarchy, and it also was a comforting sign of God's favor in the face of institutional growth and a change of leadership.

Many of Byrum's articles were biblical "proofs" of divine healing. However, he effected much of his promotion of divine healing through testimony. The following account of Byrum's ministry through the "forward move" of 1895 will show the new importance of divine healing for ministers.

Gifts of Healing

A few months after joining the Gospel Trumpet Co., Byrum began to feel that he needed the gifts of healing "but did not know just exactly what they comprised nor how to obtain them."[55] His first experience with exercising healing power came in his first year. D. S. Warner was on a preaching tour, and Byrum and Brother Mayne were the only ones available to lead a cottage prayer meeting. Near the end of the service, "Jimmy, the Office Boy" came forward for healing. Jimmy was prepared for a service following James 5: 14–15. He had a vial of oil for anointing, and he told Mayne and Byrum to proceed as "elders in the church." They did as the boy asked even though they doubted that they qualified as elders. Byrum had never preached, and Mayne had preached only four times. Yet, the boy received immediate healing.[56]

Byrum doubted his own experience, not the boy's. Even before the service was over, Byrum thought that the healing power must have come through Mayne, who had a better claim to the status of elder. However, Byrum still felt that he needed the gift of healing. He prayed for a "definite knowledge" and soon obtained it when "several people" were healed in answer to his prayers "in such a manner that there was no question as to what the Lord had given [him]."[57] He was able to exercise the gifts of healing before he ever preached and before he was ordained.

Even after he was certain that he had special gifts for healing, Byrum remained unsure about how these gifts functioned in the Church. He was in demand because of his growing reputation for answered prayers for healing; yet, a full explanation of why one person would have the gift—as opposed to the whole Church—remained to be given. Sometime between healing "Jimmy the Office Boy" and the publication of *Divine Healing of Soul and Body* (1892), Byrum challenged D. S. Warner's interpretation of 1 Corinthians 13, the classic text enumerating the "gifts of the spirit." Byrum reported attending one of Warner's Bible studies in which Warner mentioned the "gift of healing" with "gift" in the singular. Byrum pointed out that the Bible says "gifts" in the plural, and asked Warner for an explanation. Warner first suggested that one person might have power over one particular disease. This was in line with an article Warner had published in 1883 in which he asserted that no one person has all the gifts, and no gift—not even healing—is for everyone.[58] Byrum protested that sick people would then have to search for the right person, hoping that the gift for the ailment in question had been given to someone. Byrum's pressuring forced Warner to admit that he did not understand the passage.[59] Byrum could not explain it either, but at a later Bible study of divine healing the Holy Sprit revealed to him that Matthew 10:1 was the key to understanding the "gifts." From that passage, Byrum claimed that the gifts of healing were casting out evil spirits, healing sickness, and healing diseases. Further, *all* ministers had to have these gifts or they would not be able to fulfill the duties of an elder.[60]

By connecting the "gifts of healing" with anointing by elders, Byrum's new interpretation—for which he claimed biblical guidance—greatly increased the significance of divine healing for ministers. The testimonies from the Miller family showed little interest in the ministers who anointed and prayed. Healing came through the faith of the person seeking healing. Elders and ministers did not have any particular healing power but assisted with the "prayer of faith" by fulfilling the biblical plan for healing prayers. That is to say, their healing power came from their place in the Church and not the other way around. Henry C. Wickersham (E. E. Byrum's uncle) wrote, "We should not boast of laying on of hands or of any healing. We do not hear Peter, John, or any of the Apostles saying, 'I have got the gift of healing, I have got the gift of discerning, I have got the grand detecter [sic] in me.'"[61] In the early years of the movement, the focus of healing was entirely on the person healed (or not healed). Byrum's interpretation, however, increased the instrumentality of the minister. Now a healing reflected not only on the healed person but also on the person through whom the healing power came.[62] Divine healing was the physical parallel of the spiritual gift of sanctification. If the afflicted person and the Church met all the necessary conditions, then God would grant healing. Rightly applying for the promised benefits (sanctification and healing) was the "secret of salvation." Ministers had to have the gifts of healing or else they could not *demonstrate* healing. If they could not demonstrate healing, they could not effectively preach sanctification. In effect, Byrum demonstrated a gift and then testified that his gift was essential to the future of the Church.

The "Forward Move" of 1895

1895 was a watershed for the Church of God. That year, Byrum believed that "the Lord made clear to [him] in various ways that he wanted not only [Byrum], but also the church, to advance on the line of divine healing and the graces of the Holy Spirit." There were too many failed prayers and too much confusion about divine healing.[63]

Before the June camp meeting, Byrum had a dream in which he and the other Church of God preachers were wading in the lake at the campground. Occasionally someone would wade waist-deep, but the others would call him or her back with a warning. Byrum and a few others waded in up to their necks, and this produced "loud protestations against such boldness." Remarking that he had heard that swimming was easier in deep water, Byrum sprang forward off the shelf and into the deep part of the lake. He found himself on top of the water. He could run on the lake "while those on the shore stood looking on with great fear and trembling."[64] Slowly others began to join him, and then the dream ended. God told Byrum that the dream showed that the gospel workers "were only playing along the shores, and not moving out into the deep, where he wanted to show a manifestation of his power in healing the sick and with victory and power over devils."[65]

Byrum told this message to the general camp meeting. Initially the camp meeting saw a remarkable number of healings, including several cases where people were healed of terminal diseases. The last Sunday, however, a tragic case showed the limits of healing power to the Church. Two six-year-old girls who had been born blind came forward for prayer. Byrum reported that the "faith of all the ministers vanished, [his] included. The girls arose after the prayer, saying, 'Mama, we can see, can't we? Can we see?' But their eyes were not opened."[66]

Distraught and defeated, Byrum prayed for an explanation of the failure. The Lord revealed to him that this case required the gift of miracles, not the gifts of healing.[67] Byrum realized that no one in the Church of God claimed such a gift. At that point, Byrum fully understood the dream about the lake and knew that God wanted someone to seek the gift of miracles. He took this information to Warner, who, according to Byrum, said, "Brother Byrum, this is of God. He wants his church to advance on these lines and no doubt desires you to put in for that gift." After silent prayer, Warner said that God wanted him to lay hands on Byrum for the gift of miracles. There were no outward manifestations, but Byrum received an "inward consciousness that God had answered the prayer."[68]

The next morning, Byrum addressed ministers who were meeting to consider the gifts of the Spirit. He intended to discuss the disputed final chapter of the Gospel of Mark ("These signs shall follow..."). He claimed that he did not intend to mention his new consecration; however, he found that he could not speak any words other than his testimony. After he told the account of the previous night, several saints said "amen" and four other ministers claimed to receive a similar "anointing of power." One skeptical minister remarked, "I would rather see a few miracles wrought than to hear you [Byrum] tell about it."[69]

The blind girls returned for a service of prayer and anointing by Byrum and the four other ministers. It was another complete and public failure. Byrum was again confused and discouraged. He reported that "the enemy" told him that this failure proved that God had not given any human gifts of healing and miracles. The camp meeting Byrum had expected to mark the Church's forward progress on healing and miracles had instead concluded with what appeared to be the dark opposite of Emma Miller's healing.[70]

Immediately after the camp meeting, Byrum and J. W. Daughtery left for a four-month tour of Church of God camp meetings in Canada and the Western United States. Byrum experienced a constant "spiritual battle" in which he questioned his faith in healing and in the gifts he had experienced.[71] After many struggles and additional failed healings, Byrum received an answer to his prayers. God told him that there was no use "continually asking the Lord for something you have already obtained." Just as the Miller sisters had to claim their healings even when confronted with recurrent symptoms, Byrum had to claim the gift of healing in the face of failures. At the next service, instead of asking for help, he praised God for the gifts he had received and said, "Lord, now make manifest thy power to thy servant."[72] That meeting and several of the following were great successes full of healings and miracles. Byrum published several of the accounts and decided that upon his return to the office he would begin a column in the *Trumpet* devoted entirely to divine healing.[73]

Remedies vs. Divine Healing

Before Byrum returned home, D. S. Warner published an article in the *Trumpet* that recommended natural remedies instead of divine healing. Warner was responding to a request for an explanation of 1 Timothy 5:23, the passage in which Paul told Timothy to "drink no longer water, but use a little wine for thy stomach's sake, and thine oft infirmities." Warner's explanation was moderate, and he carefully warned that people should never resort to "medical help instead of to God, or in preference to God, or because they are not willing to get right with God." However, he had no doubt that the passage is "scriptural support of the use of natural remedies for the healing of the body." Faithless reliance on doctors of medicine was wrong, but the sanctified could discern their own motives and properly use "God-created remedies." Human beings should not ask

God to do what they could do for themselves with natural remedies. Moreover, Warner insisted that the use of medicine was not evidence of sin or a lack of faith. He enjoined the readers of the *Trumpet* as follows: "Let not such as use nature's virtues out of honor to the Creator judge such as do not, nor such as utterly discard all natural means judge them who employ them to the glory of God."[74]

Two months after publishing this article, Warner died. The death notice appeared in the December 12, 1895 *Trumpet*. Three issues later, E. E. Byrum refuted one of the last doctrinal articles written by D. S. Warner, the founder and leader of the Church of God movement. Byrum did not mention Warner by name, but regular readers of the *Trumpet* could not have misinterpreted the message that there was a new editor and a new approach to divine healing at the *Gospel Trumpet*.[75]

Byrum's article began, "During our absence in October an article was published in the *Trumpet*, in which the brother who wrote it lowered the standard below the Bible line, while trying to expose certain lines of fanaticism." Byrum was particularly disturbed by Warner's assertion that the saints should not seek divine healing when natural remedies exist. Referring to this particular point, Byrum wrote, "This is not the Bible standard. The Bible says that the means for healing are the prayer of faith and the elders of the church." As for Warner's warning about judging people based on their use of remedies, Byrum asserted that those who use herbs and tea are "weak in the faith."

In case any doubts lingered about the disagreement between Warner and Byrum, Byrum concluded the debate in established Church of God fashion: he provided a testimony. The February 6, 1896 divine healing page included a letter from Josephine Courtney, the sister of Emma Miller and the cousin of D. S. Warner's widow. She reported that she had been severely constipated last fall. "Following the advice of the *Trumpet*," she doctored herself with natural herbs. They did not work, so she asked God to show her the source of the problem. In a dream, God revealed that the Bible does not endorse remedies for the children of God. Courtney discarded her herbs and soon was healed. However, she quickly became sick again because of her weakened spiritual condition. Her troubles continued until she "prayed the prayer of faith, the only one God has promised to answer."[76]

Conclusion

The central message of the Church of God movement was that sanctification eradicated sinful desires and brought the saints into a Holy Spirit-directed unity. This belief made testimony the characteristic form of theological expression in the Church for two reasons. First, testimony spread the message itself. Individual saints told of their experiences of sanctification as poignantly and affectingly as possible, in hopes of attracting new converts and reinforcing the feeling of unity among the existing members of the Church. Second, testimony was the only acceptable way for individuals to assert authority in the movement. The "unity of the saints" meant that there could be no hierarchy and no human-created organizations. There could be no legitimate differences of opinion, and therefore no one asserted "opinions." In place of "I think" or "in my opinion," the writers of the *Trumpet* used such testimonial phrases as "I feel led" or "It has been revealed to me." If the point were contentious, evidence—possibly a fully developed testimony—would accompany it. The affective stories of God's marvelous dealings with the saints helped spread the Church of God movement and also helped to govern it.

Divine healing proved exceptionally important in the Church of God because it improved testimonies and because physical healing helped bridge the gap between the "telling" and the "feeling." The healing testimony of Emma Miller and her extended family created excitement among the saints who detected evidence of the reemergence of the New Testament church. These testimonies also attracted the attention of the secular media and brought new converts to the Church. They were quite simply the most miraculous stories yet to appear in the *Trumpet*. They also presented the best supporting evidence. People could *see* the healings. Unlike sanctification, there was an immediate external and physical change that the saints believed corresponded to an inward and spiritual grace. Thus, the saints embraced divine healing because it fit their hopes and expectations about how God would expand the mission of the Church. The converts in turn joined at least in part because of divine healing, and therefore they understood healing to be central to the Church's message.

The Byrum story showed how testimony could be used to assert personal authority and change the Church's message. Byrum used testimony to reinterpret divine healing so that it was as much a gift exercised by ministers as it was a grace experienced by the afflicted. The result was that ministers—and Byrum in particular—could now testify to their instrumentality in healing. This created an unofficial hierarchy of ministers who had the gifts of healing over those who did not. Since Byrum was the best-known healer, this cemented his authority in the Church. Moreover, in a radical break from D. S. Warner, Byrum taught that divine healing was the only God-appointed system of healing for the saints. Under this interpretation, the use of medicine or herbs was evidence of a poor spiritual condition. Not seeking divine healing exclusively was tantamount to declaring a lack of faith in God's power. Thus, the laity was more dependent than ever on those with the gifts of healing.

Byrum's interpretation of divine healing increased his own authority and that of several other ministers. The following chapter will show, however, that the new emphasis on divine healing created unintended consequences for the Church. Suddenly divine healing had changed from a particular instance of grace into everyone's responsibility. Failed healings could now testify against the minister or the patient. Unanswered prayers suggested divine judgment. Because divine healing was now the only option and was connected to personal holiness and even membership in the Church, the saints demanded explanations of the finer points of divine healing.

Notes

1. Testimony is difficult to define even when restricted to a religious context. At its most basic, it is an assertion of facts. A person solemnly swears—explicitly in court or implicitly in a religious service—to firsthand knowledge of some facts. For this recounting to be testimony, however, these facts and their interpretation must have some communally accepted import. Rebecca Chopp has defined testimony as "discourse that refers to a reality outside the ordinary order of things." ("Theology and the Poetics of Testimony," in *Converging on Culture: Theologians in Dialogue with Cultural Analysis and Criticism*, ed. Delwin Brown and others [New York: Oxford University Press, 2001], 61.) Thus, Christian testimony interprets the "facts" it presents as evidence of God's work in the world. Testimony also asserts the authority of the one testifying. This final aspect of testimony was particularly important in holiness meetings and the Church of God because insight into the "reality outside the ordinary order of things" reflected the internal state of the one testifying. According to Paul Ricour, "testimony is the action itself as it attests outside of himself, to the interior man, to his conviction, to his faith" ("The Hermeneutics of Testimony," in *Essays on Biblical Interpretation*, ed. Lewis S. Mudge [Philadelphia: Fortress, 1980], 130).

2. Brown, *From Infidelity to Christianity*.

3. Immediate, subjective experiences—whatever they might be—are beyond the scope of historical inquiry. Testimonies are texts. However, it is important to note that the saints themselves believed that their religious experiences of sanctification and healing could be separated from the discourses about the experiences. For an introduction to the difficulties associated with attempting to signify "inner experience" in studies of religion, see Robert H. Sharf, "Experience," chapter five in Mark C. Taylor, ed., *Critical Terms for Religious Studies* (Chicago: University of Chicago Press, 1998). For a discussion of the theological import of "respecting and protecting this gap between the named and the unnamable," see Chopp, *Converging on Culture*, 64.

4. John 1:50. For an indication of the importance of miraculous stories and experiences in promoting the Church of God, see Henry C. Wickersham, *A History of the Church* (Moundsville, W.Va.: Gospel Trumpet Co., 1900). Wickersham divided church history into four dispensations; the last began in 1880 and was "A General Reformation and a Gathering of God's People into One Church." He let the saints tell their own story with testimonies. See especially the testimonies of J. N. Howard, George L. Cole, and William G. Schell. Each of these men reported that witnessing miracles of healing in the Church of God movement convinced him that God was beginning a new dispensation marked by signs and wonders.

5. Testimony was a fundamental part of the holiness movement from its very beginning with Phoebe Palmer's Tuesday Meetings. However, when the holiness movement was interdenominational (as opposed to anti-denominational), participants were already

members of some church. Testimony spoke of a higher experience in the Christian life. With the Church of God, testimony was foundational for demonstrating membership, and was therefore extraordinarily important. For testimony in Palmer's meetings, see Dieter, *The Holiness Revival of the Nineteenth Century*, 30–32. According to Daniel Steele, an influential holiness theologian, testimony was one of the "Fruits of Perfect Love." "A confessing mouth always attends a believing heart. As in the world of matter occult forces manifest themselves in their effects, so in the world of mind an unloosed tongue is the infallible result of the hidden Transformer, the Holy Spirit" (*Love Enthroned* [New York: Nelson and Phillips, 1875], chap. 11).

6. "Handing over to Satan" is from 1 Cor. 5:5 and 1 Tim. 1:20. For an example of testimony that was rejected because the woman had been quarrelling openly in the assembly, see Jennie C. Rutty, "An Open Letter," *GT* 14:31 (Aug. 9, 1894): 2.

7. Early examples are D. S. Warner, "Faith Healing an Important Factor in Soul Saving," *GT* 6:3 (Nov. 1, 1883): 2–3; and J. W. Byers, "We Must Preach Divine Healing," *GT* 15:51 (Dec. 26, 1895): 4. In 1910, the *Trumpet* published a five-part series by John C. Blaney on "Miracles and Signs as a Means of Reaching People with the Gospel." Blaney was arguing that miracles and signs were essential for the Church's continued success. See the issues from Sept. 29 to Oct. 27.

8. For an example of how D. S. Warner used healing the body as a figure for reuniting the universal church, see his poem "Soul-Cripple City." It was originally published in Warner's *Poems of Grace and Truth* (Grand Junction, Mich.: Gospel Trumpet Co., 1890), 119–74. Thomas Fudge has reprinted it as an appendix in *Daniel Warner and the Paradox of Religious Democracy in Nineteenth-Century America* (Lewiston, N.Y.: Edwin Mellen Press, 1998).

9. A testimony in the *Trumpet* reported "The Great Physitin [sic] now is here; hallelujah, I am healed SOUL and BODY." Chloe K. Hatton, "Instantly Healed by the Lord after Six Weeks Suffering and Helpless," *GT* 5:11 (Sept. 22, 1882): 2, 5. In 1892, E. E. Byrum titled his first book on healing *Divine Healing of Soul and Body*.

10. J. C. Fisher and S. G. Odell, "The Great Physician," no. 19 in J. C. Fisher, ed., *Songs of Victory*. The hymn also appeared in *GT* 7:9 (July 15, 1885): 1. The scripture reference introducing the hymn in the songbook was Psalm 147:3, "He healeth the broken in heart, and bindeth up their wounds."

11. A. L. Byers, ed., *Two Hundred Genuine Instances of Divine Healing* (Anderson, Ind.: Gospel Trumpet Co., 1911), 272.

12. The *Gospel Trumpet* published hundreds of divine healing testimonies. The first appeared in the January 1, 1882 issue. That year there were three other healing testimonies in the *Trumpet*. In 1883, there were eleven, including one that the Gospel Trumpet Co. issued as a stand-alone tract. In 1884 there were at least twenty-two divine healing testimonies, even though there were six fewer issues that year because Warner moved to Ohio. From 1895 through the end of the period covered in this study, every issue of the *Trumpet*—now a weekly—included a divine healing page. It was extremely rare for a page to not have at least one divine healing testimony, and some pages had as many as six. Volume 28, number 24 of the *Trumpet* included a sixteen-page supplement consisting entirely of testimonies. Starting in 1891, the Church published a semi-monthly children's paper. Its "Little Letters" column included healing testimonies for children. From 1896 through 1898, J. W. Byers published a monthly paper titled *Tidings of Healing*, and it too had testimonies, although not as many as the *Trumpet*. In addition to the periodicals, many Church of God books included testimonies. E. E. Byrum's *Divine Healing of Soul*

and Body (1892) had thirty-nine testimonies that accounted for 113 of the book's 248 pages. J. W. Byers's *The Grace of Healing* (1899) had an additional forty-three healing testimonies. The title of A. L. Byers's *Two Hundred Genuine Instances of Divine Healing* (1911) speaks for itself. E. E. Byrum's *Miracles and Healing* (1919) had an additional forty-three testimonies. J. Grant Anderson's *Divine Healing* (1926) was the last large collection of healing testimonies; it had seventy-three.

13. J. S. Smurr, "Cancer Healed," *GT* 8:7 (June 5, 1886): 1; Reuben Phillips, "Healed of a Cancerous Tumor," *GT* 15:2 (March 7, 1895). J. Grant Anderson's *Divine Healing* had devoted a section to healing from cancer (56–63). For consumption and colds, see Anna E. Albright, "Healing of Cancer and Consumption," in E. E. Byrum, *Healing of Soul and Body*, 235–38; and Mrs. F. A. Hunt, "Chills and Fever Healed," in J. W. Byers, *Grace of Healing*, 308–9. Other diseases included Lizzie Clark, "How I Was Healed of Rheumatism," *GT* 14:24 (June 14, 1894): 4; Emma Tufford, "A Wonderful Deliverance from Smallpox," *GT* 22:10 (March 6, 1902): 6–7; and Lucy H. Peabody, "Pneumonia Healed," in J. W. Byers, *Grace of Healing*, 309–10.

14. Addie Coon, "Restoration of Eyesight," in E. E. Byrum, *Healing of Soul and Body*, 196–97; Minnie Chapman, "The Blind and Lame See and Walk," in Byrum, *Healing of Soul and Body*, 221–23; S. B. Kuffel, "Healed," *GT* 5:23 (Aug. 29, 1883): 2. Kuffel regained hearing after eleven years.

15. Dagmar Rasmussen, "'If They Drink any Deadly Thing it Shall Not Hurt Them'—A Living Witness to the Power of Mark 16:18," in J. W. Byers, *Grace of Healing*, 322–25; Anna Cheatham, "Healed of a Snakebite," *GT* 22:42 (Oct. 16, 1902): 8; A. J. Byers, "Rough on Rats Poison," in A. L. Byers, *Two Hundred Instances*, 44–45; L. R. Blocker, "Rattlesnake Bite," in *Two Hundred Instances*, 80–81; F. P. Dimm, "Poisoned Eating Toadstools," in *Two Hundred Instances*, 91–92. For opposition to serpent handling, see D. S. Warner, "A Snakey Religion," *GT* 12:58 (Dec. 29, 1892): 1.

16. "Faith" in J. W. Byers, *Grace of Healing*, 244–49.

17. "Wonderful Healing," *GT* 9:17 (Sept. 1, 1889): 1.

18. C. E. Woods, "An Accidental Wound in the Body," in A. L Byers, *Two Hundred Instances*, 35–36. Accidents are some of the most remarkable testimonies. See, for instance, E. A. Soules, "Head Severely Crushed," in A. L. Byers, *Two Hundred Instances*, 65–67; James A. Speelman, "Struck by a Fast Train," in *Two Hundred Instances*, 203–5.

19. "Raised to Life," *GT* 10:9 (July 15, 1888): 2; Mary Heldenbrand, "Drowned Child Resuscitated and Healed," in A. L. Byers, *200 Instances*, 172–74; Nancy (King) Taylor, "Raised from the Dead," in E. E. Byrum, *Startling Incidents and Experiences in the Christian Life* (Anderson, Ind.: Gospel Trumpet Co., 1915), 135–41. The latter testimony included a corroborating statement by E. E. Byrum.

20. Rhoda Keagy, a member of the Trumpet Family, kept a diary for 1888. Tuesday, March 6, she wrote that Sister Fisher had "corrected some testimonies for the paper." Keagy did not indicate what "correcting" entailed. (Archives of the Church of God, "Keagy, Rhoda Diary, 1888.")

21. I have based this outline on my reading of over 500 Church of God healing testimonies. See note 12 above.

22. See E. E. Byrum, "The Lord is our Physician," *GT* 12:6 (Feb. 4, 1892): 2. The article said to follow James 5:14–15 whenever elders were available. If no elders but at least one other child of God could be found, then follow Matthew 18:19–20. John 15:7 served all the isolated saints. See also E. E. Byrum, *The Great Physician* (Moundsville,

W.Va.: Gospel Trumpet Co., 1899), 67–71 for the articles "Anointing with Oil," "What to Do in Case There are No Elders," and "Promises When Alone."

23. E. E. Byrum, "Believe for Healing," *GT* 15:49 (Dec. 12, 1895): 4. From 1895 until at least the mid-1950s, the Gospel Trumpet Co. sent anointed handkerchiefs free of charge to readers who requested them. The practice was based on Acts 19:11–12 in which Paul is reported to have sent handkerchiefs and aprons to the sick. See E. E. Byrum, "Questions Answered: Sending Anointed Handkerchiefs," *GT* 20:49 (Dec. 13, 1900): 4. Sending handkerchiefs started with an experiment by D. S. Warner and J. C. Fisher in 1885, but it was not common practice until Byrum re-introduced it in 1895. See D. S. Warner, "The Power of God Sent By Mail," *GT* 8:18 (Dec. 1, 1886): 1. James Opp has identified the practice of sending handkerchiefs in the Pentecostal movement as evidence of the shift from "healing as a bodily extension of the process of sanctification" to a "power that can be exchanged, held, and embedded within material objects" ("Religion, Medicine, and the Body: Protestant Faith Healing in Canada, 1880–1930" [Ph.D. diss., Carleton University, 2000], 277). That the Church of God was sending handkerchiefs as early as 1885 suggests that this shift in the theology of healing happened before the Pentecostal outpourings of 1901 and 1906.

24. The following letter by Elsie Ethel Myers appeared in *The Shining Light* 1:2 (Feb. 1, 1891): 4. "The Lord has forgiven my sins, and I want you all to pray for me that I may be sanctified. I am ten years old. I was very sick with the Measles, and last Friday night about eight o'clock the Lord healed me, and I got up the next morning at six o'clock and was able to go to meeting on Sunday. I thank the Lord for healing my body."

25. According to C. E. Brown, "This notable miracle was a widespread subject of comment in the movement for a whole generation" (*When the Trumpet Sounded,* 111). A. L. Byers also wrote about Miller's healing. "Marvelous healings were common, but as this one was a healing of complete blindness and was one of the earliest cases, it is here mentioned" (*Birth of a Reformation,* 306–7). See also the biographical sketch of the third editor of the *Gospel Trumpet,* F. G. Smith, in *Heralds of a Brighter Day.* Smith recalled that he was a little boy when his parents took him to the meeting where Miller was healed. The shouting and rejoicing of the saints scared him so much that he would not stop crying. The meeting made a lasting impression. As he grew older and had the experience explained to him, "he never had to be convinced that God was at work among his people" (John W. V. Smith, *Heralds of a Brighter Day,* 105).

26. E. E. Byrum, *The Secret of Salvation: How to Get It and How to Keep It* (Anderson, Ind.: Gospel Trumpet Co., 1896), 359. This is the publication information in my copy, but note that the date and the place do not match. In 1896, the publication place would have been Grand Junction, Michigan,.

27. One indication of the importance of Miller's testimony for the Church of God is the number of reprints and updates published by the Gospel Trumpet Co. The first version was a letter dated July 21, 1883. It was printed under the head "A Wonderful Faith Cure" in the Sept. 15, 1883 issue of the *Trumpet* (vol. 5, no. 24, p. 1). The *Trumpet* published an expanded and updated version titled "God's Wonderful Dealings with Sister Emma Miller" on Dec. 15, 1884 (vol. 6, no. 20, pp. 1–2). This version was also printed as a stand-alone tract in 1884, and it reappeared unchanged in the *Trumpet* on Nov. 1, 1886 (vol. 8, no. 16, p. 1). Miller submitted an additional update titled "The Blind Eyes Opened" (*GT* 15:1 [Jan. 3, 1895]). Versions of Miller's testimony also appeared in three books by E. E. Byrum. See "The Blind Eyes Opened" in *Divine Healing of Soul and*

Body, 142–45; "Healing of the Blind" in *Secret of Salvation,* 359–60; and "Blind Eyes Restored to Sight" in *Miracles and Healing,* 285–86.

28. Emma Miller, "God's Wonderful Dealings with Sister Emma Miller," *GT* 6:20 (Dec. 15, 1884): 2.

29. Emma Miller, "The Blind Eyes Opened," in E. E. Byrum, *Divine Healing of Soul and Body,* 143–44.

30. Emma Miller, "God's Wonderful Dealings with Sister Emma Miller," 2.

31. Emma Miller, "The Blind Eyes Opened," in E. E. Byrum, *Divine Healing of Soul and Body,* 145.

32. J. C. Fisher, *GT* 5:24 (Sept. 15, 1883): 3–4.

33. D. S. Warner, "The Third General Assembly of the Saints in Michigan—And Grove Meeting in Indiana," *GT* 6:2 (Oct. 15, 1883): 4. One of the few critiques of divine healing testimonies was written by J. M. Buckley and appeared in *Century Magazine* in 1886. According to Buckley, these testimonies commonly displayed four fatal flaws. 1. Testimonies to the cure of internal diseases were worthless, especially without an expert diagnosis by a physician. 2. Testimonies to immediate cures do not respect the nature of disease. Symptoms often go into remission only to return later. A cure has to be observed over a long period. 3. Often, "the condition of the patient prior to the alleged cure has been greatly exaggerated in the description." 4. Testimonies frequently omit important facts, such as beneficial medical attention ("Faith-Healing and Kindred Phenomena," *Century Magazine,* June 1886, 223–25). Nothing could be done about the last charge, but the continuing report of Emma Miller's healing attempted to address the first three. It was an external healing, and follow-up testimonies showed that it was permanent. Statements by physicians and family members established that she had not exaggerated her previous condition.

34. J. C. Fisher, "Conclusion of the Michigan Assembly, More Healing Power Manifest," *GT* 6:2 (Oct. 15, 1883): 3. Between her healing in 1883 and her testimony in 1884, Josephine Miller married and changed her name to Courtney. The *Trumpet* gave no indication that Josephine Miller and Josephine Courtney were the same person. E. E. Byrum's story "Go To Bay View, Michigan" proves that Miller and Courtney were in fact the same (*Life Experiences* [Anderson, Ind.: Gospel Trumpet Co., 1928], 202–6).

35. Courtney did not attribute her insight to outside authorities; however, two divine healing evangelists were famous for the "acting on faith" doctrine. Mrs. Elizabeth Mix and Carrie Judd Montgomery were both teaching in the early 1880s that symptoms are deceptions from the devil. One must follow the command of Mark 11:24: "believe that ye receive them [gifts of healing], and ye shall have them." See Paul Chappell, "The Divine Healing Movement in America" (Ph.D. diss., Drew University, 1983), 96–97. See also R. Kelso Carter, "Divine Healing, or 'Faith Cure,'" *Century Magazine,* 780. For a criticism of divine healing testimony that focuses on the "believe that you receive" doctrine, see A. F. Schauffler, "Faith-Cures," *Century Magazine,* Dec. 1885, 274–78. Schauffler charged that the language used in testimony was unreliable because "faith healers make a distinction between disease and symptoms so marked that they claim to be healed of disease even while the symptoms continue" (276).

36. Josephine Courtney, *GT* 6:14 (Sept. 15, 1884): 4.

37. "Keagy, Rhoda Diary, 1888." Church of God Archives. See also, E. E. Byrum, *Life Experiences,* 82–83.

38. Rhoda Keagy, diary, March 4, 1888, and Dec. 11, 1888. See also Harold Phillips, *Miracle of Survival,* 36–38.

39. Belle Courtney, "Dear Children of the Shining Light," *SL* 2:1 (Jan. 1, 1892): 4.

40. "Gone to Live With Jesus," *SL* 3:23 (Dec. 1, 1893): 4.

41. Josephine Courtney, "Praise God for Healing," *GT* 16:6 (Feb. 6, 1896): 6. Internal evidence proves that Courtney wrote this article after October 1895.

42. Emma J. Billig, "The Lord is My Healer," *GT* 22:24 (June 19, 1902): 8.

43. Anna Albright's testimony identified Frankie Miller's story as the key to her own healing ("Healed by the Lord," *GT* 8:24 [March 1, 1887]). However, Frankie's testimony was not publicized as much as Emma Miller's and Josephine Courtney's, probably because it was the third.

44. Frankie Miller, "Healed, Soul, Body, and Mind" in E. E. Byrum, *Divine Healing of Soul and Body*, 155–59.

45. Frankie Miller, "Healed by the Power of God," *GT* 7:1 (June 6, 1885): 1; "The Glorious Holy War," *GT* 8:10 (Aug. 1, 1886): 1.

46. See, for example, A. K. Thomas, "How the Lord led Me," *GT* 6:20 (Dec. 15, 1884): 4. After her sanctification, the healing power came for Thomas's hands. Warner and Fisher were having a healing service, and she supposed it was for her so she requested anointing. This *interfered* with the healing, because God had already begun it and was able to complete it without help. The next day she had a fever, but worked through it in faith. By end of the day, she felt better than ever.

47. "Bless the Lord, O my soul, and forget not all his benefits; Who forgiveth all thine iniquities; who healeth all thy diseases" (Psalm 103:2–3). "Jesus Christ the same yesterday, and today, and forever" (Hebrews 13:8). "Is any sick among you? let him call for the elders of the church; and let them pray over him; anointing him with oil in the name of the Lord; And the prayer of faith shall save the sick, and the Lord shall raise him up; and if he have committed any sins, they shall be forgiven him" (James 5:14–15).

48. According to William G. Schell, in the spring of 1887, Fisher "forsook his wife and eloped with a grass-widow." The June camp meeting "was not accompanied by the usual power of God," and God revealed that the good work could not continue unless the Church renounced Fisher (Wickersham, *History of the Church*, 366–67). For a humorous account of Warner's disfellowshipping of Fisher, see "The Sanctified Saints," *Chicago Tribune*, Feb. 16, 1888, 1.

49. E. E. Byrum, *Life Experiences*, 77.

50. See chapters 17 and 18 of A. L. Byers, *Birth of a Reformation*. They are, respectively, "The Ministry of Song" and "Poetic Inspirations."

51. E. E. Byrum, *Travels and Experiences in Other Lands* (Moundsville, W.Va.: Gospel Trumpet Co., 1905), 26–27 and 30.

52. Phillips, *Miracle of Survival*, 101.

53. Strege, *I Saw the Church*, 63.

54. The ouster of Byrum's predecessor for moral turpitude underscored the necessity of a demonstrably holy life for all Gospel Trumpet workers.

55. E. E. Byrum, *Life Experiences*, 128.

56. E. E. Byrum, *Life Experiences*, 128; 94–96 for "Jimmy, the Office Boy." See also E. E. Byrum, *Travels*, 27–28.

57. E. E. Byrum, *Life Experiences*, 28. Byrum's first wife died in 1888 after only nine months of marriage. Rhoda Keagy's diary recorded that Byrum and several others had prayed for her healing, but she did not improve (Dec. 1 and 2, 1888). Byrum did not mention her death in any of his histories of how he came to his belief in divine healing.

However, it is at least plausible that his wife's death motivated Byrum to study divine healing.

58. D. S. Warner, "Healing in Christ," *GT* 6:1 (Oct. 1, 1883): 2. Warner was making the point that sanctification was more important to the Church than were the gifts of the Spirit. Everyone is promised sanctification, because sanctification was all the Church needed. Warner saw the gifts of the Spirit as an added benefit. Daniel Steele gave a similar interpretation that also emphasized the plural gifts (*Half-Hours with St. Paul and Other Bible Readings* [Boston: The Christian Witness Co., 1895], 249).

59. E. E. Byrum, *Life Experiences*, 130.

60. E. E. Byrum, *Life Experiences,* 131. See "Divine Healing: The Commission," *GT* 15:44 (Nov. 7, 1895): 4; "Divine Healing: The Will of God to Heal," *GT* 15:45 (Nov. 14, 1895): 4.

61. *Holiness Bible Subjects*, 296.

62. Byrum was always careful to note that he did not say he had the power to heal. Only God could heal. His gift was that God worked through him for healing. See E. E. Byrum, "Christ the Healer," *GT* 15:47 (Nov. 28, 1895): 4.

63. E. E. Byrum, *Travels*, 28–29.

64. Knowing his audience, Byrum insisted that God did not want the saints to walk on water.

65. E. E. Byrum, *Travels*, 29. Two versions of this dream appeared in the literature. The first was in *Travels*, and the second was a published sermon Byrum gave at camp meeting in 1926 ("Experiences—Miracles and Healing," *GT* 46:27 [July 8, 1926]: 7, 11–12). The first does not mention any names, but the second identifies J. W. Byers as one of the ministers who went with Byrum all the way into the deep. In the second Byrum neglected to mention that he walked on the water; instead, he just swam in the deep.

66. E. E. Byrum, *Travels*, 31; *Life Experiences*, 133.

67. Recall that the "gifts of healing" were for casting out devils, healing diseases, and healing sickness.

68. E. E. Byrum, *Travels*, 32.

69. E. E. Byrum, *Travels,* 33; *Life Experiences,* 135.

70. The fact that Byrum did not describe this as the opposite of the Miller healing shows how far his understanding of divine healing was from that of the earlier saints. For Byrum's story, the blind girls—not their blindness—corresponded to Miller's blindness. Their continued presence reflected *Byrum's* need for a divine gift of healing power. He later obtained this gift, but the girls disappeared from the record of the Church of God.

71. E. E. Byrum, *Life Experiences*, 136.

72. E. E. Byrum, *Travels*, 36.

73. E. E. Byrum, *Travels,* 38. From Nov. 7, 1895, until well after Byrum's term as editor was over in 1916, the back page of the *Trumpet* was the Divine Healing Page.

74. D. S. Warner, "Question," *GT* 15:42 (Oct. 24, 1895): 2. This article also appeared as "An Explanation About Divine Healing" in Warren C. Roark, comp., *Divine Healing* (Anderson, Ind.: Gospel Trumpet Co., 1945), 114–19. See also, Strege, *I Saw the Church*, 72–73.

75. E. E. Byrum, "Means used in Divine Healing," *GT* 16:1 (Jan. 2, 1896): 4.

76. Josephine Courtney, "Praise God for Healing," *GT* 16:6 (Feb. 6, 1896): 6.

CHAPTER 4

DIVINE HEALING DOCTRINE, 1890–1905

When the earth shall cease to be, And the heavens pass away,
The unchanging word of God we'll see, Just as it is today.
On the word of God I calmly rest, With a sweet assurance in my breast;
For I know it is his holy will, Each promise to fulfill.
(C. W. Naylor/B. E. Warren, "The Unchanging Word")

Bible Proofs of Divine Healing

E. E. Byrum introduced his doctrine of divine healing with the following observation: "We do not base the doctrine of divine healing upon the testimonies of those who have been healed in these last days; nor upon what has been written in many of the volumes published, for there is a more solid foundation upon which to build. The Word of God is the true basis upon which its principles are founded, and it is presented in the strongest terms from Genesis to Revelation."[1] The preceding chapter of this book suggests that Byrum was underestimating the importance of testimony to doctrinal development, and the fact that this very quote strongly resembled a passage from R. Kelso Carter's *Century Magazine* article (1887) indicates that divine healing publications were influential as well.[2] However, Byrum accurately reported the Church of God's understanding of doctrine. No matter where the opinions originally came from, they had to be compared with the Bible. If the Bible contradicted the teaching, then it had to be abandoned. If, however, the new idea proved to be a "Bible doctrine," then the origin became irrelevant. Thus, in the opinion of members of the Church of God,

91

all accepted divine healing doctrines were truly from the Bible, no matter what intermediate sources the Holy Spirit used to reveal them.[3]

A glance at any of the divine healing books or articles from the Gospel Trumpet Co. would turn up many scriptural passages. Church of God writers never strayed far from the text of the Bible. Among the extreme examples was the divine healing calendar of 1898. Every new subscriber to the *Gospel Trumpet* received a wall calendar that presented "a collection of nearly all the scriptures in the Bible which set forth the promises of divine healing."[4] For good measure, the *Trumpet* also published all 78 passages in a series of Divine Healing columns from September 8 to October 20 of 1898. By 1901, the relevant quotations were familiar enough for the editors of the *Trumpet* to publish "Thoughts on Divine Healing," a statement about divine healing pieced together entirely from unattributed biblical passages.[5] However, simply stating scripture did not make a doctrine. Even the strongest critics of the divine healing movement readily admitted miraculous healings do indeed appear from Genesis to Revelation and that Jesus and the apostles healed the sick, cast out demons, and raised the dead.[6] The problem lay at the point where the saints extrapolated from miracles of the Bible to divine healing in the present. Divine healing books and articles existed precisely to demonstrate that the Bible says that healing is available today.

The Bible contains scores of passages about miraculous healings, but very few say that divine healing should be a present reality for the reader. Even the clearest statements leave much room for interpretation and do not—on their own at least—establish divine healing as an essential part of the Christian message. The kind of doctrine the Church of God eventually developed—which proscribed medicine and obligated ministers to preach divine healing—required biblical proof. A throwaway observation by A. L. Byers said that Psalm 103:1–3 ("Bless the Lord, O my soul: and all that is within me, bless his holy name. Bless the Lord, O my soul, and forget not all his benefits: Who forgiveth all thine iniquities; who healeth all thy diseases") was the *central* verse, literally and physically, of the Bible, and thus "those who do not preach healing miss the center of the gospel."[7] Byers knew he was conflating the physical center of the book with the central meaning of the text, and he presented it as an interesting piece of trivia. However, this simple observation highlighted what the more serious arguments for divine healing were attempting to show.

Four arguments for divine healing dominated the Church of God literature. In roughly chronological order, these were: healing as a gift to the faithful, healing directly from Jesus, healing as part of the Great Commission, and healing in the atonement.[8] Each of these arguments had parallels—and probably roots—in the divine healing movement; however, the Church's distinctive soteriology and ecclesiology often shaped the articulations. Further, this order also reflects the increasing integration of divine healing into the theology of the Church of God.

Each stage brought with it more promises and more demands, both for ministers and for the afflicted.

Divine Healing as a Benefit to the Faithful

The initial foundation of divine healing in the Church of God and also in the divine healing movement was James 5:14–16:

> Is any sick among you? let him call for the elders of the church; and let them pray over him, anointing him with oil in the name of the Lord: And the prayer of faith shall save the sick, and the Lord shall raise him up; and if he have committed sins, they shall be forgiven him. Confess your faults one to another, that ye may be healed. The effectual prayer of a righteous man availeth much.

This is the clearest statement in the Bible that Christians should pray for healing. Every proponent of divine healing used this passage, and some such as Charles Cullis, the founder of modern divine healing, relied on it almost exclusively.[9] The earliest accounts of divine healing in the Church of God either quoted this passage or described anointing services that were clearly based on its instructions. James 5:14–16 convinced people of the possibility of divine healing and brought them forward for prayer and the laying on of hands. As long as people were experiencing healing, this passage, combined with the testimonies of the healed, could form the basis of the kind of successful divine healing ministry that Charles Cullis had. In a movement or a denomination, it added an option for those who were sick. However, that was about all it could do. It certainly could not serve as the sole basis of the kind of divine healing doctrine that prohibited the use of medicine, insisted that ministers preach divine healing, or associated ministerial authority with effective healing.

B. B. Warfield, professor of Didactic and Polemic Theology at Princeton Theological Seminary and an outspoken critic of the divine healing movement, went so far as to say that James 5:14–16 was irrelevant to any proof of divine healing because it gives "no promise of healing in a specifically miraculous manner."[10] He was right, of course. It is entirely possible to read the passage as offering spiritual but not physical benefits, and therefore this passage would not convince those who believed that "the day of miracles is past." Most of the folk in holiness circles, however, were willing to make the conceptual leap from "the prayer of faith shall save the sick" to "the prayer of faith shall heal—physically and immediately—the sick."

Yet, even those who read James as a statement about divine healing could interpret it as simply one option for healing among others. D. S. Warner's was the prime example of this position in the Church of God. We have seen in chapter three that he harmonized prayer for healing with the use of natural remedies. Charles Cullis too "believed medicine and the supernatural worked together without conflict."[11] In a retrospective article, purporting to tell the "History of Divine Healing Among Us," one of the Church of God's strongest supporters of divine healing in the atonement wrote that in the early years of the Church of God divine healing "was in the background as an option with remedies, medicine, etc."[12]

A common practice in Church of God divine healing material was to assert that most people acted as if James said, "Is any sick among you? let him send for the doctor, no matter if an infidel, and let him practice medicine upon you."[13] For skeptics, however, this only highlighted the fact that James did not say anything at all about physicians. R. L. Farquar, the author of several divine healing articles for the *Trumpet*, was concerned that the saints had "been too tender-footed in teaching [divine healing] as a doctrine of the Bible," and so he attempted to demonstrate that James 5:14–15 was a command. Using the "let" from Hebrews 13:1 ("Let brotherly love continue") to interpret "let the afflicted pray" and "let the sick call the elders," he argued that the Church had to be active. According to Farquar, James was commanding the Church to preach divine healing in a manner that would encourage and enjoin the afflicted to pray.[14] Even with this elaboration, however, James did not provide a theology of divine healing. Further commentary was necessary.

Divine Healing Directly from Jesus

The second argument telescoped the years between Jesus' earthly ministry and the present to say that healing power continues to come directly from a personal relationship with Jesus. Where the other three proofs of divine healing could often seem impersonal and automatic—if the afflicted would follow the rules of the Bible, then, as per God's plan, healing would come—this portrayal based healing on Jesus' unchanging will. Jesus loves his people, and therefore he heals their diseases. The most important text was Hebrews 13:8 ("Jesus Christ the same yesterday, and today, and forever"), which was often shortened to "He is just the same today." In the simplest formulation of this proof, the text functioned to make all the miracle stories from the gospels into promises for the present-day church. How did one respond to the critics who said that Jesus' miracles were not in question but also were not relevant to the present discussion? "Jesus is just the same today." Why should one expect healing when obeying James 5:14–16? "Jesus: the same yesterday, today, and forever." Is there not a fundamental difference between the stories of the gospels and the nineteenth-century church? There should not be, because "*Jesus* is just the same today." If there was a difference, then it came because the followers of Jesus had strayed from the true message.

Paul Chappell has identified the use of this argument with the "simple and literal interpretation of Scripture." Mrs. Sarah Mix, a divine healing evangelist and a pioneer of the idea that the healed had to "exercise their faith," used this passage to say that Christ is

> 'the same yesterday, and to-day, and forever' ... and that the same power that healed the Centurion's servant, that rebuked the fever in Peter's wife's mother, that cast the devils out of many, that healed the sick of the palsy, that caused the cripple to leap for joy, that gave hearing to the deaf and sight to the blind, will produce the same results to-day in answer to the 'prayer of faith.'[15]

Other divine healing advocates such as John A. Dowie used Hebrews 13:8 as a quick and easy way to deflect questions about the cessation of miracles and to provide a minimal justification for focusing on divine healing in their ministries.[16]

The "just the same today" argument was particularly important to the Church of God. By itself, Hebrews 13:8 could not carry much theological weight. However, it did not have to in the Church of God because divine healing was only a part of the larger movement. The idea of sanctification, for instance, prepared Church of God adherents for the immediate experience of the divine. Moreover, the Church's "evening light" amillennial dispensationalism explained the return of the grace of healing along with the other marks of the "morning light."[17] J. W. Byers introduced his chapter, "Divine Healing in the Life and Ministry of Christ," with this brief statement of the evening light theology:

> Prophetic inspiration tells us of this blessed period of light which has followed the gloom of the dark ages. 'But it shall be one day which shall be known to the Lord, not day, nor night: but it shall come to pass, that at evening time it shall be light'—Zech. 14:7. Thank God, the Son of Righteousness with healing in his wings is shining upon his people. The evening time has come and before the day of the gospel dispensation shall close, the inhabitants of the earth must see the brightness of the church of God shining forth in the glory of the morning.[18]

Church of God people had already accepted the conflation of the early Church with the present, so it was relatively simple to say that, among all the other similarities, Jesus still healed diseases.

This interpretation of divine healing—the affective, personal identification with Jesus—was the most common one used in hymns, and they are some of the clearest and earliest statements about healing. In 1888, D. S. Warner published "O Lord Thou Healest Me" in *Anthems from the Throne*, the second Church of God songbook. The song explained that healing comes directly from Jesus, that Jesus is the same as he always was, and that he is a compassionate healer. Verse two said, "Thy Love, O God! Abideth forever, thy might, power the same; And all thy Word declares, thou art willing to heal the sick and lame."[19] In other words, because Jesus is the same as he was in the gospels, the entire Bible (or at least the New Testament) was evidence of present-day divine healing. The third verse said that Jesus' heart is full of compassion, and verse four declared Christ the "perfect physician." The 1893 songbook, *Echoes from Glory*, reprinted "O Lord, Thou Healest Me" and added E. E. Byrum's "I Am Healed." This hymn said that ministers could get "the precious gift of healing pow'r, thro the Spirit," and so it points toward the next section on "healing in the Great Commission." However, the chorus ("I am healed, I know I am, I'm healed this very hour, For my Jesus says I am, And I feel his mighty power") fits this section and is a good reminder of how the ideas often overlapped.[20]

The 1897 songbook illustrated nicely the importance of the overall theology of the Church of God movement. By publishing them in *Songs of the Evening Light,* the Gospel Trumpet Co. literally put the divine healing hymns in the context of the final dispensation. Further, three of the hymns about healing ("I've Touched the Hem of His Garment," "O Lord, Thou Healest Me," and "I Am Healed") were in the first person and placed testimonies to a personal experience of Jesus' healing power in the mouths of the congregants. One even inserted the singers into the gospel story itself with the chorus, "I've touched the hem of his garment, And now I too am free; His healing power this very hour, Gives life and health to me."[21] The other two healing hymns were third person explanations of Jesus' work. Number 79 made its point with its title, "He is Just the Same Today."[22] "Jesus Heals" announced in the first verse that he "heals the blind and lame, And his power is just the same, as when first to earth he came." The second verse reiterated the "just the same" theme and added that you will receive healing if you "ask in faith" (James 5:15). The third verse turned to an alternative to Hebrews 13:8, Jesus' promise from Matthew 28:20, "Lo, I'm with you to the end."[23]

Every time these hymns were sung or quoted, they reinforced the notion that healing came immediately from a personal relationship with Jesus. The strongest supporters of the "healing in the atonement" position were always quick to admit that Jesus does heal isolated individuals who pray the prayer of faith. Yet, this explanation of divine healing was not close enough to the center of the Church's mission to demand a response from adherents or ministers. Healings reflected positively on the movement as they functioned as further evidence of the return of the apostolic church. As D. S. Warner wrote, "the longer we walk in the light as God is in the light, the greater still those displays of power in us."[24] Nevertheless, it did not elevate divine healing above a benefit—a bonus—that might accompany holiness.

Divine Healing as Part of the Great Commission

The next step asserted that divine healing was an essential component of the work of the Church and the role of a minister. In other words, God *always* uses divine healing to attract people to the gospel, and therefore every minister must be able to exercise the gifts of healing. The latter was an important distinction that moved divine healing from a vague mark of the Church as a whole that might be observed at a camp meeting or read about in the *Trumpet* to a mark of the Church as a local reality. D. S. Warner wrote that healing was a "necessary part of the church" in 1883, but the idea that every minister should have the gifts of healing came around 1887.[25] E. E. Byrum clearly articulated this position in *Divine Healing of Soul and Body* (1892) when he wrote, "It is the privilege and duty of every minister of the Gospel to possess and exercise the gifts of healing because that comes with the commission."[26] Further evidence of the integration of divine healing into the mission of the Church is that the motto of the *Trumpet* changed in 1892. For the first time, the stated purpose of the periodical included "the publication of full salvation, and divine healing of the body."[27]

The key text was Mark 16:15–18, in which the risen Jesus told the eleven disciples

> Go ye into all the world and preach the gospel to every creature. He that be-lieveth and is baptized shall be saved; but he that believeth not shall be damned. And these signs shall follow them that believe; in my name shall they cast out devils; they shall speak with new tongues; They shall take up serpents; and if they drink any deadly thing, it shall not hurt them; they shall lay hands on the sick, and they shall recover.

Highlighting this passage proved problematic for the Church. At first, the content of the text was not a significant problem, but that changed by the turn of the century when people started to expand their religious practices beyond divine healing into speaking in tongues, taking up serpents, and drinking poison.[28] The initial problem was with the text itself, because it was widely thought to be spurious. Critics had declared it to be a later addition not present in the earliest manuscripts of the Bible.[29]

Historical critical arguments were not enough to convince advocates of divine healing.[30] E. E. Byrum in particular went to great lengths to demonstrate that Mark 16:15–18 harmonized with the rest of the Bible. To show internal consistency, Byrum quoted Matthew 28:12, 20 and Luke 9:6, both of which indicate that divine healing was part of the commission to the original apostles. Neither of these passages, however, said that Jesus intended divine healing to continue in the church beyond the time of the apostles. Matthew and Luke both say that Jesus sent the apostles out to heal the sick, but neither includes the time-less promise of Mark that the signs would follow "them that believe." Thus, Byrum showed that the commission to heal was not only for the apostles, but also for the seventy and for Paul. There is no reason, according to Byrum, to believe that the commission to heal changed after it had been given to Paul, and so Mark 16 is an accurate statement of Jesus' plan for his ministers.[31]

Evidently, this proof was not sufficient for Byrum, because in 1904—well after the "divine healing in the atonement" argument had made Mark 16 largely irrelevant to the promotion of divine healing in the Church of God—he traveled to Europe to examine in person the earliest manuscripts of the Bible. Supplied with influential letters of introduction and blessed with remarkable good luck, Byrum managed to examine the oldest New Testament manuscripts at the Bodleian Library in Oxford, the British Museum, the Bibliotheque Nationale in Paris, a library in Venice, and the Vatican Library. With the exception of one manuscript from the Vatican's collection, each one had Mark 16:15–18 perfectly intact. The Vatican's text had a blank space where the passage should have been, and it was the only such blank space in the entire manuscript. Byrum concluded that the scribe responsible for this copy knew of this passage but chose to omit it. The scribe's reasons were lost, but Byrum extrapolated from his own observations of religious organizations and suggested this explanation: "It may be the signs and wonders promised to the church had almost ceased at that time because of the unbelief of the apostate professors, and in order to free themselves they kept the truth hid from the people."[32]

The connection between the commission and divine healing meant that people could expect—and not just hope for—miraculous physical healing in the Church. A demonstration of the gifts of healing could increase a minister's personal authority, but the absence of successful healing could also jeopardize one's position in the Church. The perception of an increase or decrease in movement-wide healings was now a barometer of the Church's faithfulness to its mission. Moreover, since Jesus himself declared that divine healing belonged to "them that believe," the pressure on Church members to demonstrate their faith by abandoning medicine and trusting Jesus was very strong. William Schell, a prominent Church of God minister and proponent of divine healing in the commission, wrote that "trusting both the Lord and the physician" was the standard under the law of Moses. However, according to Schell, Jesus brought the "better testament" so that "the perfect standard of healing is established in the church." The implication was that only a fool or an unbeliever would reject the "better standard of healing."[33] E. E. Byrum was more direct: "The use of medicine is for two classes of persons, viz.: Those who are not acquainted with God, and those of his children who are afraid to trust him."[34]

Divine Healing in the Atonement

Placing the justification for emphasizing divine healing in the Great Commission made healing a servant of the gospel. It was a spiritual gift that functioned to advertise Christianity and instruct converts about God's benefits. Proponents of divine healing frequently emphasized it to such a degree that it was effectively *the* spiritual gift; however, that was not logically necessary. That Mark 16 mentioned several other signs was not lost on the holiness movement or the Church of God. A controversy known as the Advancement Heresy arose in the Church of God in 1895–1896. A minister heeded E. E. Byrum's and William Schell's call for an advancement (a "forward step") in spiritual gifts and declared that he had the gift of discernment which enabled him to determine which ministers were in and which were out of harmony with the movement. Byrum intervened with a stern warning in the *Trumpet*, but the danger of spiritual gifts was abundantly clear to the saints.[35] George Cole reported that this controversy squelched discussion of spiritual gifts in the Church for several years.[36]

The doctrine of divine healing in the atonement solved the problem of spiritual gifts by promoting healing from a servant of the gospel to the gospel itself. The Good News was that Jesus' death on the cross bore away sin *and* sickness, and therefore "we might as well subtract salvation from the atonement as to subtract healing from it."[37]

In essence, this argument asserted that sickness originally came from sin and Jesus' atonement took away sin and its effects.[38] The key texts were Matthew 8:17 and Isaiah 53:45. The Gospel of Matthew says that Jesus fulfilled that "which was spoken by Esaias the prophet, saying, Himself took our infirmities, and bare our sicknesses." By itself, this could mean that Jesus fulfilled the prophecy by taking away the sins of the world and by performing the miracles of healing told of in the four Gospels. However, Isaiah 53:4–5 filled in the details. It says, "Surely he [Jesus—according to Matthew] hath born our griefs, and carried our sorrows; yet we did esteem him stricken, smitten of God, and afflicted. But he was wounded for our transgressions, he was bruised for our iniquities: the chastisement of our peace was upon him; and with his stripes we are healed."

For the Church of God, two additional points of clarification completed the proof; however, the practical implications still required elaboration. The first point was that King James's translators made a mistake when they rendered "griefs" for "infirmities" and "sorrows" for "sicknesses" in Isaiah 53:4. Even the opponents of divine healing admitted as much, so this was not a serious problem. This passage motivated several Church of God ministers to support the Revised Version translation of the Bible.[39] The second point was that "bore our sicknesses" had to mean "took them away" and not "endured" or "suffered."[40] Arguing from the original language was not persuasive in this case, so J. W. Byers devised an alternative demonstration using 1 Peter 2:24, which says, "Who his own self bare our sins in his own body on the tree, that we, being dead to sin, should live unto righteousness: by whose stripes ye were healed." This would not have satisfied biblical scholars or even mainline Protestant ministers, but for Byers's audience it sufficed to show that sickness was "borne" as was sin, away on Christ's own body.[41]

The Church of God ministers had a theology of sanctification that allowed them to omit an intermediate step in the proof. Once they established that Jesus took away sickness just as he took away sin, then their demonstration of present-day, immediate physical healing was complete. A critique of the atonement theory of divine healing by Marvin R. Vincent, a Presbyterian who rejected holiness doctrines of entire sanctification, shows how important the Church's soteriology was for its doctrine of healing. According to Vincent, the whole idea of "healing in the atonement" was simply special pleading. He agreed that the final redemption was undeniably for the body; however, "a vast intermediate work of cleansing takes place between conversion and final sanctification of the *soul*, and therefore we are to infer a similar intermediate work for the *body*."[42] Church of God people, of course, rejected the "vast intermediate work of cleansing" in favor of entire sanctification.[43] The immediate healing of the body paralleled the immediate cleansing of the soul, and therefore Psalm 103:2–3 ("Bless the Lord, O my soul, and forget not all his benefits; Who forgiveth all thine iniquities, who healeth all thy diseases") could stand as an additional proof of divine healing in the atonement. The belief in the visible effects of sanctification prepared the Church for a doctrine that integrated physical healing into Christ's atoning sacrifice.

Church of God people recognized divine healing in the atonement as the most radical divine healing doctrine, and that was a positive assessment. It may be difficult for readers today to understand, but between 1895 and 1905 there were strong incentives in the Church to affirm the doctrine. The natural tendency of the Church of God movement was to "raise the standard" of anything it deemed a "Bible doctrine"—including healing—to its extreme.[44] Thus, "divine healing in the atonement" became a label and a standard of orthodoxy. Being able to affirm it meant being properly radical, trusting God, and rejecting humanly devised medical systems.[45]

The social pressure to affirm the—or better, *an*—atonement doctrine was an important factor in developing the doctrine itself. The doctrine did not stretch very far, and, at the very least, affirming it meant that one believed that sickness was somehow related to sin, that healing of the body was an essential aspect of the gospel, and that every faithful Christian could expect to receive divine healing. Several authors who were self-identified preachers of the atonement doctrine carefully avoided some of the most radical implications of this doctrine. This was especially true after 1900. The more common caveats were that sickness was only *indirectly* related to sin, and therefore illness in no way implied spiritual deficiency; that healing and salvation were both in the atonement, but salvation was primary and necessary, while healing was a secondary benefit; and that every Christian who prays for healing can expect *an answer* that may or may not include physical restoration.[46]

For every nuanced argument, however, there was one asserting that healing and salvation were in the atonement "to the same extent," that ministers had to both preach and exhibit divine healing, and that it was the duty of all afflicted Christians to get the faith necessary for healing.[47] The fact that several ministers worked hard to define an acceptable doctrine under this umbrella term rather than rejecting the atonement concept altogether is a good indication of how important divine healing was to the Church of God around the turn of the twentieth century.

Bible Problems for Divine Healing

Divine healing fit the Church of God perfectly—at least as a theory. The immediate experience of Jesus' healing power harmonized with the opposition to hierarchy and "man rule." The grace of healing confirmed the belief in the reemergence of the signs of the apostolic church. Gifts of healing attracted new converts and provided a symbol of authority for ministers who could not rely on ordination but had to show the "fruits of the spirit." The cleansing from the effects of sin was a parallel with entire sanctification. The fact that mainline denominations repudiated divine healing only served to confirm its importance for Church of God people. Thus, the doctrine and practice of divine healing were more securely integrated into the Church of God than a few proof texts from the Bible might indicate. However, the Bible was one of the best resources for establishing or contesting doctrine, and the biblical witness for the continuation of miraculous healing was less than ideal. Skeptics and critics found texts that seemed to undermine the whole idea of faith-based healing. Such critics did not write articles that the *Trumpet* published, but they did send questions to the editor. These same objections appeared year after year, and, for the most part, the editors gave the same answers. The texts fit in three broad categories: passages that recommended remedies, medicines, or anything other than faith for healing; texts that spoke well of physicians or indicated that medical care was part of God's plan for humanity; and texts that indicated that a prayer for healing could be a prayer against God's will. Proponents of divine healing had to explain away these Bible problems.

Medical Means

Several biblical texts described the use of something for healing other than a simple prayer of faith or the touch of a minister. These aids to healing were not necessarily medicines or remedies—although both of those were included in the debate—so the divine healing movement called them "medical means" or just "means" for short.[48] J. W. Byers labeled the cluster of texts the "Hezikiah's figs, the blind man's clay, and Timothy's wine" challenge, for the three most troublesome texts. These three stories and several others—including the passages that used the word "medicine," the account of the healing of Naaman, and the parable of the Good Samaritan—demanded at least passing attention for two reasons. First, divine healing doctrine rested on a few biblical verses about healing bolstered by the assertion that the entire biblical witness ("from Genesis to Revelation") supported divine healing. A few clear counterexamples could have brought down the entire construction. Therefore, defenders of the doctrine had to argue that—their literal meanings notwithstanding—these texts supported healing through faith not means. The second reason was that neither the divine healing movement nor the Church of God had a definition of "medicine" to guide its argument. Every example was a potential medicine, because no clear reason existed for the rejection of figs or wine or anything else. With these explanations, the working definitions of such ideas as "medicine," "hygiene," and "food" began to emerge. Within the period covered in this chapter, the Church of God was able to answer the challenges posed by these texts. However, even relatively straightforward biblical interpretation exposed the fact that the Church had to expand divine healing doctrine beyond the Bible.

Occasionally someone would assert that the Bible recognized medicine because the word "medicine" appeared in the English translation. This was an uncommon argument, probably because two of the four references (Jer. 30:13 and Jer. 46:11) clearly said that medicine was not useful. When the argument did arise, it was the easiest to answer because there were no questions of definition. The point was to determine what the Bible said about "medicine," whatever that was. Proverbs 17:22 said, "A merry heart doeth good like a medicine," and Ezekiel 46:12 said, "And the fruit thereof shall be for meat, and the leaf thereof for medicine." Divine healing proponents dismissed the verse from Proverbs as a poor translation. J. W. Byers noted that his Bible had a marginal note indicating that a more accurate rendering was "doeth good *to a medicine*, showing that a merry heart is better than a medicine."[49] Several years later, J. C. Blaney used the American Standard Version's translation ("A cheerful heart is a good medicine") to show that the point was that a merry heart is good for health. "The assumption of usefulness of medicine is not part of the Bible."[50] Biblical interpretation explained the passage from Ezekiel. As can be seen from a parallel with Revelation 22:2, it was about the tree of life and could not possibly be mistaken for a "material remedy" such as an herb.[51] Further, because the leaves of the tree of life in Revelation refer to Jesus Christ, "this scripture is about the Christ *as the means of healing*."[52] Thus, all the "medicine texts" properly understood denounced medicine. The one from Ezekiel even pointed to divine healing in the atonement.

The parable of the Good Samaritan (Luke 10:30–37) was slightly more problematic. In the story, the Samaritan found the battered man and "bound up his wounds, pouring in oil and wine" (Luke 10:34). Jesus concluded the story by telling his audience to "go, and do thou likewise." Some critics of divine healing interpreted this as a command to not only "show mercy" but to give medical attention. An example from the *Bible Expositor* said with regard to this parable, "Had a Mormon, Doweite, or a Saint (?) of the 'Gospel Trumpet' clique been there they would have objected to medicine and said, 'We will pray over him.' Some of them would have wanted to lay on their saintly (?) hands and pray. But Jesus Christ endorsed the use of medicine."[53]

As one would expect, the advocates of divine healing rejected this interpretation. Moderates, such as William Boardman, granted that the Samaritan gave the injured man "medicine" but denied that the point of the story was to promote medicine.[54] Boardman insisted that the parable was only incidentally about medicine. The most one could reasonably say was that "whenever, as in this case, [giving medicine] is the best thing one can do, it is both right and lovely." Divine healing was much better if it was an option. Further, Boardman noted that it simply would not have made sense in the story for a Samaritan to have the gifts of healing.[55] Church of God authors were more concerned about medicine than Boardman was and were not willing to concede that the wine and the oil were medicinal. According to Byrum, "the Samaritan bound up the wounds of the unfortunate man and made him as comfortable as possible, but gave him no drugs nor poisonous medicines to take."[56]

Byrum's use of the word "poisonous" indicated that he believed that medicine had verifiable physiological effects. The application of wine and oil was perfectly acceptable because they were benign substances. They did not really *do* anything other than make the injured man more comfortable. This raises the question, how does one's belief about medical means affect divine healing? Moreover, how should the historical development of science and medicine relate to biblical interpretation? How would it change the story if oil was "well-nigh the universal remedy in the medical practice of the day"?[57] What does the parable say about divine healing if the Samaritan and the injured man thought the treatment was the height of medical care? Do the standards of acceptable behavior for the saints (the definition of "medicine") change with advances in science?

To my knowledge, no one in the divine healing movement or the Church of God directly addressed these questions. It would be surprising to find that kind of historical sense in a primitivist movement. They did attempt to refute the specific charge that oil had medicinal or curative power, but not that the Samaritan *thought* that it did.[58] No well-formulated definition of medicine existed in the literature of the Church of God. However, the explanations of the remaining texts showed that—explicitly stated or not—faith for divine healing was related to the belief in the efficacy of medicine.

Three of the four remaining examples of "medicine" in the Bible were stories.[59] In the first, Naaman had leprosy and consulted Elisha, the prophet of the Lord, who told him to wash seven times in the Jordan. Naaman was angry because he had expected a spectacular cure from Elisha; however, he followed the instructions and was made clean (2 Kings 5:1–14). The second story was about Hezekiah who was "sick unto death" when he prayed to the Lord for healing. God sent Isaiah to him to report that God would answer his prayers on the third day. Then Isaiah told Hezekiah to lay a lump of figs on his boil. He did and recovered (2 Kings 20:1–7). The final story was of Jesus' healing of the man born blind. Jesus "spat on the ground, and made clay of the spittle, and he anointed

the eyes of the blind man with the clay." After the man washed off the mud, he
was able to see (John 9:6–7).[60]

A variety of responses to these stories existed in the Church of God. J. W.
Byers, for instance, admitted that the Old Testament examples appeared to recommend medical means, but he claimed they were irrelevant because they had
"nothing to do with the New Testament means of healing."[61] As for the clay
Jesus used, Sarah Smith wrote that it too was an instrument of healing. This led
her to ask if *Jesus* still uses clay to heal. Indeed he does, she concluded. Just as
Jesus purified the clay of the ground to open the eyes of the blind, he now "puri-
fies clay [by which she meant human beings] with his own precious blood, and
the regeneration of the spirit and the renewing of the Holy Ghost; and we must
be partakers of His flesh and blood."[62] These two examples show how the belief
that Jesus brought a better standard of healing explained these stories, even if
they did show the use of medical means.

The most common and most interesting explanation, however, denied that
water, figs, and mud were medicinal. Instead, these stories told of how men rejected the medical knowledge of their time and obediently and faithfully submitted to God's command. Internal evidence—especially Naaman's doubts about
the efficacy of the river Jordan—supported this interpretation.[63] J. W. Byers
wrote of the Hezekiah story, "it is very evident that the figs did not heal him; but
God said, 'I will heal thee.'"[64] It is also evident that none of the advocates of
divine healing seriously considered water, figs, or mud to be possible medicines.
Byrum said that no physician prescribed the figs for Hezekiah, and, without the
prayer, "they might have put on the figs by the wholesale" and he still would
have died.[65] The introduction of physicians into the debate suggests the association of "medicine" with the medical profession. However, the absence of a prescription was not the only reason Byrum discounted the figs; nor did the story
itself say that the figs had no curative powers. Rather, he simply did not believe—no matter what the Bible said—that a bunch of figs would heal a boil.[66]
Similarly, Byers wrote, "No one has heard of born blindness being healed by the
use of clay as medicine since then, or even before. It is evident that the spittle
and clay were used as a requirement of submission and obedience from the blind
man."[67]

There is no denying that these stories asserted that God is the ultimate
source of healing. One could easily deduce, however, that they show that God
works through means, and that God's power and the created means are so inter-
mingled that sorting them out is beyond human comprehension.[68] That was not
how proponents of divine healing read them. They were committed to a division
between healing through faith and healing through medicine. Faith could—and,
for the sake of clarity, it should—work on its own. Medicine too had physiological effects on human beings, effects that were independent of belief. These
stories were about things that did not qualify as medicine because they would
fail any scientific test. Therefore, looking at these stories through an interpretive

lens colored with the divine healing doctrine showed that these "means" were a test of faith. Naaman, Hezekiah, and the blind man could not reasonably have believed that the means were going to cure them. God demanded that they submit to a "treatment" that contradicted the medical knowledge of the day. The lesson for contemporary believers was just the same: reject medicine and trust God for healing. In the Bible, God presented various tests of obedience, but now one only had to follow the requirements of James 5:14–15.[69]

The final text was the most difficult to explain, Paul's advice to Timothy to "Take no longer water, but use a little wine for thy stomach's sake and thine oft infirmities" (1 Tim. 5:23). Paul and Timothy were undeniably faithful Christians, so no one could argue that Paul was counseling a remedy Timothy could use until he had enough faith for healing. It was advice given after Pentecost, so no dispensational argument explained it away. The verse said that Paul—not God—intended the wine as a remedy, and there was no reason to think it was a test of Timothy's obedience. Everyone knew of the physiological effects of fermented wine, and unfermented grape juice was a plausible remedy.[70] Thus, this passage was the most serious biblical challenge for the radical anti-medicine divine healing position.[71] It appeared in questions to the editor more frequently than any other passage, probably because the explanation for it was the least convincing.

The prevailing explanation was that grape juice was *food*, not medicine.[72] Before he decided that Paul's advice to Timothy was "scriptural support of the use of natural remedies for the body," D. S. Warner wrote two articles about the classification of grape juice. The New Testament, according to Warner, never counseled the use of medicine, but it recommended "temperance and a healthful use of diet, even the special adaptation of food and drink to our particular physical condition, even the use of a 'little wine,'—pure unfermented grape juice—in case of physical infirmities."[73] It is anyone's guess what that distinction would have meant in practice. When pushed for a further definition by a man who insisted that the use of "any means for the restoration of the body from affliction, save faith and prayer to God" was faithless, Warner decided there was no functional difference between a food with healing properties and a remedy.[74]

Warner's article appeared in the *Trumpet* in 1895. The next *Trumpet* article to identify Timothy's wine as a remedy was J. D. Ferrill's 1912 article about "fanaticism" in dress, healing, and behavior.[75] In between were numerous tortured arguments intended to show that Paul's advice was for health but not for healing. The wine was good food, not good medicine. Byrum noted that Paul "was not a physician, neither did he go about practicing medicine," and therefore he gave Timothy "some instructions from the standpoint of health, and not from a medical standpoint."[76]

This sounds like the assertion, "Paul did not doctor because he was not a doctor." That was part of the argument but not the main point. The operative distinction was between healthful living and medicinal healing, and the key was the condition of the water in Palestine. Timothy lived where the water was full of alkali, and was nothing less than a mild poison.[77] Therefore, Paul was not telling Timothy to drink wine for its healing properties. Timothy had to stop ruining his health with the limewater, and drinking grape juice would remove the cause of his infirmity. Just as one had to abandon alcohol, tobacco, coffee, and tea before claiming divine healing, Timothy had to stop drinking the local water.[78] The message of Paul's advice for members of the Church of God was that eating good food "for the maintenance of health is justifiable and to be commended." However, in the case of illness, one must not "resort to medicine beyond ordinary hygienic principles" but should call the elders for prayer and anointing.[79]

Physicians

In the Church of God, practicing medicine was tantamount to being an unrepentant sinner. D. S. Warner was the most charitable commentator in that he allowed that doctoring could bring relief to those who were without faith. However, the saints did not need medicine, and the profession was full of ungodliness. Warner advised "saved physicians to aspire to a calling more free from the appearance of evil."[80] Fred Hahn also granted the outside possibility of a good doctor other than the Great Physician, but he focused on the sins, saying that physicians "as a class, are godless men, probably on account of the tendency of their profession to make them materialists, and with their female patients too often lustful."[81] No true saint could abide the appearance of evil, so this effectively excluded practicing physicians from the Church.

Warner and Hahn wrote their articles before the Church established a reputation for divine healing. Stronger denunciations of physicians came from Church of God writers who had first-hand experience competing with and debating doctors. J. W. Byers had a divine healing home in Oakland and espoused the atonement doctrine. He believed that the growing cultural authority of orthodox physicians threatened the Church's ability to preach divine healing. Where Warner and Hahn thought that physicians primarily harmed themselves—doctoring excluded them from salvation just as did smoking and drinking—Byers thought physicians interfered with the Church:

> The M.D.'s have set up images of drugs and medicine and made decrees that all must bow down before them, but ... [let us] declare that we will not serve their medicine gods, nor worship the images they have set up.[82]

George Cole's position in Chicago was similar to Byers's in Oakland, but he claimed that medical doctors were actually satanic influences. Cole was an advocate of the atonement doctrine of healing and was the superintendent of the Chicago healing home; he claimed that he had met with "blasphemy and threats of vengeance from the hand of the law by the venders of the medical system." From this conflict, he discovered that "with the practice of medicine there is an infernal spirit of devils accompanying that system that foams and writhes, carrying those affected thereby to wish vengeance wreaked upon the saints of God."[83] A third Church of God minister, L H. Morgan, held an M.D. from the Battle Creek Sanitarium and was a successful physician and an Inspector for the Illinois Board of Health before he experienced divine healing and became a Church of God minister.[84] He brought an insider's view of medical practice and the zeal of a convert to show that the Hippocratic oath demanded obedience to "Apollo—the devil—Satan."[85]

All but one of the biblical passages about physicians harmonized with the belief that medical practice and a saintly life were mutually exclusive, either because doctoring was no longer necessary or because it was harmful.[86] The one problem was that Paul called Luke "the beloved physician" (Col. 4:14). Church members believed Luke to be the author of the Gospel according to Luke and the book of Acts, a friend and colleague of Paul, and one of the seventy commissioned by Jesus to preach the gospel and heal the sick.[87] If he practiced medicine as part of his ministry, then the whole opposition to medicine was untenable.

The passage from Colossians is the only statement in the Bible indicating that Luke was a physician, and it does not say if Luke was working as a physician or just keeping the title. The question for the divine healing debate, therefore, was "Did Luke ever practice medicine after he began to preach?"[88] Opponents and advocates of the use of medicine both looked to the Bible for clues about Luke's ministry. Specifically, they examined the two books attributed to Luke himself to see if he described healing as a minister or as a physician would.

The strongest opponents of divine healing placed a lot of faith in this one passage. In it they found the key to proving that Luke not only continued to practice medicine, but was also Paul's personal physician. Marvin Vincent and Daniel Steele said that an accurate translation of Colossians 4:14 said "my" and not "the" beloved physician. Vincent said that no one could read Second Corinthians and deny that Paul was a sick man, and thus "Luke was not only his friend but his physician."[89] Steele insisted on calling Luke "Dr. Luke," and he produced an involved "inference from Holy Scripture" showing that Luke gave medical attention to Paul. In brief, Paul first preached in Galatia because an "infirmity of the flesh" prevented him from traveling (Gal. 4:13). Then, from the change of pronoun from "they" to "we" in Acts 16:7–10, Steele concluded that Luke—the author of Acts—joined Paul in Galatia. Why would Paul have sent for Luke? Steele said it was because Paul "was in need of [Luke's] professional services."[90] Thus, men like Vincent and Steele who were searching for a biblical justification for the use of medicine created a medical career for Luke from meager evidence.

William Boardman wrote the moderate, pro-divine healing interpretation of Luke the beloved physician. Boardman's belief that divine healing and medical care could peacefully coexist put him in the enviable position of not having to prove or deny that Luke practiced medicine. He took Paul's words literally (*"the* beloved physician"*) and assumed that Luke never repudiated his training or his profession. God's calling of Luke showed "that a physician may be a very good man" and "that the Lord has nothing against physicians, as such."[91] No one should despise doctors or condemn those who rely on medicine for healing. However, Boardman's commitment to divine healing colored his interpretation of Luke's ministry. The overarching message, he said, was that a physician had recognized that divine healing was superior to medical care. Luke wrote two books, "and the feature of healing, not by medical skill, but by the power of God through faith, is a great one in both." Thus, Luke embodied the truth that medical healing was good and divine healing was incomparably better.[92]

The most radical proponents of divine healing denied that Luke practiced medicine—or even thought of himself as a "physician"—after his conversion. All the Church of God writers who published an opinion about Luke's medical career were in the radical camp. Notable non-Church of God radicals were R. Kelso Carter, A. B. Simpson, J. A. Dowie, and Carrie Judd Montgomery. Simpson, for example, took Boardman's argument about Luke's authorship of the Gospel of Luke and Acts one step further: "if God had wanted to guard us against the fanaticism of Divine Healing, how easy it would have been for him to record a single instance in which the early believers sent for Luke." The silence about medicine from a physician proved that Luke left doctoring behind forever.[93]

In response to those who asserted that Luke was Paul's physician, this group simply said that the Bible said *"the* beloved physician," not *"my* beloved physician."[94] In contrast to their work with Isaiah 53, the King James translators got this word correct. Paul was not suggesting that Luke had doctored him. Further, "the beloved physician" implied—as did "the Great Physician"—that there was only one such physician. Instead of commending the medical doctors, it was a condemnation. As with "The Good Samaritan," the adjective did not normally fit the noun. In this interpretation, Luke was no more a physician after he began to preach than Matthew was a publican or Simon was a Zealot.[95]

Merely denying that Luke was Paul's physician appears to have sufficed as a response to Vincent's or Steele's proof that Luke practiced medicine. No longer responses to Paul's statement appeared in the literature. The saints did produce a biblical proof that Luke did not use medicine when he had the chance. The standard argument was as follows: In Acts 20:9, Eutychus fell to his death from a window because Paul's preaching lulled him to sleep. Verses 6 and 7 proved that Luke was at the meeting, but verse 10 said that only Paul went down to heal Eutychus through prayer. Thus, after Paul had called Luke "the beloved physician" (or even "my beloved physician"), Luke and Paul both recognized that Paul's prayers had more healing power than Luke's medicine.[96] According to Byrum, Luke was not anyone's physician after his conversion; "he did not carry his apothecary's shop with him, nor practice medicine while on his evangelistic tours." He left his medical career behind with all other sinful behavior.[97]

"Why Some are Not Healed"

The question that underlay all of the wrangling over biblical texts was why some people who appear to have met all the conditions of holiness are not healed. One possible answer was that a belief in modern divine healing was simply a mistake. As Marvin Vincent said, "An economy of miracle was for the Church's infancy. The Church which is hungry for miracles is in her second childhood."[98] Mature Christians should have understood that God wanted them to use medicine and follow the advice of physicians. The sections above have discussed how the ministers of the Church of God refuted—or at least rejected—that argument. They believed that the Bible precluded the use of medicines. Further, the evening light was a rebirth, not a second childhood. The second explanation for the absence of healing was that, in the vast majority of cases, the afflicted only *appeared* to have met the conditions for healing. Church of God proponents of divine healing favored this explanation. To maintain it, however, they had to refute the third option, that divine purposes are inscrutable to human beings. God heals whom God wishes to heal, but physical infirmity may very well be necessary for God's purposes. This did not challenge the possibility of divine healing, nor did it recommend medicine.[99] It did break the link between divine healing and holiness. If healing—or at least an explanation of God's refusal to heal—did not reliably follow from fulfilling a set of conditions, then divine healing could not stand at the center of the Church's ministry.

Several biblical stories showed that God either imposed sickness on a person or refused to grant healing. The simplest cases for advocates of divine healing were those in which God used physical suffering as a reproof of sinful behavior. Miriam, for instance, contracted leprosy because she complained about Moses' marriage (Num. 12).[100] David's infant son died because David had an affair with Bathsheba and killed Uriah (2 Sam. 12:1–24). These and other passages like them implied that physical infirmity could come directly from God; however, they in no way challenged the divine healing doctrines. Holiness had to precede healing. Miriam and David did not meet the basic requirements for the "prayer of faith." Further, Miriam and David both understood exactly why they were suffering. These examples showed that God sent a clear message when using illness for punishment or discipline. Thus, no one should use these texts to avoid praying for healing or meeting the conditions of holiness. An afflicted person should pray the prayer of faith expecting either healing or an explanation of God's refusal to grant the request.

The story of Job was slightly more problematic because Job was a righteous man (Job 1:1). The afflictions were a test of Job's faithfulness imposed by Satan and permitted by God. This story showed that sickness did not automatically imply sin. Job was not punished for anything—not his own sin or anyone else's. Sickness could simply be a temptation from Satan. Granting that, however, changed divine healing very little. It was an important, though seldom heeded, warning to the congregation against rushing to judgment based on the presence of illness. The useful models for the saints were Job's three friends who thought Job must have offended God somehow. As for the afflicted person, however, Job's story did not significantly change the prescribed reaction to illness. If sickness came as a temptation from Satan, that did not suggest that God wanted the person to accept it. Following Job's example, he or she was expected to be faithful to God, trusting that—as with Job—passing the test of faithfulness would bring perfect healing.

The most difficult biblical challenges for divine healing were two post-resurrection texts in which God did not grant healing. In 2 Timothy 4:20, Paul reported having to leave Trophimus behind due to illness. Further, and most important, Paul himself suffered from something he described as a "thorn in the flesh, the messenger of Satan to buffet me, lest I should be exalted above measure" (2 Cor. 12:7). Three times Paul asked God to remove the thorn, but God said, "My grace is sufficient for thee: for my strength is made perfect in weakness" (2 Cor. 12:8–9). According to critics of divine healing, these passages showed that God refused to heal Paul and his closest associates.[101] Therefore, those who advocated divine healing were claiming to "know the mind of the Lord" and saying that God promised healing even when faced with the biblical evidence that God's purpose could be "better served by infirmity, as it was with Paul's thorn."[102] Daniel Steele said that these texts proved that there is no way to know if God intended to heal or not. Ministers had to teach the sick to pray to God for healing with the phrase "if it be thy will."[103]

E. E. Byrum was particularly offended by the "if it be thy will" prayer. He thought it showed an inherent lack of faith in God's promises and was itself responsible for many failed healings.[104] The saints did know the mind of God regarding healing, because of God's self-revelation in the Bible. Nothing could be clearer, according to Byrum, than God's willingness to heal those who pray in faith "doubting nothing." Jesus' mission was as much to heal the body as to save the soul.[105] The fact that some were not healed had nothing to do with God's will; the Bible very plainly said that "any" might be healed if they "lived up to the promises." Byrum admitted that God occasionally delayed healing as a lesson, but delays usually resulted from a lack of faith or the presence of an obstacle to healing.[106] Thus, a person could be sick for a long time without sinning, but "unless God has some special motive, a long affliction does not live up to the privilege."[107] The delay was finite as well, for God promised healing in this lifetime. Just as no one should die without entire sanctification, no one should die without healing. The Bible said, "it is appointed unto men once to die"; and therefore immortality was out of the question. However, no one should die of disease. According to the divine healing literature of the Church of God, God's willingness to heal was transparent in the scriptures. God might not heal at the very moment of the prayer, but there could be no doubt that God would eventually heal everyone who met the conditions of holiness. The vast majority of people who believed that their afflictions stemmed from God's special purpose for their lives were simply using the "if it be thy will" prayer as an excuse for their lack of faith.[108]

Advocates of divine healing had to explain why the examples of Paul and Trophimus did not challenge the doctrine. There were three possibilities. First, the infirmities could have come from sin. That was out of the question with Paul, but Carter said, "it is perfectly possible that Trophimus made a mistake, or that he did not absolutely follow the leading of the Holy Ghost."[109] Casting aspersions on one of Paul's chosen evangelists was a difficult position to take, and the Church of God did not adopt it. Second, these texts could be irrelevant because they were not about sickness or because the conditions were temporary. The Bible said Trophimus was "sick," so that argument did not work. However, it never said that Trophimus *was not* healed. According to William Boardman, we likely would have heard of Trophimus's healing if Paul had lived to write a third letter to Timothy or a second letter to the Ephesians.[110] In contrast, God told Paul that the thorn in his flesh was a permanent condition; however, no one knew for sure what it was. There were several attempts to prove that Paul did not have a disease.[111] The third and most important option was to assert that these were very special cases of God's direct intervention for the spread of the gospel, and therefore they did not apply to the average saint. Trophimus's sickness had the special purpose of preventing him from accompanying Paul to his martyrdom in Rome. No doubt, said the common explanation, God had further work for Trophimus and used sickness to save him from "the trap Satan [had] set for him, the clutches of the terrible Nero."[112] Paul's thorn in the flesh, whatever it was, kept Paul humble and demonstrated that God could bring power out of weakness. None of the other apostles had such a thorn. Equating Paul's experience with modern sickness did not work, because "none of us has ever had an abundance of revelations to the extent that Paul had, so that we should require a 'thorn in the flesh' like his."[113]

Thus, the Church of God had completely reversed the assumptions of the opponents of divine healing who believed that the miraculous healings in the Bible were unusual and performed for a specific purpose in the promotion of Christianity. For the Church of God, divine healing was God's normal activity. The Bible so clearly revealed God's willingness to heal that the average member of the Church should *expect* divine healing. The aberration in God's activity was not healing, but the refusal to heal. Paul and Trophimus were examples of a special revelation. Therefore, members of the Church of God who suffered afflictions and were not confident that God was using that affliction for a very specific reason needed to examine their lives and their spiritual conditions. According to the tract *Why Some are Not Healed*, a failed prayer usually "indicates that you have not done your best."[114]

Conclusion

In 1905, the *Gospel Trumpet* published an article by George Cole, the superintendent of the Church of God's missionary and healing home in Chicago, that purported to tell the "History of Divine Healing Among Us."[115] The article had so few details that it would have been of little use to anyone who did not already know the Church's history. Cole's intent was to show that the Church's doctrine of divine healing had grown closer and closer to the will of God, and that, as of 1905, "divine healing in the atonement is here to stay." In a sense Cole was correct; it is still possible to find members of the Church of God who claim that Jesus' atonement for sin and sickness made divine healing possible. However, that belief bears little resemblance to what Cole intended by "healing in the atonement." He meant the conglomeration of beliefs about healing covered in this chapter. For Cole, Byrum, and the other Church of God ministers who focused on divine healing, healing was a sign of personal holiness, ministerial authority, and the return of the True Church. As we have seen, divine healing was an essential aspect of the gospel, and every minister had to preach and demonstrate healing. Every faithful Christian had to have faith for healing and rely on it exclusively. Using medicine showed a lack of faith, and practicing medicine was sinful. Protracted illness was not in and of itself proof of sin, but it certainly raised suspicions among the saints. Further, the Bible so clearly stated God's will to heal, that those who were not immediately healed needed to examine themselves closely for a lack of faith or unholy behavior that created an obstacle for healing.

This precarious doctrinal construction began to crumble before Cole's ink was dry. Chapter six will show the challenges that came from, among other things, failed prayers for the healing of children and beloved ministers, lawsuits against parents who refused to give their children medicine, the smallpox epidemic, and mandatory inoculations for schoolchildren. Before turning to these direct challenges, however, chapter five will explore how the connection between holy behavior and health introduced preventive medicine into the Church of God.

Notes

1. Byrum, *Divine Healing of Soul and Body*, 49–50. The Gospel Trumpet Co. also published this chapter as a tract titled *The Doctrine of Divine Healing*.

2. R. Kelso Carter was an important leader in the divine healing movement. Carter experienced entire sanctification and divine healing in 1879 and left the Presbyterian Church for the Methodist Episcopal Church. He wrote, "Individual cases of healing, or phenomena, are absolutely worthless as to the question before us. All the cases in the world have nothing whatever to do directly with the doctrine of Divine Healing, for the very simple reason that they are not and never have been made the basis or ground of that doctrine. The only foundation is the Word of God, and hence the examination of cases per se has no direct bearing upon the subject" ("Divine Healing, or 'Faith Cure,'" 777). For information about Carter, see "Carter, R(ussell) Kelso" in Kostlevy, ed., *Historical Dictionary of the Holiness Movement.*

3. Tracing the origin of doctrines in the Church of God beyond the movement itself is very difficult. The belief described here made all truth the common property of all Christians, and therefore attribution of sources was unnecessary. Because writers in the Church did not want to expose readers to the errors of sect Babylon, they avoided mentioning non-Church of God sources. Finally, the problem was aggravated because they did have a sense that word-for-word copying was plagiarism, and therefore they restated things in their own words. Several direct connections between members of the Church of God and the wider divine healing movement do exist in the literature, and the parallels in the teachings are too close to attribute to anything other than mutual influence.

4. Advertisement, "Wall Roll and Divine Healing Calendar" *GT* 18:8 (Feb. 24, 1898): 7. The calendar was 13 x 20 inches, and continuing subscribers could purchase one for 50 cents.

5. George E. Berg, "Thoughts on Divine Healing," *GT* 21:49 (Dec. 11, 1901): 8.

6. See the first page of Marvin R. Vincent, "Modern Miracles," *Presbyterian Review* 4, no. 15 (July 1883): 473–502. See also Benjamin B. Warfield, *Miracles: Yesterday and Today: True and False* (New York: Scribner's, 1918; reprint Grand Rapids, Mich.: Eerdmans, 1965), 173. (The title of the original publication was *Counterfeit Miracles.* The page refers to the reprint edition.)

7. *Two Hundred Genuine Instances of Divine Healing,* 296–97.

8. I say "roughly" chronological because the arguments all co-existed. Examples of "divine healing in the atonement" appeared in the *Trumpet* as early as 1883, and "divine healing as a gift to the faithful" continued to appear throughout the period covered in this study. However, each of the arguments was largely eclipsed by its successors.

9. Charles Cullis was an Episcopalian and a homeopathic physician. He experienced entire sanctification in 1862 and established a home for consumptives in Boston. Through his healing homes, his Faith Training College, and his publishing efforts (the periodical *Times of Refreshing* and the Willard Tract Repository), Cullis became the central figure in the mid-nineteenth-century divine healing movement in America. See "Cullis, Charles" in Kostlevy, ed., *Biographical Dictionary of the Holiness Movement.* For a biography of Cullis by one of his most influential students, see William E. Boardman, *Faith-Work; or the Labours of Dr. Cullis, in Boston* (London: Daldy Ibister, 1875). On the specific issue of Cullis's reliance on the passage from James, see Paul Chappell, "The Divine Healing Movement in America," 138; and Donald Dayton, *Theological Roots of Pentecostalism,* 123.

10. B. B. Warfield, *Miracles,* 169.

11. For Warner, see D. S. Warner, "Question," *GT* 15:42 (Oct. 24, 1895): 2, and the discussions in chapters three and five of this book. The quote about Cullis is from Chappell, "The Divine Healing Movement in America," 282.

12. George Cole, "The History of Divine Healing Among Us," *GT* 25:28 (July 20, 1905): 8.

13. J. W. Byers, *Grace of Healing*, 222; E. E. Byrum, "Faith and Prayer," *GT* 15:1 (Jan. 3, 1895): 2–3. At the national camp meeting in 1913, E. E. Byrum said that the modern version of James apparently read, "Is any sick among you, let him send for the best doctor in town, and let him give medicine until he gets well or dies" (*Camp-Meeting Sermons* [Anderson, Ind.: Gospel Trumpet Co., 1913], 472). In a related case, a woman wrote to the *Trumpet* about her experience with Christian Science. She said "God does not say, If there is any sick among you let him call for a Christian Science mind-healer, and let him argue against the disease" (Frances Palmer, "Christian Science," *GT* 18:17 [April 28, 1898]: 3).

14. R. L. Farquar, "The Doctrine of Healing," *GT* 17:19 (May 13, 1897): 4.

15. Mrs. Edward Mix, "Faith in God," *Triumphs of Faith* (June, 1881): 84. Quoted in Paul Chappell, "Divine Healing Movement in America," 96. Chappell mistakenly identified Sarah Mix as "Elizabeth." For this error and several others in Chappell's dissertation, see Baer, "Perfectly Empowered Bodies," 40, n. 55.

16. See, for example, John Alexander Dowie, "God's Way of Healing," *Leaves of Healing* 1:1 new series (Aug. 31, 1894): 7. Dowie preached "divine healing in the atonement," but he also used Hebrews 13:8 extensively. In this particular article, he asserted, "Because He is unchangeable, and because He is present, in spirit, just as when in the flesh, He is the healer of His people." For more about Dowie, see Grant Wacker, "Marching to Zion: Religion in a Modern Utopian Community," *Church History* 54 (1985): 496–511; and E. L. Blumhofer, "Dowie, John Alexander" in Burgess and McGee, eds., *Dictionary of Pentecostal and Charismatic Movements*.

17. See Merle Strege, "Apocalyptic Identity," chapter five of *I Saw the Church*.

18. J. W. Byers, *Grace of Healing,* 43. The "Son of Righteousness with healing in his wings" refers to Mal. 4:2.

19. D. S. Warner/B. E. Warren, "O Lord, Thou Healest Me," no. 72 in *Anthems from the Throne*, 2d ed., ed. D. S. Warner and B. E. Warren (Grand Junction, Mich.: Gospel Trumpet Co., 1888).

20. E. E. Byrum/B. E. Warren, "I Am Healed," no. 170 in *Echoes From Glory; for the Sunday-School and for Prayer, Praise, and Gospel Meetings with Primary Instruction in Music,* ed. B. E. Warren and D. S. Warner (Grand Junction, Mich.: Gospel Trumpet Co., 1893).

21. "I've Touched the Hem of His Garment," no. 125 in *Songs of the Evening Light; for Sunday-Schools, Missionary and Revival Meetings, and Gospel Work in General,* ed. B. E. Warren and A. L. Byers (Moundsville, W.Va.: Gospel Trumpet Co., 1897). The reference is to Matthew 14:36. ("And [they] besought [Jesus] that they might only touch the hem of his garment; and as many as touched were made perfectly whole.") See also Matt. 9:20–26; Mark 5:25–36; and Luke 8:43–48 for the story of the woman who touched Jesus' clothes and was healed.

22. J. W. Byers/A. L. Byers, "He is Just the Same Today." This song is number 442 in *Worship the Lord: Hymnal of the Church of God* (Anderson, Ind.: Warner Press, 1989).

23. J. E. Roberts, "Jesus Heals," no. 62 in *Songs of the Evening Light.* In the King James Version, the wording was "Lo. I am with you always, even unto the end of the world." It frequently served to bolster Hebrews 13:8 or to add a bit of variety. The passage from Matthew had the advantage of being from Jesus himself, but Hebrews does a

better job of making the point that Jesus not only remains with his church but remains without change.

24. D. S. Warner, "Healing in Christ," *GT* 6:1 (Oct. 1, 1883): 2. See also D. S. Warner, "Anointing for Healing," *GT* 10:6 (June 1, 1888): 1, in which Warner said that the "gifts were meant to stay in the church, but Babylon has left His Church. They return when people come out of sects."

25. See chapter three for a discussion of E. E. Byrum's changes to the doctrine of divine healing. For evidence of Warner seeking the gifts of healing, see D. S. Warner, "Power of God Sent by Mail," *GT* 8:18 (Dec. 1, 1886).

26. E. E. Byrum, *Divine Healing of Soul and Body*, 102. For the authority-granting function of divine healing, see Jonathan R. Baer, "Redeemed Bodies: The Functions of Divine Healing in Incipient Pentecostalism," *Church History* 70, no. 4 (2001): 735–71.

27. The old motto said, "DEFINITE, RADICAL, ANTI-SECTARIAN. Sent Forth in the name of the Lord Jesus Christ. For the Purity and Unity of His Church, the Defence of ALL His Truth, And the Destruction of Sect Babylon." The new motto was: "DEFINITE, RADICAL, ANTI-SECTARIAN. Sent forth in the name of the Lord Jesus Christ. For the Publication of full Salvation, and Divine healing of the body. The Unity of all true Christians in "the faith once delivered to the saints." It first appeared in the Jan. 7, 1892 issue and remained substantially unchanged until Nov. 4, 1915.

28. D. S. Warner (unsigned editorial), "A Snaky Religion," *GT* 12:58 (Dec. 29, 1892): 1; J. W. Byers, "The Gift of Tongues," *GT* 18:25 (June 23, 1898): 1–2; James S. M'Creary, "The Baptism of Fire," *GT* 18:6 (Feb. 10, 1898); Thomas Carter, "The Fire-baptized Holiness Association of America," *GT* 20:11 (March 15, 1900): 3; G. W. Carey, "Wild-fire Demonstration," *GT* 20:42 (Oct. 25, 1900); Jennie C. Rutty, "The Gifts of Tongues," *GT* 22:28 (Sept. 18, 1902): 3; J. E. Forrest, "The Health of the Body," *GT* 25:23 (June 15, 1905): 8; E. E. Byrum, "A Craze for Tongues," *GT* 27:3 (Jan. 17, 1907): 8–9.

29. See B. B. Warfield, *Miracles*, 167–69.

30. A. J. Gordon's revised edition of *The Ministry of Healing* included a brief appendix about this passage (245–46). Gordon concluded that the doubts were so ill-founded that "it was hardly worth while to disturb the reader's mind with them" (245). Gordon referred the interested reader to "the fresh and able Commentary of Morrison." J. W. Byers quoted a large section of this appendix in *Grace of Healing* (164–65).

31. See E. E. Byrum, *Secret of Salvation*, 298–303. A brief synopsis of this argument is as follows. Acts 5:12–16 shows that the apostles did in fact heal the sick in fulfillment of the commission. In Luke 10:1–20, Jesus sent out seventy others and told them to heal the sick. This they did. Finally, Paul, who became a follower of Jesus only after the crucifixion, healed the crippled man at Lystra (Acts 14:8). See also E. E. Byrum, *The Great Physician* (Moundsville, W.Va.: Gospel Trumpet Co., 1899), 17–30.

32. E. E. Byrum, *Travels and Experiences in Other Lands*, 101–9. The quote is from page 108.

33. William G. Schell, *The Better Testament; or, The Two Testaments Compared* (Moundsville, W.Va.: Gospel Trumpet Co., 1899), 364–69. Schell was also making a distinction between the promise of healing in the Old Testament, which was only for "sicknesses," and the standard Jesus brought, which included "all sicknesses, all diseases, and all imperfections of the physical body." See 367–68.

34. E. E. Byrum, *Divine Healing of Soul and Body*, 112.

35. See E. E. Byrum's four articles about "Truth and Error" in the April 9, 17, 23, and 30, 1896 issues of the *Trumpet*.

36. George Cole, "A History of Divine Healing Among Us," *GT* 25:28 (July 20, 1905): 8.

37. J. W. Byers, *Grace of Healing*, 38.

38. The first systematic discussion of the atonement theory of divine healing appeared in Otto Stockmayer's *Sickness and the Gospel* around 1878. R. L. Stanton, *Gospel Parallelisms: Illustrated in the Healing of Body and Soul* (Buffalo, N.Y.: Offices of Triumphs of Faith, 1883) and R. Kelso Carter, *The Atonement for Sin and Sickness* (Boston: Willard Tract Repository, 1884) were the most complete expositions of this doctrine. See also Carter's repudiation of the doctrine in *"Faith Healing" Reviewed after Twenty Years* (Boston: Christian Witness Co., 1897). The first hint of this argument in the Church of God appeared in an article by D. S. Warner in 1883, but he did not use the phrase "in the atonement," nor did he draw the radical conclusions that became the mark of this doctrine. E. E. Byrum's *Divine Healing of Soul and Body* (1892) put salvation and healing in parallel but emphasized the commission more than the atonement. Fred Hahn's 1894 article and pamphlet was the first in the Church of God to assert that "the atonement of Christ" is the foundation of divine healing doctrine. J. W. Byers published the first systematic explanation in *The Grace of Healing* (1899). At the Moundsville camp meeting in 1902, "about eighty" ministers signed a lengthy statement detailing how "divine healing is in the atonement." This statement appeared in the *Trumpet* and as a tract.

39. See pages 66–67 of R. L. Stanton, "Healing Through Faith," *Presbyterian Review* 5:17 (March 1884): 49–79. For the opposing view, see page 315 of Marvin R. Vincent, "Dr. Stanton on 'Healing Through Faith,'" *Presbyterian Review* 5:18 (April 1884): 305–29.

40. In the divine healing movement, a few authors turned to the Hebrew roots of "borne" to prove that it meant "taken away." This argument was not successful.

41. J. W. Byers, *Grace of Healing*, 145. R. Kelso Carter gave this argument in outline in "Divine Healing, or 'Faith Cure,'" 778.

42. Marvin R. Vincent, "Modern Miracles," *Presbyterian Review* 4:15 (1883): 473–502. The quote is from page 474. A. J. Gordon also asserted that there is "a vast intermediate work of cleansing and renewal effected for the soul." For this reason, Gordon would only say, *"in its ultimate consequences* the atonement affects the body as well as the soul of man" (*The Ministry of Healing* [Boston: Howard Gannett, 1883], 18). Certain promises of present-day healing lay in the commission and in James 5:14–15. See *Ministry of Healing*, 16–38.

43. This was true of the divine healing movement as well, with some modifications. According to Paul Chappell, "during the early years of the healing movement, acceptance of the holiness doctrine preceded and prepared the way for faith healing" ("Divine Healing Movement in America," 72).

44. Mary Hildenbrand, "Raise the Standard," *GT* 18:47 (Nov. 24, 1898): 8.

45. The statement on healing from the 1902 camp meeting indicates how important this doctrine (or at least this phrase) became for judging orthodoxy. Apologies from those who initially rejected the doctrine were further evidence of the pressure. For examples of the latter, see A. B. Palmer, "Christ our Sufficient Physician," *GT* 26:31 (August 9, 1906): 4, and Lena Shoffner, "Our Life and Strength from Jesus," *GT* 22:30 (July 24, 1902): 8.

46. C. W. Naylor, for instance, said that sickness had no bearing on the moral condition, and, therefore, Christ could not have atoned for sickness. Yet, healing was *in the atonement*, because healing comes through redemption, which in turn came through Jesus' sacrifice. ("Questions Answered," *GT* 29:23 [June 17, 1909]: 10.) See also John C. Blaney, editorial note, *GT* 22:45 (Nov. 6, 1902): 4. Blaney wrote, "God has no use for ministers who do not preach healing and practise [sic] trusting God for their bodies. He demands of all his ministers to so live before him that they can pray the prayer of faith for the sick. The preacher who dopes himself with medicine, and is afraid to trust his body wholly in the hands of the Lord, can not pray the prayer of faith for others."

47. F. G. Smith, "Christ's Atonement Includes Soul and Body," *GT* 23:37 (Sept. 10, 1903): 6–7. Smith initially rejected the atonement doctrine but came to believe that "our bodies are included in the atonement of Christ *to the same extent* that our souls are."

48. SAPOLIO, a patent medicine, had the advertising slogan "Use the Means and Heaven Will Give You the Blessing...Never Neglect a Useful Article Like SAPOLIO." *Fairmont (Indiana) News*, Friday, September 3, 1897, p. 7.

49. J. W. Byers, *Grace of Healing*, 273.

50. J. C. Blaney, "The Bible and the Use of Medicine: Some Difficult Texts Explained" *GT* 34:30 (1914): 7–8.

51. J. W. Byers, *Grace of Healing*, 273.

52. J. C. Blaney, "The Bible and the Use of Medicine," 8.

53. Quoted in J. C. Blaney, "The Bible and the Use of Medicine," 8. The question marks are from the original.

54. See pages 99–100 of William Boardman, *The Great Physician (Jehovah Rophi)* (Boston: Willard Tract Repository, 1881) for an extensive discussion of this parable. Boardman was a Presbyterian and a member of the Keswick Movement. He got his start in divine healing with Charles Cullis and took a moderate approach to medicine and physicians. This is evident not only in his use of the parable of the Good Samaritan but also in his argument that Luke's experience as a physician made him a more compassionate author than the other Gospel writers (103–4).

55. Boardman, *Great Physician*, 99–100.

56. E. E. Byrum, *Miracles and Healing* (Anderson, Ind.: Gospel Trumpet Co., 1919), 150.

57. B. B. Warfield, *Miracles*, 171. Warfield was arguing that the anointing in James 5:14–15 might be about medical care.

58. R. Kelso Carter, *Atonement for Sin and Sickness*, 152–57; E. E. Byrum, *Miracles*, 157. Some critics also suggested that James 5:14–15 was about medical care because of the anointing. Byrum denied that oil had any curative properties outside the context of prayer, but the charge did not bother him. Following Carter, it was just fine with him to say that James is about the use of means, because that meant that the "means for healing" were prayer, anointing oil, and the laying on of hands. See, E. E. Byrum, "Means used in Divine Healing," *GT* 16:1 (Jan. 2, 1896): 4; "Some Hiding Places Uncovered," *GT* 16:2 (Jan. 9, 1896): 4; "Reviewed from a Bible Standpoint," *GT* 18:12 (March 24, 1898): 4; "The Medicine Question," *GT* 23:44 (Oct. 29, 1903): 8.

59. The fourth was Paul's advice to Timothy (1 Tim. 5:23). This chapter will discuss it below.

60. For an example of a critic's use of these stories, see A. F. Schauffler, "Faith-Cures," *Century Magazine*, Dec. 1885, 274–78.

61. J. W. Byers, *Grace of Healing*, 272.

62. Sarah Smith, "Does Christ Use Clay?" *GT* 10:4 (May 1, 1888): 1.

63. E. E. Byrum, *Great Physician*, 62–63. Byrum first thought that the Naaman story was self-evidently about overcoming doubts and trusting the Lord. He included it without comment as an example of the "Works of Faith." In his next book on healing, *Miracles and Healing* (1919), he explained that the water was not a remedy.

64. J. W. Byers, *Grace of Healing*, 272.

65. See E. E. Byrum, "Some Hiding Places Uncovered," *GT* 16:2 (Jan. 9, 1896): 4 and *Secret of Salvation*, 377. See also J. W. Byers, "Fifteen Objections Answered," *GT* 18:31 (Aug. 4, 1898): 8.

66. In an interesting aside, Byrum asked rhetorically why none of the critics of divine healing dip in the Jordan or rub figs on themselves if they think they are such good medicines (*Secret of Salvation*, 377).

67. J. W. Byers, *Grace of Healing*, 272.

68. Marvin Vincent was more subtle than most. Rather than citing Jesus' use of means in healing, he referred to his use of ordinary things in other miracles. "[Jesus] never despised natural agencies, but used them freely. He alone could change water into wine, but the servants could fill the jars and were bidden to do so. He alone could bring into the net the miraculous draught of fishes, but the disciples could cast the net and bring it to shore" ("Modern Miracles," 500).

69. J. E. Forrest, "Healings of Christ and His Followers," *GT* 35:9 (July 1, 1915). According to Forrest, "since no physician's compound was used, [this was] a means of reproving the medical profession of the day."

70. The idea that Paul would have told Timothy to drink alcoholic wine was beyond the limits of credulity. E. E. Byrum said, "there is no chance for winebibbers or medicine toppers to hide behind even the literal application of this [passage]" (*Secret of Salvation*, 380).

71. An example of this position comes from Viannah Crites's testimony. She proudly reported that her family had not used "medicine or simple remedies" even though they had suffered a rusty pitchfork injury, rheumatism, catarrh, bronchitis, typhoid, spinal meningitis, heart trouble, measles, dysentery, and pneumonia ("Increase of Faith," *GT* 21:10 [March 7, 1901]: 8).

72. William Boardman was among the first to suggest this interpretation. He simply asked the rhetorical question, "Is it not the province of diet, not of medicine?" (*Great Physician*, 105).

73. D. S. Warner, "The Ministers of God See Eye to Eye," *GT* 14:1 (Jan. 4, 1894): 4; "Questions," *GT* 15:3 (Jan. 17, 1895): 3. The quote is from the first article, but the second has a similar statement.

74. D. S. Warner, "Questions." See also Roark, *Divine Healing*, 115. For more about the debate over this passage, see chapter three.

75. J. D. Ferrill, "Fanaticism," *GT* 32:26 (July 4, 1912): 12. Ferrill was concerned that fanatical behavior was hindering the cause of Christ, and his primary example was divine healing. He was bothered that some saints refused such simple remedies as salt water for an inflamed eye. Ferrill noted that "people in such an 'iron jacket' rule of fanaticism have quite a difficulty explaining 'Timothy's wine' or 'Hezekiah's figs.'"

76. E. E. Byrum, "Some Hiding Places Uncovered," 4; *Secret of Salvation*, 379–80.

77. Byrum testified that he saw places in Palestine where every pool and stream had warning signs declaring the water unsafe for consumption (*Secret of Salvation*, 379).

78. "Questions Answered," *GT* 25:15 (April 13, 1905): 4. However, Paul's prescription was specific enough that only those with exactly the same problem as Timothy should use it as justification for (unfermented) wine.

79. A. L. Byers, "Questions Answered," *GT* 20:20 (Aug. 2, 1900): 4. It is also worth noting that an unnamed editor of the *Trumpet* observed that the Bible does not say that Timothy *was not* healed ("Questions Answered," *GT* 25:18 [May 4, 1905]: 4).

80. D. S. Warner, "Question," *GT* 15:14 (April 4, 1895): 2.

81. Fred Hahn, *Hints on Healing* (Grand Junction, Mich.: Gospel Trumpet Co., 1894), 4.

82. J. W. Byers, *Grace of Healing,* 148. In another part of the book, however, Byers said that the real problem came from the Doctors of Divinity and not the Medical Doctors. As scientists, the M.D.s at least had to admit that they were often ineffectual; the D.D.s would admit nothing (278).

83. George Cole, "Doctors and Medicine Opposed to Faith in God," *GT* 22:17 (April 24, 1902): 2.

84. L. H. Morgan, "A Doctor's Experience with Divine Healing," *GT* 27:14 (April 11, 1907): 16. At least two other physicians, George Achor and S. G. Bryant, quit their practice to become advocates of divine healing in the Church of God. Both wrote extensively for the *Trumpet.* See, for example, George Achor, "Why People are Not Healed," *GT* 18:46 (Nov. 17, 1898): 8; and S. G. Bryant, "God's Means of Healing," *GT* 26:9 (March 1, 1906): 8.

85. L. H. Morgan, "Medical Practice, Its Relation to Christianity" in *Two Hundred Instances,* 475–91. The quote is from page 482.

86. The passages are: Gen. 50:2; 2 Chron. 16:12; Job 13:4; Jer. 8:22; Matt. 9:12; Mark 2:17; Mark 5:26; Luke 4:23; Luke 5:31; and Luke 8:43. Job 13:4 ("But ye are forgers of lies, ye are all physicians of no value") was a particular favorite. The Old Testament passages were no problem, because Jesus had brought a better standard of healing. The New Testament sayings (Matt. 9:12; Mark 2:17, and Luke 5:31) that said, "they that are whole have no need of the physician, but they that are sick" were interpreted as referring to a spiritual condition. The sanctified were "whole" and had no need of a physician.

87. E. E. Byrum, *Secret of Salvation,* 388–89. Byrum noted that the Bible does not say that Luke was among the seventy. Further, if he was, Jesus certainly did not choose him because he was a physician: "it is not likely the Lord picked out seventy physicians and sent them forth, giving them the command."

88. E. E. Byrum, *Secret of Salvation,* 386–89. It was reprinted as "Luke, the Physician," *GT* 18:46 (Nov. 17, 1898): 8.

89. Marvin R. Vincent, "Dr. Stanton on 'Healing Through Faith,'" 320. For the details of the Greek translation, see Daniel Steele, *Half-Hours with St. Paul and Other Bible Readings* (Boston: Christian Witness Co., 1895), 250–54. Steele said, "it is grammatical to express the unemphatic possessive pronoun by the article in Greek as it is in English, 'the doctor' meaning 'my doctor.'" A parallel with Col. 1:1, in which the KJV translates "Timotheus the brother" as "Timotheus our brother" supported his point.

90. Daniel Steele, *Half-Hours with St. Paul,* 253–54.

91. William Boardman, *Great Physician,* 101.

92. William Boardman, *Great Physician,* 101 and 106.

93. A. B. Simpson, *Inquiries and Answers,* question 26.

94. E. E. Byrum, "Luke, the Physician," *GT* 18:46 (Nov. 17, 1898): 8.

95. George P. Tasker, "Luke the Physician," *GT* 34:36 (Sept. 10, 1914): 9. See also E. E. Byrum, "Luke, the Physician," *GT* 18:46 (Nov. 17, 1898): 8.

96. This story became the standard response to the "Luke the Physician" argument. See E. E. Byrum, *Secret of Salvation,* 387; and J. W. Byers, *Grace of Healing,* 223.

97. E. E. Byrum, "Luke, the Physician," *GT* 18:46 (Nov. 17, 1898): 8.

98. Marvin R. Vincent, "Dr. Stanton on 'Healing Through Faith,'" 329.

99. According to J. W. Byers, it was strange that "nearly all, if not all who make such an excuse for sickness will spare neither pains nor money in the employment of physicians and material remedies" (*Two Hundred Instances,* 411).

100. Byrum, *Doctrine of Healing,* 6. Besides, Miriam was healed when Moses prayed for her.

101. A third text occasionally appeared in the arguments over divine healing. Epaphroditus, one of Paul's companions in ministry, was "sick nigh unto death." However, God "had mercy on him," and Paul sent him as a minister to Philippi (Phil. 3:25–29).

102. Marvin R. Vincent, "Modern Miracles," 500. Otto Stockmayer wrote the first statement of the atonement theory of divine healing, *Sickness and the Gospel.* He was certainly a proponent of divine healing; however, his interpretation of these texts aligned with the critics of divine healing. According to Stockmayer, "If an apostle had to submit to this, how canst thou refuse unconditionally, and in all circumstances to bear sickness and pain, relying on the fact that Christ has borne them for us?" (34).

103. Daniel Steele, *Half-Hours with St. Paul,* 247.

104. E. E. Byrum, *The Power of Healing* (Anderson, Ind.: Gospel Trumpet Co., nd), 4. See also "God's Willingness to Heal" in *Two Hundred Instances.* 365–67.

105. E. E, Byrum, "Important Points," *GT* 17:18 (May 6, 1897): 8.

106. E. E. Byrum, "Divine Healing: The Will of God to Heal," *GT* 15:45 (Nov. 14, 1895): 4. See also E. E. Byrum, "Divine Healing: How People are Healed," *GT* 16:28 (July 2, 1896): 4.

107. E. E. Byrum, "Points on Healing," *GT* 23:15 (April 9, 1903): 8.

108. G. P. Tasker, "If It Be Thy Will," *GT* 24:27 (July 14, 1904): 8. See also E. E. Byrum, "His Great Compassion," *GT* 26:15 (April 12, 1906): 8.

109. Kelso Carter, *Atonement for Sin and Sickness,* 123.

110. William Boardman, *Great Physician,* 111. Church of God authors also adopted this argument.

111. See especially E. E. Byrum, *Secret of Salvation,* 380–86; and J. W. Byers, "A Thorn in the Flesh," *GT* 18:37 (Sept. 15, 1898): 1–2. Byrum and Byers both attempted to refute the prevailing hypotheses about the thorn (disease, weak eyes, speech impediment, and deformed body). Byrum thought the thorn was not physical at all, but "the persecutions which he had to meet." Byers offered that it might have been the "wounds and bruises" from when Paul was left for dead at Lystra. See also question 11 in A. B. Simpson, *Inquiries and Answers Concerning Divine Healing* (New York: Christian Alliance Pub. Co., nd). Simpson's analysis was not as extensive but showed that "we have every reason to believe that it was not sickness."

112. Boardman, *Great Physician,* 110.

113. J. W. Byers, "Paul's Thorn in the Flesh" in *Two Hundred Instances,* 413.

114. E. E. Byrum, *Why Some are Not Healed* (Anderson, Ind. and Kansas City, Mo.: Gospel Trumpet Co., nd), 8.

115. George Cole, "The History of Divine Healing Among Us," *GT* 25:28 (July 20, 1905): 8.

CHAPTER 5

BEHAVIOR AND HEALTH REFORM

Let a holy life tell the gospel story.
I am a child of God.
(B. E. Warren, "A Child of God")

When the saints of the Church of God examined the Bible for a description of sanctified behavior, they found few useful details. The guiding principle for the sanctified was "whatsoever ye do, do all to the glory of God" (1 Cor. 10:31), but that begged the question "What *can* one do to the glory of God?"[1] Further, what behavior was appropriate for children and others who had not yet experienced sanctification? Could one, for example, use tobacco, wear a corset, or read a novel? These specific activities did not exist in the Holy Land when the books of the Bible were written, and yet the Church of God included each on its list of things no saint could do without the appearance of sin, and no child could be allowed to do if he was to be trained "in the way he should go" (Prov. 22:6).

At first glance, there is nothing particularly interesting about the Church's behavioral strictures. It is a commonplace that holiness people did not use tobacco, drink alcohol, dance, wear jewelry, attend "amusements," or even smile. As an outgrowth of the holiness movement, the Church of God inherited much of its behavioral code from the holiness and temperance movements. Historians of the Church of God have suggested the radical proscriptions stemmed from competition with other sects. According to legend, the Church's opposition to neckties began when D. S. Warner tried to convert a Free Methodist. The man reportedly offered to give up his membership in the Free Methodist sect if Warner would give up his tie. Warner removed it and never wore one again.[2] As this story suggested, the desire to be the holiest of the holy undoubtedly contributed to the emerging definition of a holy life. However, this example (and the histories that have used it) underestimates the significance of behavior—as if behavior could be *just* for the benefit of the spiritually weak—and misses the fact that Gospel Trumpet Co. literature justified behavioral proscriptions in terms of holiness and physical health. Another interpretation swings too far in the other direction by suggesting that these practices were only for the spiritual benefit of the saints themselves. C. E. Brown, the fourth editor of the *Trumpet*, understood the Church of God as part of the continuum of movements in "radical Christianity," and he designated the behavioral practices of the Church "ascetic disciplines." The members of the Church of God definitely believed they were avoiding the pleasures of the world for spiritual benefit. However, the term "asceticism" implies a mortification of the flesh that does not quite fit in the Church of God. The saints believed that their practices would improve their spiritual *and* their physical conditions. Further, at least in theory, sanctification should have made these practices second nature, and not "disciplines" at all.[3] The Church's own explanations came from health reform literature.[4] As such, these articles and ideas represented much more than common sense advice. They introduced an ideology of health that formed an alternative to divine healing in the Church of God.[5]

James Wharton has characterized health reform movements as "hygienic ideologies," "professions of physical Arminianism." By this, he meant they taught that "bodily happiness is intended by nature (God), but each person must assume responsibility for his physical salvation and earn it by physiological rectitude."[6] This fit well with the Church of God's emphasis on pursuing sanctification. The connection extended even further, however, because health reformers taught that physiological rectitude was a practice necessary to overcome "deranged appetites." Human beings were killing themselves by doing and eating things they thought they wanted. Through generations of wrongheaded behavior, humans developed a taste for such things as alcohol and tobacco, and they passed these appetites to their children who then suffered through no fault of their own. Health reformer programs promised—through practice—to restore the natural appetites. A vegetarian Graham diet, for instance, was initially bland and unsatisfying but it soon became delicious and life-giving. The desire for sweets, red meat, and white bread disappeared; so maintaining the reformed appetite required no effort at all.

The parallel with inbred sin and sanctification is obvious. Both inbred sin and deranged appetites were corrupt desires that led people to act against their own best interests and violate God's laws of holiness and health. Through the pursuit of holiness, sanctification removed inbred sin; and health reform eradicated corrupt appetites through the practice of healthful living. The ideas were so close that Church of God appropriations of health reform frequently identified sin with deranged appetites and holiness with natural desires.[7]

An important difference, however, was that the definition of particular deranged appetites (as opposed to "deranged appetites" as a general term) came
from health reform experts such as Sylvester Graham, Langdon B. Coles, John
Harvey Kellogg, and Orson S. Fowler. The reformers were as strongly opposed
to the medical establishment of the time as were the members of the Church of
God—and that is likely why they were given a hearing in the *Trumpet*—but
there was nothing inherently religious about their articles. Warner and the
Church of God baptized them into the fold by adding sanctification as the ultimate goal of all behavior, but the health reform articles remained advice from
human experts.[8] Unlike the Seventh-day Adventists, no divine revelations supported these behavioral proscriptions and recommendations.[9] When a better
method for promoting health came along, many of the saints of the Church of
God were able to change their behavior. Therefore, the use of health reform literature as a guide to a holy life provided a precedent for the sanctified use of
remedies and medicines.

The Health Department

D. S. Warner brought his interest in health into the *Gospel Trumpet*. The first
issue to publish a divine healing testimony was also the first to excerpt an article
about healthful living, a description from the *New York Tribune* of the debility
incurred from using coffee, tea, or opium.[10] Subsequent issues included articles
about a variety of health-related subjects written by nationally recognized experts. A series of "health hints" from Dr. J. C. Jackson, frequent contributor to
the *Water-Cure Journal* and the proprietor of "Our Home on the Hillside" health
institute, said, "Study yourself. Find out what your own organization demands,
obey the law thereof, and you will no more be sick."[11] John Harvey Kellogg, the
superintendent of the school of hygiene in the Battle Creek Sanitarium, was
quoted about the importance of fresh air.[12] Langdon B. Coles's analysis of the
dangers of tobacco appeared in several places in Gospel Trumpet Co. literature.
Coles was an Adventist, and his book was extremely successful. His thesis was,
"it is as truly a sin against Heaven, to violate the law of life, as to break one of
the Ten Commandments."[13] The section about tobacco said, "that man who
chews and smokes his tobacco is doing that to himself which should be called
gradual suicide, and that for his offspring should be denominated manslaughter."[14]

It is worth noting that the *Trumpet* attributed these articles to their authors,
in contrast to the practice with divine healing arguments. Divine healing was a
religious doctrine ultimately rooted in the Bible. Attributing an interpretation to
an author who had not yet experienced entire sanctification would not have advanced the doctrine among the saints, and it might have led someone away from
the Church of God. Health reformers, however, were important for their own

personal knowledge. This is why the *Trumpet* identified J. C. Jackson and O. S. Fowler as "doctors," although its editors were generally opposed to honorific titles.

Another possible reason for the attributions was that they provided a defense against unwanted associations. It is curious that none of the Gospel Trumpet literature mentioned Ellen G. White, the Seventh-day Adventist "prophetess of health." From 1884 to 1896, the Trumpet Home was a mere sixty-two miles from Battle Creek, the home of White and the center of Seventh-day Adventist health reform. That the Church was aware of the Adventists is clear from testimonies and polemics.[15] Warner, H. M. Riggle, and Henry C. Wickersham all wrote extensive refutations of Adventist eschatology. The most notable, begun by Warner and completed by Riggle, was *The Cleansing of the Sanctuary*, a 541-page response to *The Sanctuary and its Cleansing* by Uriah Smith, professor of Biblical Exegesis at Battle Creek College.[16] Therefore, the similarities between the health advice works of the Church of God and the Seventh-day Adventists likely reflected a direct influence of the SDA on the Church, not just that both groups relied on the same sources. The Church of God and the SDA were competing for members, and Warner believed in health reform and wanted to present it in the *Trumpet*. However, he had to avoid any association with Ellen White's revelations or the religious convictions of the reformers themselves. He did so by emphasizing the scientific foundation of health reform.

In 1892, the same year the Gospel Trumpet Co. published E. E. Byrum's *Divine Healing of Soul and Body*, D. S. Warner felt that the Lord gave him "the duty of still more closely adhering to health and life promoting and preserving habits."[17] Warner did not elaborate how he came to this new commitment; however, in the months before he began the new column, he had a severe attack of rheumatism on his trip to the western United States. His report from Denver indicated that the thin air in the mountains had aggravated his condition and he had thought he was going to die, but anointing and prayer brought relief. Leaving Denver, he visited several health spas, notably Iron Springs in Manitou, Colorado (where he found the natural soda water "electrifying to the system"), and the hot springs of Glenwood Springs, Colorado. His declining physical condition combined with the effects he felt from air and water may have directed his interest to health reform.[18] In any case, his new discipline included a desire to share the laws of health with readers of the *Trumpet*. On February 11, 1892, Warner began the "Health Department," a weekly column devoted to health reform initiatives. It ran for just over a year.[19]

Warner wrote the first Health Department article himself with long citations from George Combe's *Moral Philosophy, or The Duties of Man*, and several unnamed works by R. T. Trall, E. B. Foote, Dr. Galen, and Dr. Hoffman. After justifying the new column as a guide to God's natural laws, Warner offered a lengthy explanation of how daily cold water baths could improve the constitution and prevent sickness.[20] The final column recommended faith for healing but, in lieu of the proper consecration, also listed several good remedies. The author, George Achor, had been a physician but left the practice of medicine to become a Church of God minister. He had consulted Trall's *Hydropathic Encyclopedia* (1852) but claimed most of the information came from his experience as a doctor.[21] Between Warner's introduction and Achor's conclusion, the Health Department presented a wide variety of topics, including the dangers of warm feet and dirty clothes, the importance of cold baths and proper ventilation, the correct technique for chewing food, the function of saliva, and the perils of corset-wearing.

By far the most common topic was eating—what, how much, when, and even how to eat. Food was a special concern of Warner's ever since he read O. S. Fowler's *Physiology Animal and Mental* on Thanksgiving Day, 1876.[22] The second most common topic was cleanliness and bathing. These were relatively safe topics for discussion. A heavy diet and infrequent bathing were normal practices in the rural United States in the late nineteenth century. Warner was trying to redefine them as health violations—even sin—but there was no inherent stigma attached to them, as there would have been with drinking, smoking, or the other staples of health reform literature, sexual sins. The articles that did mention tobacco and alcohol frequently connected them with a poor diet and presented them as the ultimate dissolution that could result from improper eating. An example was Warner's discussion of chewing, or "the slow and unconscious process of suicide...the hoggish habit of swallowing food unmasticated." In short, people who did not chew enough used water to wash down their food. The water diluted the saliva and forced the stomach to work hard to digest the food. This in turn exhausted the system and produced a desire for beer, wine, tobacco, tea, and coffee.[23] None of the Health Department articles mentioned sexual sins; however, several did refer to the "animalizing" effects of a meat diet. In the book that converted D. S. Warner to a reformed diet, O. S. Fowler stated his Fundamental Dietetic Law: "Man has only to live on the natural diet of the tiger, or the horse, or the monkey, to develop in himself, only to a far higher degree, the particular faculties which predominate in these respective animals."[24] Eating meat increased passions and eroded self-control.[25] The dangers should have been obvious to the saints of the Church of God.[26] Thus, the Health Department portrayed the laws of nature as the keys to the delicate balance that promoted physical health and spiritual holiness.

Not everyone in the Church appreciated health reform articles in the *Trumpet*. Some saw no compelling reason to change their menus, obtain new wardrobes, and spend more time scrubbing clothes and cleaning the house. One man boldly told Warner to stick to publishing testimonies and quit denouncing tea and coffee. Warner called the man an addict and accused him of making an idol of tea.[27] Subsequent columns included testimonies from readers who had benefited from health reform. Jennie C. Rutty—who later wrote several tracts and three advice books for boys and girls—told how her former diet had reversed the benefits of divine healing. Then she had read the articles on health in the Health Department, adopted a "two meal system," and was "free from all digestive disorders and disease." A. B. Guildersleeve, a reader from Pittsburgh, testified to his own improved health and wanted to counter those who thought Warner's efforts "to promote good health unprofitable." Moses Thompson wrote because the Health Department of September 22 had enabled him to overcome his desire for meat. He also wanted to thank God for giving "[Warner] the courage and wisdom to handle this delicate subject."[28]

The subject of health reform was delicate both for the effort it demanded from Church members and for the challenge it presented to divine healing. One Church member complained about Warner's articles because "Christ did not lay down any direct legislation concerning food." Further, ever since the man's wife had attended a camp meeting that served a menu based on Warner's Health Department, she and "a large portion of the people in that place were down sick with fevers." Another correspondent reported that the "Spirit showed [him] that our afflictions resulted from our precautions to preserve our health, which led to our speaking of the kind of food we should furnish to our stomach."[29] Associate editor and business manager E. E. Byrum shared some of the concerns about Warner's emphasis on health reform. Byrum wrote only two of the fifty-eight Health Department columns, and both prominently featured divine healing.[30] Of particular interest was an editorial note he appended to J. H. Hanaford's article from May 12, 1892. According to Hanaford, health was neither mysterious nor miraculous, and so, "as free moral agents, we determine and control our physical conditions by our conduct in accordance with our constitution and the laws which our kind heavenly Father has constituted." Hanaford said that this was the proper way to obey the epistle of James and "combine prayer with works." Byrum feared that some readers might get the wrong idea about "faith and works" from Hanaford's article. Byrum agreed that breaking known laws of God was detrimental to health, but James's teaching about works, faith, and health did not include diet and hygiene. James 5:13–15 was perfectly clear that the only works for healing were prayer, anointing, and the laying-on of hands.[31]

The Health Department concluded with the March 30, 1893 issue, and health reform articles for adults largely disappeared from the *Trumpet*. Gospel Trumpet Co. records offered no explanation for this change. E. E. Byrum's growing influence over the *Trumpet* must have been a contributing factor, as was the increased interest in divine healing in the Church of God movement as a whole. A highly symbolic change occurred in 1895 when Byrum christened the final page of the *Trumpet* the Divine Healing Page, the first regular column to take the place of Warner's Health Department. However, the changes in the *Trumpet* did not mean that divine healing had vanquished health reform. Health reform ideas temporarily disappeared as a guide to adults, but reemerged in advice to mothers and children, places that ultimately were more influential for the development of the Church of God.[32]

Train Your Children for Heaven

Children were a problem for the early Church of God. The movement taught that sanctification broke all the bonds of the world, making one a member of the body of Christ. Jesus was the model, and he said that his biological relatives were of no consequence when compared with his true brothers and sisters in the Lord (Matt. 12:48–50). Further, the saints took Galatians 3:28 as proof that sanctification removed gender differences and propelled both men and women into the ministry. "Mother" Sarah Smith, one of the first members of D. S. Warner's evangelistic team told her husband in the early 1880s, "I am done cooking for farming."[33] The ideal, therefore, was to shake the dust from one's feet and pursue holiness.[34] In practice, however, many of the saints were not as free as Jesus and Mother Smith. Leaving a husband to cook for himself was one thing, but leaving babies was entirely different. More to the point, an "unequally yoked" saint could leave his or her spouse's spiritual condition up to the Holy Spirit, but it was completely unacceptable to do the same with children. There had to be a way to bring children up into the Church, and—no matter what calling they felt—women had to do it. To help with the production of young Church members and to define childrearing as a holy vocation, the Gospel Trumpet Co. began to publish a children's newspaper and advice literature for mothers in the early 1890s.

This literature drew heavily from works on health reform, and it influenced the Church's approach to health in at least two ways. First, they presented a mechanistic explanation of health. In articles that were longer and more detailed than any of those from the Health Department, children learned to control their bodies by regulating their diets and their behavior. This expert advice came with the imprimatur of the Gospel Trumpet Co., and children learned that healthful living was holy living. The second influence was subtler. The health reform literature solidified the ideals of domesticity in the Church of God and changed the understanding of sanctification and sin. The role of a sanctified mother was now to create a clean, holy home that was separate from the dangers and temptations of the world.[35] This home could promote the sanctification of the children and preserve that of the adults. In contrast to the earlier concept of sanctification shielding the individual from the world, one now had to protect the home from corruption and temptations in order to protect the spiritual condition of the family. Thus, spiritual purity was under siege by every form of corruption, from dirt to germs to lust.

The Church's first published advice to parents was D. S. Warner's *Train Your Children for Heaven* (c. 1890). Warner was alarmed that many of the parents in the Church of God spent less effort training their children than "a horse trainer does on a horse."[36] He assumed that the saints knew the difference between holy and sinful behavior in a child, so the only explanation for this negligence was that they did not understand that parenting could lead children into holiness. The key was that Proverbs 22:6 ("Train up a child in the way that he should go; and when he is old he will not depart from it") was "based upon sound physiological principles." In other words, both health reform and Proverbs taught that repeated behaviors produced habits and appetites that could prevent spiritual awakening or ease the child into a life of holiness.[37] The parents' duty, therefore, was to study the particular make-up of a child, ask God for the wisdom to adopt the best means, and not stop until the child was fully trained.[38]

The single most important factor in childrearing was oversight by a parent who set a good example. However, Warner's excursus on food said that the internal states produced by a diet could aid the training or destroy the parent's efforts. He said that Paul's counsel to the Corinthians ("I have fed you with milk and not with meat; for hitherto ye were not able to bear it, neither now are ye able" [1 Cor. 3:2]) was another biblical passage founded on physiological truths. Children protected from "animalizing" meat diets were less restless, peevish, and ill-natured. Thus, a proper diet produced receptivity to correction.[39] Eating meat unnecessarily complicated childrearing, but many children had overcome their diets and grown into a life of holiness. Tea, coffee, and white bread, on the other hand, were so pernicious that the saints could not allow their children to consume them. These substances deranged the stomach and produced a feverish state that in turn created a restless mind and an irritable nature. Satan used this irritable nature to make a child self-willed. The self-willed child who used coffee, tea, and white bread would end in "drunkenness, misery, death and hell."[40] Training a child according to phrenological principles was so important that Warner counseled parents to quit their jobs rather than neglect their children.[41]

The Church of God advice that followed Warner's tract continued to use health reform ideas as a guide to childrearing. However, the focus changed to specific behaviors and added a concern with sexual sins that Warner had not mentioned. The stimulation of the sexual organs was a common theme in the works of Sylvester Graham, O. S. Fowler, and others.[42] Moreover, concern about the physical dangers of illicit sexual relations increased in the 1880s and 1890s because of the emergence of the germ theory of disease. The pathogen responsible for gonorrhea was one of the first to be isolated (1879), and syphilis followed soon after. In 1894, *Syphilis in the Innocent* made venereal diseases everyone's concern by saying that one could contract syphilis through mere association with an infected person.[43]

E. E. Byrum's *The Boy's Companion, or a Warning Against the Secret Vice and other Bad Habits* (1893) was the first work in the Church of God to address this delicate topic. It began with four testimonies from prisoners who had all started on the wrong path at least partly due to masturbation and the lack of parental oversight. The first prisoner stated the theme of the book:

I truly believe if someone could have obtained the right sort of influence over me, and pointed out the consequences of my way of living, I would have been saved long before I had given my youthful life to sin and wickedness.[44]

After the testimony, the rest of the book attempted to gain just that kind of wholesome influence over boys by showing that masturbators would end up in prison or a "consumptive's grave."[45]

Two concerns lay behind the attack on the secret vice. First was a physiological theory based on the idea of a vital force. This came directly from health reform literature and was a special concern of Sylvester Graham's.[46] The idea was that the body contained a limited "vital force" that gave life to every organ in the body. One excited organ pulled the vital force from the others. Habitual excitement of the sexual organs could deprive the heart, brain, lungs, and stomach to a degree that the person suffered dementia, consumption, and an overpowering appetite for stimulants. The excess vital force in the sexual organs would demand release and likely lead to sexual sins other than masturbation. The Boy's Companion recommended a daily bath and carefully regulated diet to properly distribute the vital force and thereby reduce the temptation of the secret sin.[47]

The second concern about masturbation was that it was a *secret* sin learned from "bad boys" and brought into the home. Secret vices were supposed to be impossible in the Church of God. A holy life was its own best evidence, and sin always showed. The Boy's Companion said that, in fact, masturbation was not completely secret. Boys needed to know that Isaiah 3:9 ("the shew of thy countenance doth witness against thee") was true.[48] However, the warnings to mothers from the Trumpet belied this confidence and showed the fear that evidence would appear only after it was too late. Saints had to face the possibility that they did not know their children's spiritual conditions. God only knew what worldly corruption had entered the family. Vigilance and separation from all evil influences were necessary, but sanctification offered the only certain protection.[49]

After the publication of the Boy's Companion (1893), open discussion of sexual sins and problems increased in the Church of God. Soon Church members began to worry about women and girls as well. In 1894, a Church member from Danville, Illinois, with the improbable name of Mary Housekeeper founded a rescue home for "fallen women."[50] The following year the Gospel Trumpet Co. began publishing tracts and books designed to prevent Church of God girls from "falling" themselves.[51] The arguments resembled those of the Boy's Companion but were fraught with much more importance. Girls would eventually become mothers, in both the biological and social senses. Physical infirmity could have impaired their offspring, and moral turpitude would have imperiled their homes.[52]

Everything relating to sex was dangerous, but the Church of God rejected the "marital purity" doctrine, which held that sanctification removed all sexual desire, and therefore that all sexual congress was a sign of sin. D. S. Warner's second wife adopted this idea in the early 1880s and received severe chastisement for it.[53] Sex did have a place in marriage, but it was scary and required careful control. The argument about vital force that Byrum used against masturbation also applied to sex within marriage, so any form of sexual excitement threatened to "undermine the constitution...[and produce] a weak and sickly mass of feminine humanity."[54] Girls who practiced the secret sin became physically unfit for marriage and motherhood. Married women who indulged in the "unbridled exercise of amativeness" did the same.[55]

A similar argument said that corsets could produce many of the same problems as excessive venery. Because of the pressure applied to the internal organs, a corset wearer "not only brings disease upon herself, but deprives her offspring of a robust constitution, and implants disease and brings them forth to grow up puny and dwarfed in body."[56] The Church of God authors supported their opposition to corsets with quotes from health reformers. W. J. Henry's *The Evil Effects of Tight Lacing* had a particularly extensive collection of references, including *The Journal of Health*; B. O. Flower; Lyman B. Sperry, M.D.; Joel Dorman Steele, M.D.; Mrs. P. B. Sauer, M.D., author of *Maternity*; Alice B. Stockham, M.D., author of *Tokology*; and the ubiquitous O. S. Fowler. As with the discussion of the physical consequences of sexual sins, the anti-corset material relied on health reform experts from outside the Church of God.

The moral dangers of sexual sins and corset wearing did not require the same kind of expert testimony as did the physical dangers, although one author did assert that "statistics of prostitution" showed that many girls became prostitutes through their "love for fashion and dress."[57] Secret sin, unbridled amativeness, and a love for fashion and the admiration of the world separated a girl from the Church of God and put her closer to the fallen women than to the saints. Such a girl threatened to contaminate the Church rather than purify the home. As Jennie C. Rutty wrote to girls, "Woman's sphere is home. It is her kingdom, and she is queen in it, guiding it well to the honor and glory of God."[58]

Near the end of the nineteenth century, a contributor to the *Trumpet* asserted that "self abuse" had overtaken drunkenness as the "greatest, most accursed, and most destructive crime in our land."[59] Another focused on dirty homes as symptoms of sinful hearts and said that those who are not clean could not dwell with Christ.[60] The ideal of the home as a sanctuary from the world was now firmly entrenched in the Church. The fear of corruption, disease, and debility—the physical contamination of the world—led Church members to turn to expert health advice, another influence from the outside world. Medical doctors and scientists (filtered through ministers, of course) told Church members how to eat, dress, and rear their children. The influence of medical science continued to grow in the Church in the early twentieth century. As the Church of God changed from a band of flying evangelists to a collection of congregations comprised of families, separation from the world meant separation from the bad parts of the world, and the saints needed to know what to keep out of their homes.

Health, Home, and Success

Private Lectures

D. Otis Teasley (1876–1942) was one of the more progressive ministers in the Church of God. He entered the ministry in 1896 and served for several years as a traveling evangelist. In 1904, he moved to New York City to superintend the missionary home. After six years, he moved to Anderson as the general editor of the *Missionary Herald*. In 1917, he assumed the chair of the board of directors for the Gospel Trumpet Co. As a writer and speaker, Teasley addressed many topics other ministers would not. He was responsible in large part for the introduction of Sunday school and Christian education in the Church, an important step toward acceptance of ideas and practices from denominational Christianity. He also wrote the Church of God's first book devoted entirely to hermeneutics.[61]

In 1904, while still based in New York, Teasley presented a series of lectures on sexual physiology and related topics to the women and girls of the Gospel Trumpet Family. The lectures were so successful that he expanded them and published them later that year as *Private Lectures to Mothers and Daughters on Sexual Purity: including love, courtship, marriage, sexual physiology, and the evil effects of tight lacing*. The next year he published a similar series for men and boys. Teasley's justification for these talks differed for the two sexes, but for both he said that Christian conduct demanded laying aside false modesty. For boys, the reluctance to speak of sexual sins was "a relic of superstition; and the sooner we discard it and instruct ourselves, the sooner we shall be able to discern the wisdom of God in the creation of the human body."[62] For girls, there was a dire need to address the dangers of life: "Never in the history of the world was there a time when uncleanness and sexual impurity were more prevalent than at the present."[63]

True to his word, Teasley's lectures were frank. He used scientific language to present the most detailed work on health and physiology the Gospel Trumpet Co. had yet published. For instance, Teasley explained the changes associated with puberty to boys and girls, and in so doing, he mentioned the scrotum, testes, vas deferens, ovaries, menstruation, and menopause. This is not to say that the lectures were the best possible source of physiological information. A course on music composition was the extent of Teasley's formal education, and much of the material in his lectures was at least a generation old. Yet, Teasley's lectures were an important step for the Church, no matter how dubious the content. They said that the saints needed to know about their bodies. Every parent and minister was duty bound to study sexual physiology and teach it to the children, because knowledge of the fragility of the human system would prevent nine-tenths of all violations of natural laws.[64]

The book for men and boys shared many concerns and some sources with E. E. Byrum's *Boy's Companion*. Three of the five lectures were about mastur-bation—its dangers, how to detect it, and how to prevent it with diet, exercise, and baths. The focus on physiology and the intended audience of boys *and* men gave these lectures a more clinical tone than Byrum had used. The implications were as alarming, but the stories were more believable. According to Teasley, masturbation led to disease and unhappy marriages rather than to prison. He granted that the immediate effects of the secret sin had "sometimes been over-drawn by patent-medicine pamphlets and quack doctors," but this in no way diminished the long-term dangers. Boys who did not immediately experience the warning symptoms often gained a false sense of security until it was too late.[65] Teasley did assure his audience that night emissions were not a disease so long as they occurred no more than once a week and were not accompanied by poor health.[66]

The remaining two lectures departed from earlier addresses to men and boys by emphasizing that personal holiness and moral rectitude were for the good of the family, not just the individual. One entitled "Illicit Sexual Intercourse and Its Attendant Ills" was the first to broach this subject in the Church of God. By em-phasizing the perils of social decay and disease, Teasley artfully discussed adul-tery without implicating the saints. Even if none of the men in the Church were tempted by extramarital sexual intercourse, they needed to know that adultery was destroying families and thereby undermining the United States.[67] Moreover, sexual sins had unleashed venereal diseases that threatened everyone. Syphilis was a particular concern because Teasley believed it could spread by "combs, hair-brushes, towels, drink-cups, water closets, knives and forks, a kiss, and, when the skin is broken, by an ordinary handshake."[68] Men and boys needed protection that only a stable family could provide. In case anyone missed that point, the final lecture—"Love, Courtship, and Marriage"—reiterated it.

The lectures to mothers and daughters were even more focused on family life, as the relational terms "mothers" and "daughters" indicated. The five lec-tures were "Social Purity" parts one and two, "Love, Courtship and Marriage," "Sexual Physiology and Maternity," and "Tight Lacing and Dress." In contrast to earlier advice to girls by the Church of God, these lectures barely mentioned masturbation. It was one of the possible activities in the second of the "three degrees of unchastity": mental impurity, secret adultery, and prostitution. Moreover, neither the causes of unchastity nor the means of its prevention were physical. Teasley did not prescribe diets, baths, or exercise. Girls needed protec-tion from novels, romance magazines, and bad company. Just as a parent should warn a boy that the first sip of alcohol led to the gutter, a girl should hear that "the first approach of mental impurity" led to the brothel.[69]

The best protection for girls was pure religion and plain truth as interpreted by the Church. Lectures on sexual physiology by their parents and ministers would keep them close to home, satisfy their curiosity, and inoculate them from the lies of unsaved boys. A clear exposition of the physical effects of wearing corsets would protect the girls both from internal organ damage and from wearing fashionable clothes. Lessons in cleaning the home protected the family from dirt and gave the girls a vocation. Tales of loveless marriages to unsaved men would counter the allure of prurient literature and other worldly temptations.

Both series of lectures, therefore, taught that holiness, health, and happiness were inextricably intertwined. Only the "saints of the Living God" had understood this and lifted "the standard of sexual purity and matrimony to its original plane."[70] As the saints saw it, science, God, and experience agreed that spiritual and physical health depended largely on the behavior that was characteristic of Church of God family members. This concord reflected the cultural conditioning of the movement. The Church of God developed in the context of nineteenth-century health reform—as well as holiness, domesticity, and other religious and cultural influences—and used the science and advice of the time to describe and prescribe the aspects of a holy life.

Home, Health, and Success

Several health columns appeared in the *Trumpet* after Teasley published his lectures. A fifteen-part series by George Tasker ran in 1905, and a twenty-three-part series by Robert Rothman appeared in 1907. The *Missionary Herald* began in 1910 with D. O. Teasley as the editor. One of its primary selling points was the Health Department column in each issue.[71] The topics in the *Trumpet* and the *Missionary Herald* ranged over the standard themes of food, exercise, fresh air, tobacco, alcohol, and the functions of various internal organs. The significance of most of the articles was the return of health advice to the *Trumpet* after several years of absence, but two are worth noting for their content. First was the *Missionary Herald*'s exploration of remedial foods. This was the closest thing to an endorsement of medicine the Church had seen since before Warner died. Going beyond a mere discussion of how certain diets promoted drinking and smoking, this article recommended foods that would correct specific ailments.[72] The second interesting article was Rothman's reprinting of some of D. S. Warner's writings about food, air, and water. Rothman had already covered these topics in earlier articles, but, by using Warner, he showed that health advice enjoyed the best possible pedigree in the Church of God.[73]

The Gospel Trumpet Company's next major book about healthful living was *Home, Health, and Success: or, A Guide to a Happy Home and a Successful Life* (1908) by Thomas Nelson.[74] The premise would have been familiar to readers of the *Trumpet*'s advice literature: God's immutable laws "are so arranged as to bestow blessings or punishments, accordingly as we obey or disobey." However, Nelson departed from previous works by emphasizing the blessings more than the punishments and describing the transformation of the world rather than the separation from it:

> If every husband, every wife, every parent, and every child that makes up all the homes in this wide world would arise in all the strength imparted through nature and through grace, to know and obey all the laws of home, the foul fountain of home misery would soon cease to pour out its miry contents over the home and the nation, and the sweet pure fountain of home joys and pleasures would flow like a mighty stream, gladdening and beautifying our homes and lives.[75]

This differed from the idea that behavioral proscriptions would protect children from evil and help them pursue sanctification. It was much different from the belief that the sanctified—"God's little ones"—had to suffer persecution from the world.

Nelson's book added little if anything to the Church's health advice. His sources were the same nineteenth-century health reformers Warner had used in the 1880s and 1890s, and Nelson's discussion of sexual physiology paralleled Teasley's. It is important to note, however, that Nelson was thorough; he compiled advice on every health topic the Church had discussed. Moreover, the collection of these laws and recommendations in a single volume for the whole family may have given them a stronger place in the lives of the saints. It certainly reminded Church members that natural laws underlay their code of conduct.

The true significance of *Home, Health, and Success* for the development of health reform in the Church of God, however, lay in the sections on home and success. Nelson's chapters on "Industry," "Economy," and "Business management of Home Affairs" showed that professional life had become the model for men in the Church of God. The home was a refuge for a man returning from his career in the business world. The saints had adopted the professional ideals of the progressive era that the American Medical Association successfully exploited to establish the prestige of orthodox medicine.[76]

The saints did not immediately move from embracing business models and scientific management to calling doctors. Strong opposition to medicine existed in the Church and in Nelson's book. The final two chapters in the Health section of *Home, Health, and Success* recommended divine healing for those who became sick.[77] Medicine was not "a true science" because no single theory of medicine existed and doctors did not revise their assumptions when confronted with failures. Doctors more often poisoned than cured their patients.[78] Nelson hoped "for the sake of home, property, life, and health, that people will take better care of their bodies by learning and heeding the laws of nature, and that when sick, they will search for a better way of healing than that of resorting to drugs and doctors."[79] Nelson supported his condemnation of doctors and medicine with divine healing scripture and testimonies, but the argument was essentially practical. When medicine itself became "a better way of healing," it fit well with home, health, and success.

The Necktie Controversy

That does not mean, however, that all the saints accepted medicine or Nelson's description of home, health, and success. Using advice literature to describe the Church of God risks overstating both the influence of the advice and the uniformity of opinions in the Church.[80] A debate that disrupted the Church of God from about 1909 to 1915 revealed deep divisions about behavior, worldliness, and professionalization. Everyone in the Church agreed that behavior was the outward sign of holiness, but they differed on exactly why this was so. One side asserted that the marks of holiness were set in the 1880s and any changes were signs of compromise. The other side said that the original behavioral codes developed for specific reasons—health, competition with particular religious movements, and economics—and could change with the cultural context.

The main topic of the debate was the necktie. Ever since Warner removed his tie to convert a Free Methodist, Church of God men wore plain collars without neckties.[81] The importance of this custom is clear from the effort men expended in conforming to it. In particular, removing the tie often exposed an ornamental collar, so the Gospel Trumpet Co. obtained a shipment of plain buttons and sold them at cost.[82] In 1903, the man who later became the leader of the anti-necktie faction, C. E. Orr, wrote, "Any article of dress put on merely for adornment can only be the fruit of pride in the heart." Article after article in the *Trumpet* repeated this opinion over the first decade of the twentieth century.

However, the movement was expanding into cities and was gaining converts who no longer worked on farms. The anti-tie custom caused a problem for the new members and for ministers who believed that the dress code hindered their evangelization efforts among businessmen. By 1910, "two or three [unnamed] ministers had put on the tie and worn it into the pulpit, even at a camp meeting, and they had proceeded to label as 'fanatical' those who would not do the same."[83] The controversy grew and threatened to split the Church. In an attempt to avoid division, twenty-five ministers signed the following resolution at the 1911 Anderson camp meeting:

> 1. That there is no good reason for a change in what for years has been the general attitude of the church in this country in regard to the matter, namely that the wearing of the tie is a thing to be discouraged as being unnecessary and as tending to the spirit of the world.

2. That liberty be given to its being worn by those whose consciences do not forbid their doing so on occasions when their business or other extreme circumstances require it.[84]

The debate continued, and the June 1913 camp meeting saw the adoption of another resolution condemning necktie wearing. It proved ineffective, and the leading ministers divided into the "liberal" and "radical" camps. D. O. Teasley, author of the *Lectures to Men and Boys*, was a notable member of the former camp, and C. E. Orr led the latter.[85]

In December 1913, the split was complete. The *Trumpet* no longer listed Orr as a contributing editor, and he had begun his own periodical, *Herald of Truth*, in Aberdeen, Scotland. Several ministers and readers of the *Trumpet* followed Orr out of the Church of God. After a series of leadership changes and relocations, those who split from the Church of God (Anderson) formed the Church of God (Guthrie, Oklahoma).[86]

The commentary on the schism by the "liberal" ministers demonstrated the complicated interrelations of behavior and health in the Church. The movement retained a strong streak of primitivism, so these ministers could not simply say that neckties were good for the Church's business. Rather, they argued that these changes put the Church in better alignment with true holiness. H. M. Riggle did so by saying that the only significant change over the past thirty years in the Church of God was the increase in divine healing. The proof of the reformation was that "thousands are now being healed." J. W. Byers took a different approach. He said that the standard of behavior for the Church was the primitive church of the New Testament, not the practices of the founding generation of this movement. One of his examples was that Warner had imposed his dietary standards on the Trumpet Home. Warner strongly opposed fine flour (he called it "Babylon bread") and "preached against the extravagance of two spoonfuls of sugar in mush." Byers said that the saints of the twentieth century knew better and should not make a "human creed" of Warner's diet or any other practices.[87]

The necktie controversy showed that many Church members were willing to change behavioral standards for a good reason, such as business or evangelism. Nelson's book on home, health, and success reflected a growing professionalism in the Church. Further, many of those who opposed this drift left the movement over neckties. At least some who remained recognized that practices from health reform had shaped the standards of holiness in the Church of God.

Sex Life and Home Problems

The final advice book published by the Gospel Trumpet Company in this time period was J. Grant Anderson's *Sex Life and Home Problems* (1921). Anderson (1873–1927) was one of the "liberal" ministers in the necktie controversy. A graduate from the State Normal School in Edinboro, Pennsylvania, Anderson entered the ministry in 1903 after experiencing a miraculous healing. Anderson never lost his interest in divine healing; in fact, he wrote the Church of God's last major book on that subject.[88] However, presenting a series of lectures on the "Ethics of Moral Action Relative to Individual Character Building" led him to begin "combining social and moral problems in [his] sermons." Because of this new interest, he became the editor of a department in the *Trumpet* devoted to "Home Problems" in 1917. Anderson received over 5,000 letters in the first three years. Readers clearly were interested in this topic, so the editor of the *Trumpet* asked Anderson to assemble the material from his columns into a book. The result combined the Church's behavioral proscriptions with a growing (or rediscovered) acceptance of health advice, sectarian or orthodox.[89]

The theme of the book was the same as that of the previous Church of God advice literature: God rewards perfect obedience to the laws of health and punishes any violations. Therefore, it explained the laws and imposed behavioral guides to prevent people from breaking the laws.[90] The sections about the "formative periods of life" repeated the shrill warnings of the *Boy's Companion* and *Save the Girls* about masturbation, corsets, and bad company. Anderson's choice for an eleventh commandment, for instance, was, "Thou shall not flirt, for it is the road that leads to lust, regret, and awful death."[91]

However, the advice to adults was less alarming. Reading thousands of letters from concerned Church members and people earnestly pursuing holiness convinced Anderson that many of the health warnings could not possibly have been correct. Corsets were bad, but the physical dangers had been exaggerated for non-pregnant adult women. Sex during pregnancy was not ideal, but "it happens and the race survives."[92] Moreover, Anderson determined that if thirty percent of the warnings to men and boys were true, then there would have been few men living in the United States over thirty years of age. Seminal losses not more than once a week did no harm, "whether voluntary or involuntary."[93]

Anderson blamed the myths about masturbation on "unscrupulous quack doctors" who designed advertisements to sell remedies to the uneducated. This shows that there remained considerable skepticism about the medical profession in the Church of God, but evidence suggests that the modifiers were necessary because many Church members believed many doctors were neither "unscrupulous" nor "quacks." This was particularly true with concerns about venereal diseases and pregnancy. The poster advertising the annual national camp meeting for 1919 announced that—in addition to the daily services and meetings for children, divine healing, and baptism—"Assistant Surgeon W. F. King, of the U.S. Public Health Service, will address the assembly at 2:15 P.M., June 17, in the interests of the campaign against venereal disease."[94] Opening camp meeting to a surgeon was a big step toward acknowledging the legitimacy of the medical profession. Another indication of the trend was that many of the saints thought that the Gospel Trumpet Co. should have had a medical doctor write *Sex Life and Home Problems*. Anderson defended his qualifications but admitted that the objection was reasonable and to be expected.[95] Finally, in the book itself, Anderson said that a doctor or a nurse was absolutely necessary for childbirth. Not only should "the family physician" deliver the baby, he should also examine the mother a few weeks before the due date. The casual use of the term "family physician" shows that Anderson's readers no longer feared the "medicine gods" of twenty years previous.[96]

Yet, Anderson did not confine himself to reevaluating behavioral proscriptions and recommending medical care. He wanted to help the saints have better lives and homes. In an interesting interpretation of natural selection, he said, "the physical balance in brute creation is preserved by deadly combat, but in the human family it is maintained by instinctive selection and education."[97] Because the appetites were deranged to the point that "instinctual selection" no longer proved a sure guide, Anderson supplied the education. Marriage partners should be chosen—not by love, parents, or law—but by the rules of "physiology."[98] To this end, he returned to D. S. Warner's interest in physical perfectibility and—in 1921—gave the most complete phrenological argument ever to appear in Gospel Trumpet Company literature. Anderson described the four temperaments (lymphatic, sanguine, volitive, and encephalic) along with their physical characteristics and their compatibility with one another. Some combinations should never join in marriage, because they would produce "civil war," "legalized licentiousness," or sickly children. Others were certain to create happy homes and well adjusted children.[99]

Conclusion

The idea that the saints could obtain physical health by obeying the laws of nature existed throughout the history of the Church of God. At first this approach to health was presented as a blessing of sanctification. D. S. Warner and other early leaders adopted health reform literature into the Church because it fit the general idea of the physical perfectibility of humanity, and because it gave specific direction for healthful and holy behavior. As divine healing grew in importance to become *the* health-promoting blessing of sanctification, health advice to adults temporarily became less prominent and behavioral proscription lost much of its connection with health. The marks of holiness (diet, dress, etc.) were simply signs of separation from the world. Behavioral proscriptions for children based on principles of health reform continued to have a strong influence in the Church. By the early twentieth century, the concerns for cleanliness, germs, sexual purity, and a happy home expanded beyond warnings to children and parents, and the Gospel Trumpet Co. began to publish lectures to adults about home, health, and success. The increased acceptance of professionalization combined with fears about venereal diseases and germs led the saints to greater comfort with expert medical advice. However, this chapter has shown that this was not as radical a departure as it would have seemed to those who listened only to the divine healing rhetoric of the Church. The sanctified use of material means to promote health offered an alternative to divine healing in the Church from the very beginning.

Notes

1. One might reasonably ask why this question remained after sanctification. The answer was that sanctification removed the desire to sin but did not impart perfect knowledge. Thus, one could innocently continue to disobey God's natural laws—not to damnation but with negative physical consequences. Warner addressed this question in "Unreprovable" (*GT* 7:16 [Nov. 1, 1884]: 2). He said, "the use of stimulants [such] as coffee, tea, tobacco, opium, stimulating liquors, and carnal amusements, etc., are the result of the fall of man." Sanctification would take them away, "assuming the appetite has not been perverted." See also George Tasker's thirteen-part series on "Christian Liberty and Divine Guidance" in the 1905 volume of the *Trumpet*.

2. John W. V. Smith, *The Quest for Holiness and Unity,* 194–95.

3. See C. E. Brown, "The Ascetic Discipline of the New Reformation" in *When Souls Awaken: An Interpretation of Radical Christianity* (Anderson, Ind.: Gospel Trumpet Co., 1954); and Dwight Latimer Dye, "The Asceticism in the Church of God Reformation Movement from 1880 to 1913" (Master of Religious Education thesis, University of Tulsa, 1963).

4. Even opposition to neckties had a physiological justification. This argument was not in the *Trumpet* itself but is in O. S. Fowler, *Physiology, Animal and Mental: Applied to the Preservation and Restoration of Health of Body, and Power of Mind* (New York: Fowlers and Wells, 1951), a book Warner owned and frequently quoted. Fowler thought neckties could impede air and blood and thereby lead to bronchial infections (207).

5. Historians have noted the large number of health reform-related articles and books published by the Gospel Trumpet Co.; however, no one has recognized them as a significant challenge to divine healing. It is easy to overlook the coherence of the nineteenth-century health reform movement and thereby miss its potential power. See Strege, *I Saw the Church,* 43–52 (on dress reform) and 68 (on phrenology and medical advice). The influence of health reform on the holiness movement in general remains unexplored.

6. Wharton, *Crusaders for Fitness,* 4–5. See also Abzug, *Cosmos Crumbling*; Nissenbaum, *Sex, Diet, and Debility in Jacksonian America*; Albanese, *Nature Religion in America*, chapter four; Numbers, *Prophetess of Health*; Ronald D. Walters, *American Reformers 1815–1860* (New York: Hill and Wang, 1978); idem, *Primers for Prudery.*

7. For example see A. L. Byers, "Care for Your Bodies," *GT* 12:9 (Feb. 25, 1892): 4. According to Byers, "health of the body is connected with salvation of the soul from sin and its depraving tendency." God forgave sins against laws of health just as God forgave other sins. However, after the forgiveness, the message was the same, "Go and sin no more!"

8. D. S. Warner's article "Be Strong in the Lord" (*GT* 11 [Aug. 15, 1891]) discussed the proposition that "the measure of our physical strength is the measure of our ability to glorify the Lord." After asserting that there is no need for a special revelation about health because reason and simple cause and effect teach us all we need to know, Warner

quoted several experts. Thomas Low Nichols—an M.D., a hydropath, and a proponent of free love and spiritualism—showed that health was the natural state of every living creature. Dr. R. T. Trall, the founder of the New York Hygeio-Therapeutic College, said that all natural foods agree with all people in a pure state of nature. O. S. Fowler, the premier popular phrenologist in America, said that suffering and pain were unnecessary. To these Warner added two caveats. First, sanctification was necessary for perfect obedience to God's laws. Second, God could and did suspend laws of nature for divine healing.

9. More than one reader of the *Trumpet* observed that Warner had no biblical or divine justification for his health articles. For the Seventh-day Adventists, see Ronald L. Numbers and David R. Larson, "The Adventist Tradition," in *Caring and Curing: Health and Medicine in the Western Religious Traditions*, ed. Ronald L. Numbers and Darrel W. Amundsen (New York: Macmillan, 1986): 447–67.

10. The issue was January 1, 1882, and the articles were "Cured by Faith" (page 3) and "Tobacco and Scholarship" (page 4).

11. "Health Hints," *GT* 5:15 (Feb. 15, 1883): 1. Jackson was an influential author, lecturer, and water-curist. Among his works were a book entitled *How to Treat the Sick without Medicine* and a tract on "How to Raise Beautiful Children." Both Ellen G. White and the noted divine healing evangelist Carrie Judd Montgomery visited his health institute. For more about Jackson, see Numbers, *Prophetess of Health*, 72–101. For Carrie Judd Montgomery's experiences at Our Home on the Hillside, see Carrie Judd Montgomery, *"Under His Wings": The Story of My Life* (New York: Garland, 1985; original publication Oakland, Calif.: Office of Triumphs of Faith, 1936), 32.

12. "Fresh Air," *GT* 5:22 (Aug. 15, 1883): 3 and "Pure Air," *GT* 5:22 (Aug. 15, 1883): 4. The first explained how to properly ventilate the dangerously airtight mass-produced homes. The second explained how poison air could lead to mental debility and ill temper that in turn prevented spiritual awakening.

13. Quoted from Numbers, *Prophetess of Health*, 60.

14. L. B. Coles, "Tobacco," quoted from *Philosophy of Health*, *GT* 6:1 (Oct. 1, 1883): 1. See also D. S. Warner, *The Great Tobacco Sin* (Grand Junction, Mich.: Gospel Trumpet Co., n.d.). Page 25 of Warner's tract relied on Coles for the argument that the only creatures that use tobacco are human beings and worms.

15. See Sarah Carr, "Healed from the Plague of Sin, Disease, and Adventism," *GT* 6:20 (Dec. 15, 1884); and H. M. Riggle, "Adventism Refuted," *GT* 19 (July 27, Aug. 3, and Aug. 24, 1899).

16. See D. S. Warner and Herbert McClellan Riggle, *The Cleansing of the Sanctuary; or, the Church of God in Type and Antitype, and in Prophecy and Revelation* (Moundsville, W.Va.: Gospel Trumpet Co., 1903) and Uriah Smith, *The Sanctuary and its Cleansing* (Battle Creek, Mich.: Steam Press, 1877). For further details see John E. Stanley, "Unity Amid Diversity: Interpreting the Book of Revelation in the Church of God (Anderson)," *Wesleyan Theological Journal* 25:2 (Fall 1990): 74–98; Smith, *Quest for Holiness and Unity*, 97–100 and Strege, *I Saw the Church*, 95–96.

17. D. S. Warner, "Is it to the Glory of God?" *GT* 12:28 (July 14, 1892): 4.

18. A. L. Byers, *Birth of a Reformation* (Anderson, Ind.: Gospel Trumpet Co., 1921), 375–79. Byers reprinted Warner's dispatches from his trip to California.

19. Roger Glenn Robins has noted health tips in other holiness journals. His examples were "Health Hints" columns in *Evangelical Visitor* (March 1, 1897) and a regular feature titled "Holiness and Health" in *Pentecostal Herald* (Indianapolis, 1894–1901). These began after the *Trumpet* column had ended. See Robins, "Plainfolk Modernist: the

Radical Holiness World of A. J. Tomlinson" (Ph.D. diss., Duke University, 1999), 81, n. 49.

20. "Avoiding Sickness," *GT* 12:7 (Feb. 11, 1892): 4. George Combe introduced phrenology to America when he toured the eastern United States in the 1820s. See Davies, *Phrenology Fad and Science*. R. T. Trall was a leader in the water cure, as were the other men mentioned in the article.

21. George Achor, "Temperance Chapter XIII: Medicine continued," *GT* 13:12 (March 30, 1893): 4. Achor's was an interesting case. He frequently wrote about health reform but was a staunch supporter of divine healing. In 1898, Achor, his wife (a midwife), and Church-member William Johnson were charged with manslaughter in Marion, Indiana. Johnson's wife died from childbirth-related complications. The Achors and William Johnson prayed but did not give her medicine. See chapter six for more information about divine healing trials. See also E. E. Byrum, "Charged with Murder: Three of the Saints Unjustly Cast Into Prison at Marion, Indiana: Enemies of the Cause of Christ Make a Desperate Effort to Put a Stop to the Work of Divine Healing," *GT* 18:23 (June 9, 1898): 4–5.

22. Warner, journal, Thanksgiving 1876.

23. Warner, "Mastication and Insalivation," *GT* 12:8 (Feb 18, 1892): 4.

24. Fowler, *Physiology, Animal and Mental: Applied to the Preservation and Restoration of Health of Body, and Power of Mind*, 164–67.

25. The most complete statement of the "animalizing" theory in the Health Department was Dr. J. H. Hanaford, "A Meat Diet," *GT* 12:22 (May 26, 1892): 4. According to Hanaford, eating only lean meat makes a person "ferocious." Hanaford was a Church of God minister who had medical training of some sort. Further, flesh eaters have not accomplished much and are prone to acts of cruelty. See also D. S. Warner, "Is it to the Glory of God?," *GT* 12:29 (July 21, 1892): 4; "Scientific Facts Respecting Food," *GT* 12:30 and 31 (July 28 and Aug. 4, 1892): 4; "Is it to the Glory of God?," *GT* 12:38 (Sept. 22, 1892): 4; Selected from *Human Science*, "Regulation of Animal Heat by Food," *GT* 12:41 (Oct. 13, 1892): 4; D. S. Warner, no title, *GT* 12:46 (Nov. 17, 1892): 4.

26. The Gospel Trumpet Co. issued two pamphlets that discussed excessive venery. See W. A. Haynes, *Social and Sexual Purity* (Grand Junction, Mich.: Gospel Trumpet Co., [1895]) and Jennie C. Rutty, *The Faith of Hannah* (Grand Junction, Mich.: Gospel Trumpet Co., n.d.). Several clarifications of Haynes's pamphlet appeared in the *Trumpet*. See W. A. Haynes, "Explanation," *GT* 15:34 (Aug. 29, 1895): 4; editor, "Social and Sexual Purity," *GT* 15:36 (Sept. 12, 1895): 2–3; and J. L. Green, "A Warning," *GT* 21:35 (Sept. 5, 1901): 4.

27. D. S. Warner, "What is in the Tea-pot?" *GT* 12:16 (April 14, 1892): 4. The short answer to the question posed by the title was "poison."

28. Jennie C. Rutty, "An Experience," *GT* 12:42 (Oct. 20, 1892): 4; A. B. Guildersleeve, *GT* 12:44 (Nov. 3, 1892): 4; Moses Thompson, *GT* 12:46 (Nov. 17, 1892): 4.

29. Quoted in Warner, "Is it to the Glory of God?," *GT* 12:28 (July 14, 1892): 4.

30. In contrast, George Achor, a former physician, wrote fifteen of the columns, and Warner wrote eleven. Byrum's articles were "Little Bits," *GT* 12:39 (Sept. 29, 1892): 4; and "Tobacco as an Evil," *GT* 13:6 (Feb. 16, 1893): 4. The first was a collection of short sayings, such as "Jesus was a Temperance Teacher," followed by a discourse on divine healing. The second argued that the Bible's condemnation of filthiness included the use of tobacco, and prayer could heal a tobacco addiction.

31. Dr. J. H. Hanaford, "Health," *GT* 12:20 (May 12, 1892): 4. Byrum's note followed immediately.

32. When I say that health reform disappeared as a guide for adults, I do not mean that behavioral standards changed. The change was in the argumentation. Far fewer articles quoted experts or *explained* the physical effects of meat eating or impure air. Without the explanations, these were simply behavioral proscriptions, not a theory of health.

33. "Experience of Mother Sarah Smith" in Noah H. Byrum, *Familiar Names and Faces* (Moundsville, W.Va.: Gospel Trumpet Co., 1902), 214–18. Smith was 61. She had asked God about the propriety of leaving her husband at home, and she received assurance that her children and the Lord would take care of her husband. Only after she had the "victory of consenting to break up housekeeping" did she tell her husband. Note that the title "Mother" indicated that she was not abandoning a proper gender role but was assuming a more important place in the Trumpet Family.

34. For an extended analysis of sanctification, testimony, biography, and gender in Wesleyan holiness movements, see Susie C. Stanley, *Holy Boldness: Women Preachers' Autobiographies and the Sanctified Self* (Knoxville: University of Tennessee Press, 2002). In the *Trumpet* see, for example, Jennie C. Rutty, "Without Natural Affection," *GT* 18:5 (Feb. 3, 1898): 1. Rutty was concerned about the changes sanctification could bring to a marriage. She insisted that women united to unsaved men had to remain in their marriages and continue to act in a loving manner. However, she ended with an address to the men. If only men would yield to their wives' wishes and get saved, there would not be any problem.

35. According to Regina Morantz, "Elevating the art of domesticity to a science, [female health reformers] restored to their followers a sense of purpose and direction, while they preserved in a new form traditional assumptions about woman's role which were deeply imbedded in the culture. The health reform regimen established new standards by which ordinary women could measure their own respectability and worth" ("Making Women Modern: Middle Class Women and Health Reform in 19th Century America," *Journal of Social History* 10:4 [1977]: 490–507). See also Richard L. Bushman, "The Early History of Cleanliness in America," *Journal of American History* 74:4 (March 1988): 1213–38. For studies showing how health reformers both adopted and challenged traditional gender roles, see Gayle Veronica Fischer, "Who Wears the Pants? Women, Dress Reform and Power in the Mid-Nineteenth-Century United States" (Ph.D. diss., Indiana University, 1995); and Barbara Leslie Epstein, *The Politics of Domesticity: Women, Evangelism, and Temperance in Nineteenth-Century America* (Middletown, Conn.: Wesleyan University Press, 1981).

36. D. S. Warner, *Train Your Children for Heaven* (Grand Junction, Mich.: Gospel Trumpet Co., n.d.), 16.

37. Warner, *Train Your Children*, 1. According to J. H. Kellogg, a wrong act made others easier, and a good one strengthened the resolution to do more good. See his *Second Book of Physiology and Hygiene* (New York: n.p., 1894), 223; quoted in Anita Fellman and Michael Fellman, *Making Sense of Self: Medical Advice Literature in Late Nineteenth-Century America* (Philadelphia: University of Pennsylvania Press, 1981), 123–24.

38. Warner, *Train Your Children*, 12. This was the idea behind phrenologically-based health reform. Warner used a phrenological reading of his daughter Levilla Modest to design a proper diet for her. See Warner's journal for June 18, 1878. See also chapter two.

39. Warner, "Train Up Your Children by the Aid of a Proper Diet" in *Train Your Children*, 38–43.

40. Warner, "Train Up Your Children by the Aid of a Proper Diet" in *Train Your Children*, 41–42.

41. Warner was talking to fathers as well as to mothers. The idea of separate spheres was nowhere in evidence.

42. Sylvester Graham, *A Lecture to Young Men* (New York: Arno Press, 1974; Providence, R.I.: Weeden and Cory, 1834), 24. For discussions of advice about sexual practices, see R. P. Neuman, "Masturbation, Madness, and the Modern Concepts of Childhood and Adolescence," *Journal of Social History* 8:3 (Spring 1975): 1–27; and Robert H. MacDonald, "The Frightful Consequences of Onanism: Notes on the History of a Delusion," *Journal of the History of Ideas* 28:3 (July–Sept. 1967): 423–31. For primary sources in addition to Graham, see Joseph W. Howe, M.D., *Excessive Venery Masturbation and Continence: the etiology, pathology, and treatment of the diseases resulting from venereal excess, masturbation, and continence* (New York: E. B. Treat, 1887; reprint New York: Arno Press, 1975); R. T. Trall, *Sexual Physiology: A Scientific and popular Exposition of the Fundamental Problems of Sociology* (New York: M. L. Holbrook, 1881; reprint New York: Arno Press, 1974); Dio Lewis, *Chastity; or, Our Secret Sins* (Philadelphia: George Maclean & Co., 1874).

43. Tomes, *Gospel of Germs*, 107–8. Concerns about germs led to campaigns for individual communion cups in the mid-1890s. Ellen Wallace of the Women's Christian Temperance Union argued that individual cups were necessary to restore the spirit of unity in the churches because sharing was offensive and interfered with worship (133).

44. Byrum, *The Boy's Companion, or a Warning Against the Secret Vice and other Bad Habits* (Grand Junction, Mich.: Gospel Trumpet Co., 1893), 34.

45. Byrum, *Boy's Companion*, 65. According to Anita Fellman and Michael Fellman, masturbation "was both an actual and a symbolic repudiation of adult authority" (*Making Sense of Self*, 85).

46. Orson Fowler's *Sexual Science* explained this theory and was in the possession of the Gospel Trumpet Company. It was also part of Sylvester Graham's teachings. For more information see Wharton, *Crusaders for Fitness*, 42–43; John Money, *The Destroying Angel: Sex, Fitness & Food in the Legacy of Degeneracy Theory, Graham Crackers, Kellogg's Corn Flakes & American Health History* (Buffalo, N.Y.: Prometheus Books, 1985); Stephen Nissenbaum, *Sex, Diet, and Debility in Jacksonian America: Sylvester Graham and Health Reform*, Contributions in Medical History no. 4 (Westport, Conn.: Greenwood Press, 1980). For the use of "vital force" theories in the 1870s and 1880s by regular physicians to discourage the education of pubescent girls, see Carroll Smith-Rosenberg and Charles Rosenberg, "The Female Animal: Medical and Biological Views of Woman and Her Role in Nineteenth-Century America," *Journal of American History* 60:2 (Sept. 1973): 332–56. For a more complete statement of "vitalism" in Church of God literature, see Haynes, *Social and Sexual Purity*, 8.

47. Byrum, *Boy's Companion*, 82–84.

48. Byrum, *Boy's Companion*, 65.

49. Byrum, *Boy's Companion*, 85.

50. Mary Housekeeper, "Woman's Faith Home," *GT* 14:28 (July 19, 1894) and *GT* 14:43 (Nov. 8, 1894).

51. In 1895, the Gospel Trumpet Co. published *Little Things* and *Startling News to Mothers* by E. E. Byrum, and *Social and Sexual Purity* by W. A. Haynes. According to

C. E. Brown, these tracts were more disturbing to those outside the Church than to the saints. In 1895, the Pittsburgh, Pennsylvania police ran Church of God ministers out of town for distributing indecent tracts about masturbation, and "Riggle and Cheatham were ordered out of Emlenton (PA) with their tent for the same reason" (*When the Trumpet Sounded*, 172–73). Brown did not specify the tract, but it could have been either *Startling News* or *Social and Sexual Purity*.

52. According to W. A. Haynes, "when the soul of woman becomes blackened by sin and vice, there is no greater terror to civilization" (*Save the Girls*, 8–9).

53. See "Conflict and Crisis in the Kingdom of God in Ohio," in Thomas A. Fudge, *Daniel Warner and the Paradox of Religious Democracy in Nineteenth-Century America* (Lewiston, N.Y.: Edwin Mellen Press, 1998).

54. Haynes, *Save the Girls*, 1–2.

55. Haynes, *Social and Sexual Purity*, 7.

56. Byrum, *Little Things*, 11. See also Jennie C. Rutty, *Letters of Love and Counsel for "Our Girls"* (Moundsville, W.Va.: Gospel Trumpet Co., 1899), 161.

57. Haynes, *Save the Girls*, 3.

58. Jennie C. Rutty, *Letters of Love and Counsel for "Our Girls,"* 287. On separate spheres of influence, see Linda K. Kerber, "Separate Spheres, Female Worlds, Woman's Place: The Rhetoric of Women's History," *Journal of American History* 75:1 (June 1988): 9–39.

59. Nora De Bolt Dodge, "Information and Kindly Advice for Parents," *GT* 19:11 and 12 (March 16 and 23, 1899): 2 and 3 respectively.

60. Myrtle Duncan, "Filthiness," *GT* 19:9 (March 2, 1899): 3.

61. Strege, *I Saw the Church*, 138–40.

62. D. O. Teasley, *Private Lectures to Men and Boys* (Moundsville, W.Va.: Gospel Trumpet Co., 1905), 12.

63. D. O. Teasley, *Private Lectures to Mothers and Daughters* (Moundsville, W.Va.: Gospel Trumpet Co., 1904), 12.

64. Teasley, *Private Lectures to Men*, 34 and 44.

65. Teasley, *Private Lectures to Men*, 65.

66. Teasley, *Private Lectures to Men*, 71. Teasley adopted an argument against masturbation that differed slightly from Byrum's. For Teasley, the loss of vital power resulted from ejaculation rather than from excitement. Therefore, night emissions were a serious concern. If they proved to be a problem, Teasley offered several remedies, including cold baths before bed and sleeping with a knotted sheet in the small of the back (86).

67. Teasley, *Private Lectures to Men*, 98–99. This is further evidence of the "embourgeoisement" of the Church of God. An earlier generation would not have worried about the foundation of the United States because all institutions and governments were merely impediments to holiness. See Robert Walter Wall, "The Embourgeoisement of the Free Methodist Ethos," *Wesleyan Theological Journal* 25:1 (1990): 117–29.

68. Teasley, *Private Lectures to Men*, 106. Teasley's lectures about home life and the sin of adultery became sadly ironic in 1919 when he "resigned from the Gospel Trumpet Company under heavy suspicion of adultery" (Strege, *I Saw the Church*, 162 n. 15). For more about the syphilis scare, see Nancy Tomes, *Gospel of Germs* (Cambridge, Mass.: Harvard University Press, 1998), 106–8.

69. Teasley, *Private Lectures to Mothers*, 22.

70. Teasley, *Private Lectures to Mothers*, 68.

71. The advertisement for the *Missionary Herald* in the *Trumpet* promised that the monthly column on "The Science of Healthful Living" would cost at least $25 from a reliable school of dietetics. It said that health is "of special importance to every minister of the gospel, upon the length of whose life and upon the efficiency of whose mind and body depends to a great extent, the amount of good he may do in the world." The *Herald's* column would not cover fads or athletic stunts, only "Food and feeding. Exercise and recreation. Respiration and ventilation. Rest and sleep." See "Special Features of the Missionary Herald for 1911," *GT* 30:44 (Nov. 10, 1910): 10.

72. D. O. Teasley, "Scientific Dietetics," *Missionary Herald* 2:9 (Sept. 1911): 286–88.

73. Robert Rothman, "From D. S. Warner's Writings," *GT* 28:21 (May 21, 1908): 5. This column also included a section "From G. R. Achor's Writings."

74. Thomas Nelson founded the Scandinavian parallel to the Gospel Trumpet Co., Den Evangeliske Basun Publishing Co. around 1900 in Muscatine, Iowa. The publishing house moved to St. Paul Park, Minnesota, in 1903, where it remained for twenty years before moving to Denmark. Nelson's book *Hejm, Helbred, og Lykke* was such a success in Dano-Norwegian that the Gospel Trumpet Co. published an English language version as *Home, Health, and Success*. See Strege, *I Saw the Church*, 68; and Smith, *Quest for Holiness and Unity*, 173–77.

75. Thomas Nelson, *Home, Health, and Success: or, A Guide to a Happy Home and a Successful Life* (Anderson, Ind.: Gospel Trumpet Co., 1908), 13.

76. According to Paul Starr, "the triumph of the regular profession [of medicine] depended on belief rather than force, on its growing cultural authority rather than sheer power." Moreover, "to see the rise of the profession as coercive is to underestimate how deeply its authority penetrated the beliefs of ordinary people and how firmly it had seized the imagination even of its rivals" (*The Social Transformation of American Medicine*, 229). See also Steven J. Diner, *A Very Different Age: Americans of the Progressive Era* (New York: Hill and Wang, 1998), 176, 179, and 199; Markowitz and Rosner, "Doctors in Crisis," 83–107; Rothstein, *American Physicians in the Nineteenth Century*; Robert H. Wiebe, *The Search for Order, 1877–1920* (New York: Hill and Wang, 1967), 112.

77. Most sickness could have been avoided by following the advice of the rest of the chapter, but Nelson granted that inherited weaknesses, unsanitary surroundings, and ignorance of the laws of health ensured that there would always be some sickness in the world (491).

78. Nelson, *Home, Health, and Success*, 476–77.

79. Nelson, *Home, Health, and Success*, 488.

80. A problem with using advice literature comes from the failure to note that it was prescriptive rather than descriptive. However, in this project I am interested in advice precisely because it prescribed behavior and provided a justification for that prescription. See Lynn Z. Bloom, "'It's all for Your Own Good:' Parent-Child Relationships in Popular American Child Rearing Literature, 1820–1970," *Journal of Popular Culture* 10:1 (1976): 191–98; Jay E. Mechling, "Advice to Historians on Advice to Mothers," *Journal of Social History* 9:1 (Fall 1975): 44–63; and Carl N. Degler, "What Ought to Be and What Was: Women's Sexuality in the Nineteenth Century," *American Historical Review* 79:5 (Dec. 1974): 1467–90.

81. See *Doctrine and Discipline of the Free Methodist Church* (Chicago: Free Methodist Publishing House, 1905). The third chapter was about dress. It said the Free Methodists would not receive any into fellowship until "they have left off superfluous

ornaments." It also instructed every minister in charge of a circuit to preach Wesley's sermons on dress once a year in each assembly (25).

82. The advertisement for the plain buttons in the editorial note by E. E. Byrum, *GT* 21:36 (Sept. 12, 1901): 4. The only other product advertised in the *Trumpet* was a flour mill for producing whole wheat bread (Warner, "Save Your Health and Your Wheat," *GT* 11:16 [Aug. 15, 1891]: 2).

83. Smith, *Quest for Holiness and Unity*, 197.

84. Quoted in Smith, *Quest for Holiness and Unity*, 198.

85. E. E. Byrum assigned the labels. Byrum attempted to stay out of the debate but believed that the tie could be worn for business. See *GT* 33:36 (Sept. 11, 1913): 2–4, 11–12. In a letter to his brother, E. E. Byrum reported that several of the ministers in California were "extreme on the necktie issue, claiming to hold to the faith of thirty years ago." However, he observed that their wives wore corsets and they compromised on nearly every other issue. See "E. E. Byrum to N. H. Byrum, Heinly, Phelps, and others. L. A., Calif. 1–13, '14," Church of God Archives b650, E. E. Byrum Papers, 2. Correspondence File.

86. E. E. Byrum, "A Warning to the Church," *GT* 34:7 (Feb. 19, 1914): 3–4. For more about the split, see Smith, *Quest for Holiness and Unity*, 204; and Kostlevy, ed., *Historical Dictionary of the Holiness Movement*, "Church of God (Guthrie, Oklahoma)." The Church of God (Guthrie) has experienced growing pains similar to that of the Church of God (Anderson), only on a smaller scale. In the late 1980s, a radical faction split from the Church of God (Guthrie) to form the Church of God (Sumas, Washington) and begin publishing *The Gospel Trumpet*.

87. H. M. Riggle, "30 Years Ago," *GT* 34:10 (March 5, 1914): 6; J. W. Byers, "30 Years Ago," *GT* 34:10 (March 5, 1914): 6.

88. Strege, *I Saw the Church*, 69–70. See the introduction by H. M. Riggle in J. Grant Anderson, *Divine Healing* (Anderson, Ind.: Gospel Trumpet Co., 1926), 5–6. For more about Anderson's *Divine Healing*, see chapter six.

89. J. Grant Anderson, *Sex Life and Home Problems* (Anderson, Ind.: Gospel Trumpet Co., 1921), 5.

90. Anderson, *Sex Life and Home Problems*, 90.

91. Anderson, *Sex Life and Home Problems*, 53.

92. Anderson, *Sex Life and Home Problems*, 76.

93. Anderson, *Sex Life and Home Problems*, 133.

94. The original poster is in the Church of God archives. It has been reprinted in Merle D. Strege, *A Look at the Church of God for Children, Vol. I, 1880–1930* (Anderson, Ind.: Warner Press, 1987), 16–17.

95. Anderson, *Sex Life and Home Problems*, 5–6.

96. Anderson, *Sex Life and Home Problems*, 82. Divine healing testimonies frequently bragged that the "family physician" was Jesus Christ. For example, see Pearl Owens, "Jesus is my Physician," *GT* 21:12 (March 21, 1901): 8; and W. J. Henry, "The Best Family Physician," *GT* 26:2 (Jan. 11, 1906): 8. The medicine gods reference is to J. W. Byers, *Grace of Healing* (Moundsville, W.Va.: Gospel Trumpet Co., 1899), 148. It is also worth noting that earlier condemnations of physicians often accused male doctors of taking sexual liberties with their female patients. There is no hint of that here.

97. Anderson, *Sex Life and Home Problems*, 63.

98. Anderson, *Sex Life and Home Problems*, 64.

99. Anderson, *Sex Life and Home Problems*, 66. Anderson added that no one should ever marry a person afflicted with venereal disease. I have not determined the exact source of Anderson's four temperaments; he may have put them together from several sources. However, Lorenzo Fowler's types (mental, motive, sanguine, and lymphatic) were similar [*Marriage: Its History and Ceremonies; with a phrenological and physiological exposition of the functions and qualifications for the happy marriage* (New York: Fowlers and Wells, 1847), 177–78]. D. S. Warner said that marriages between two people of the same temperament were "often attended with sad results" (*Marriage and Divorce* [Grand Junction, Mich.: Gospel Trumpet Co., [1896]). For the variety of humoral theories, see John S. Haller, *American Medicine in Transition 1840–1910* (Urbana: University of Illinois Press, 1981), 3–35.

CHAPTER 6

TRIALS AND TRANSFORMATIONS OF DIVINE HEALING

God's way is best, I will not murmur,
Although the end I may not see;
Where'er he leads I'll meekly follow.
God's way is best, is best for me.
(C.W. Naylor/C. E. Hunter, "God's Way is Best")

The Church of God witnessed the dissolution of the radical doctrine of divine healing in the first quarter of the twentieth century. At first glance, this was not at all obvious. The *Gospel Trumpet*'s new motto for 1917 proclaimed that divine healing was a core emphasis, and the testimony pages frequently included miraculous stories of physical healing. E. E. Byrum left the editor's chair to become a traveling evangelist. His healing revivals drew huge crowds and garnered positive attention from secular periodicals. Every camp meeting had at least one divine healing service, and the Gospel Trumpet Company published *Miracles and Healing* in 1919 and *Divine Healing* in 1926. However, the promises, expectations, and demands associated with the doctrine changed radically. By 1926, divine healing in the Church of God no longer stood alone as a healing system.

At the height of the atonement doctrine (1895–1905), divine healing in the Church of God was impervious to refutation. If a person was not healed and did not know why, then he or she lacked sufficient faith to claim the healing or to know God's will. If divine healing did not convince doctors and devotees of other healing systems, then the problem lay with their stubborn delusions and prejudices, not with the quality of evidence for healing. There could be no doubt that God was perfecting the bodies of the saints and the Body of Christ. Unsatis-factory results could only mean a failure to meet the conditions for healing.

In the twentieth century, failed healings truly became failures of divine healing. Legal prosecution and charges of religious fanaticism were external challenges. Deaths and prolonged infirmities of saints and their children strained the practice of divine healing from inside the Church. Some of the saints began to question the doctrine itself and increasingly looked to medical science for definitions of disease and health. Church members attempted to escape the cul-tural stigma of divine healing by insisting that the doctrine of divine healing *as taught by the Church of God* was as reasonable and reliable as medicine. In so doing, they were acknowledging medical science as the standard of healing. Once they began asking God to kill disease-causing germs instead of praying for relief from mysterious afflictions like cancer, consumption, and catarrh, divine healing as an independent system had ended. The prayer of faith became an al-ternative or a supplement to medical therapeutics—an optional route to the re-sult prescribed by medicine—not the only acceptable treatment for a saint.

In Prison for Christ's Sake

Between 1897 and 1917 the rejection of secular medicine in favor of divine healing led to at least nine criminal trials of members of the Church of God.[1] They were in Fort Wayne, Indiana (1897); Marion, Indiana (1898); Vincennes, Indiana (1899); Butler, Pennsylvania (1903); Bluefield, West Virginia (1905); Ironton, Ohio (1905); Beaver Co., Oklahoma (1909), and Oklahoma City (1911); Pocahontas, Arkansas (1912); and Oran, Missouri (1917). There also was an arrest—but no trial—for manslaughter in Riverview, Ontario (1905), and a case of Health Services workers removing children from their parents' custody to administer medicine in Jersey City, New Jersey (1910). The Marion, Indiana case was the odd one. Three Church of God ministers attended a fourth when she died from complications related to childbirth. The three were charged with murder and practicing obstetrics without a license. The grand jury reduced the charge to involuntary manslaughter, the trial jury failed to return a verdict, and the judge dismissed the case.[2] The other trials and arrests were of lay members accused of refusing to give medicine to their sick children. Three (Butler, Penn-sylvania; Bluefield, West Virginia; and Pocahontas, Arkansas) were for involun-tary manslaughter, and the remaining five were for child endangerment or neglect. Interestingly, the only two cases not decided in favor of the defendant or overturned on appeal were also the only cases in which the children lived. In the Fort Wayne case of 1897, the child suffered hearing loss, and in the Okla-homa case of 1909/1911, the child had a full recovery.

The leaders of the Church initially believed that the trials were part of God's plan to promote holiness. They predicted that these examples of Church members voluntarily suffering legal prosecution for their faith in divine healing would attract new members and strengthen the faith of those already belonging to the Church of God. However, court trials proved to be a poor vehicle for the promotion of religious doctrines. Instead of attracting new converts to divine healing, the trials exposed Church members to ridicule and legal penalties, created dissension in the Church of God, and contributed to a reformulation of the doctrine of divine healing that did not challenge health laws.

Gospel Trumpet Reports

The first trial was held in 1897 in Fort Wayne, Indiana, less than two years after the camp meeting that marked the "forward move" on miracles and healing. The divine healing page had been running for about a year, and J. W. Byers had just begun publication of *Tidings of Healing* in California. A Church member named Henry Smith was charged with child endangerment for refusing to give his twelve-year-old daughter medicine for her "typhoid pneumonia." The girl suffered hearing loss and possibly some brain damage. The doctor who testified on behalf of the county was reasonably certain that orthodox medical treatment would have prevented these effects. The court found Smith guilty and fined him $5.00 plus court costs, $17.50 in all. He chose to go to jail instead of paying the fine.

The *Fort Wayne Weekly Sentinel* and the *Fort Wayne Weekly Gazette* both reported extensively on Smith's arrest and trial. They printed court reports, arrest reports, and editorials about divine healing, child rearing, and public safety.[3] The *Trumpet* devoted an entire page to this trial. Under the heading "In Prison for Christ's Sake," the *Trumpet* published Smith's letter from jail recounting his arrest and asking the editor: Must the saints be subject to human laws that conflict with God's laws?[4] After a reprint of the account from the *Fort Wayne Weekly Gazette*, E. E. Byrum took up Smith's case and his question. Byrum's article "The Lord or Doctors, Which?" was a strong assertion that medical healing was not compatible with God's means of healing. It said that God's laws always took precedence over human laws, but, in the United States, human laws and God's laws were actually in accord. According to Byrum, the Constitution's protection of the free exercise of religion logically extended to divine healing, and therefore the law itself was on the side of the saints. However, the "opinions and make-beliefs of ungodly lawyers and doctors" often were not. Because there was no law that required taking medicine, the saints could practice divine healing confident that they were following God's laws and the laws of the land. If they had to go to jail for that, it was unfortunate and painful, but was part of God's plan to spread holiness. As Byrum wrote, "When a person is arrested and put in prison, if without compromise he stands true to God and acts as [God] directs in accordance with the word, although it may seem at the time, perhaps, to many, that it would be an awful disgrace upon the cause of Christ, yet the

Lord will get glory out of it in spreading his truth."[5] Thus, at the beginning of its experience with divine healing trials, the Church believed that the trials would spread the gospel and promote holiness.

The *Trumpet* followed closely the next three trials (Marion and Vincennes, Indiana; and Butler, Pennsylvania), interpreting each as a sign that the Church was doing something right. Just as Peter and John were incarcerated after drawing a crowd by performing miracles of healing (Acts 3:1–4:22), the Church was experiencing the persecution that followed naturally from making a bold stand for the truth.[6] Commenting on the Marion trial, Byrum wrote, "The time is here now for apostolical work and to be sure apostolical persecution will follow the same."[7] At this early stage, *persecution* was a sign to the church that it was properly offending the world by spreading the message of holiness, and *prosecution* was literally an opportunity to gain a hearing from the world. The saints "must expect now and then to be arrested for Christ's sake."[8]

This positive theological interpretation of prosecution did not mean, however, that the Church relished all opposition. Much of the commentary from the popular press never made it into the *Gospel Trumpet*. One example was an article from Vincennes, Indiana, about the arrest of Church of God member Thomas Wilson in connection with the death of his child. The *Trumpet* reprinted the story but omitted two important points. First was that Wilson's wife had also been very ill until her father came with a shotgun and insisted that she take medicine. After taking the medicine, her health improved. The other omission was that this child was the "third or fourth person that these people [meaning the congregation in Vincennes] have let die on account of their fanatical practices."[9] The *fact* of opposition to divine healing fit the Church's expectations and its stated desire to stand against the world. The *details* of that opposition, however, were often problematic. The readers of the *Gospel Trumpet* who saw only the edited report would have thought that the *Western Sun* had presented a much more positive testimony than was the case. The early articles in the *Gospel Trumpet*, therefore, presented these cases as simple contrasts between divine healing and human medical systems. They said that such a contrast would eventually work to spread the message that divine healing was far superior to human medical practice.

In addition to the overarching argument that divine healing was God's will for God's people, the articles in the *Trumpet* made more mundane cases for the legal protection of divine healing. The theological position was that divine healing was inherently superior to any possible kind of medicine and that the saints had to follow God's will no matter what the law demanded. In reality, the arguments said that any objective observer could see that divine healing was at least as effective as the medicine of the time, and, further, that no federal or state law banned divine healing.

The details in the *Trumpet* indicated that the Church's interaction with the medical establishments was complex. Medical science was still quite primitive at the end of the nineteenth century. Competing schools of thought, such as homeopathy and allopathy, prescribed radically different treatments for illnesses, and many of these treatments proved harmful. The editorials in the *Trumpet* and some of the arguments made on behalf of Church of God defendants in the courts noted that the states licensed doctors who practiced mutually contradictory systems. If any one of the medical practices were right—and the Church said none was—then the others logically had to be wrong. Thus, according to the Church of God, choosing one medical system over the others was an act of misplaced faith that had no more scientific basis than any other faith commitment.[10]

Moreover, many of the Church of God people involved in the divine healing trials abandoned medicine only after it did not work for them. The defendant in the Fort Wayne trial had suffered chronic indigestion for many years until he stopped taking the medicine given him by his physician and turned to prayer. When his children became sick, he prayed and also called a minister who was formerly a "regular practicing physician."[11] That divine healer may have been George Achor, one of the defendants in the Marion, Indiana trial. Achor had been a regular physician for twelve years before he entered the ministry and had even lectured on anatomy at the college in Marion. His wife, another of the defendants in the childbirth-related death case, was a midwife. The Achors had many connections with the medical establishment in Marion, and, according to the testimony, they did call a physician. That physician testified that the medicine he had prescribed aggravated the woman's condition and may have hastened her death.[12] In the Butler, Pennsylvania case, the defendant had called a doctor from the Board of Health who had misdiagnosed the child and said the boy was in no danger.[13] In the Missouri case of 1917, the reports conflict, but the defendant said that he had called a doctor but could not obtain medicine for his children.[14]

There were many connections between the Church of God people and doctors. The message of avoiding medicine notwithstanding, the reports of these trials indicate that Church of God people had tried medicine and continued to seek medical opinions even after affiliating with the Church. In the later cases, people called doctors and the Board of Health officials because it was required by law that they determine that the disease was not a danger to the community. The *Trumpet* followed the laws closely and published reports on exactly what the law required regarding medical attention. After the Marion case, E. E. Byrum wrote to all the Secretaries of State in the United States asking if their state had a law forcing a sick person to take medicine. None did.[15] Follow-up reports in 1902 explained that recent decisions in Ohio, Indiana, and California could not force the saints or their children to take medicine.[16]

Newspaper Reports

Newspaper coverage of the divine healing trials proved a serious obstacle to the spread of the Church's message. The idea that God was using these trials to publicize the truth about divine healing relied on the press to report accurately on the trials. In many cases, the newspapers reported only the arrest and the trial date. This was particularly a problem with dropped cases or cases decided in favor of the defendant.[17] When the newspapers did report, they were frequently inaccurate. Articles in Vincennes and Butler misidentified the Church of God as Christian Science.[18] Another newspaper in Vincennes correctly reported that the defendant was an "Evening Light Saint" but followed with the editorial comment "he is cranky on religion."[19] A few of the articles described how the Church members called the elders, anointed with oil, and followed James 5:13–15. Only the *New York Times* mentioned the Church of God, the *Gospel Trumpet,* or anything else that would have enabled a reader to learn more about the Church.[20]

In many instances, the Church found newspaper reports hostile or dismissive. According to the *Trumpet*, the editor of the *Marion Chronicle* was a chief instigator of the prosecution who "would love to see all the saints serve a term in the penitentiary, and doubtless would love to see them burned at the stake."[21] An editorial in a Fort Wayne newspaper suggested it was the other way around in that town. The judge merely fined the defendant who was "no doubt disappointed that he had not been condemned to the stake."[22] The mutual recrimination in the press and the *Trumpet* made it very difficult for the Church to spread its message.

The medical and legal reports were no better than those on religion. Most simply said that the defendants refused to use medicine of any kind. Some suggested that the practice of divine healing could pose a serious health risk for the community, although none of these cases involved diseases requiring quarantine.[23] The one editorial that did discuss medicine at length unintentionally demonstrated the primitive state of popular medical knowledge of the time. It argued that "these religious fanatics" confounded the body with the soul. However, the writer also told the story of an itinerant "Red Man" who had given a local man the secret of curing diphtheria. That knowledge unfortunately was lost. Still, human beings through medical experimentation had learned "all the functions of all the organs, excepting the Spleen." The Church of God people, according to this editorial, were returning to the "darkest of ages" by refusing to use science and medicine to discover the secrets of nature that were once known by Native Americans.[24]

Reports on legal decisions frequently noted only the crime charged, the court schedule, and the final decision of the court. In a few instances, the newspapers accurately reported that the courts had declared that the state could regulate behavior, even when that behavior related to religious belief. The Fort

Wayne, Indiana, and the Beaver, Oklahoma, papers both said that the court had declared that nothing restricts the *beliefs* of the Church members, just their *actions*. This missed the subtle point that restricting behavior did restrict belief, but the courts had ruled that the state could do so to protect the general welfare.[25] Another report from Fort Wayne added overzealously, "Deputy Thomas quoted Supreme Court decisions which say that faith cure attendance is not proper for sick people."[26]

Legal Decisions

The verdicts in most of these trials favored the defendants, but the trials themselves seldom progressed as the Church of God members had hoped. In order for the trials to set forth the Church's teachings about divine healing, the judges would have had to allow testimony about religion. This happened in only two of the reported cases.[27] In a third, the judge might have permitted testimony, but the counsel for the defense rested without argument because it thought the prosecution had not made the case.[28] Thus, the legal strategy for winning the case took precedence over testifying about divine healing. The charge to the jury in the Butler, Pennsylvania trial asserted that the case was "in no sense whatever a question of Christian faith or the efficacy of prayer," and therefore religious testimony was irrelevant and out of place.[29]

Defense lawyers did manage to introduce testimony about divine healing in the Butler case by finding a member of the Church who had studied with a regular physician and had a diploma for physiology and hygiene. However, the attempt to challenge the privileged status the court gave to expert medical testimony failed. The medically trained Church member explained to the court that the members of the Church of God followed James 5:14–15, which said that elders should be called to pray for the sick.[30] The judge undermined this testimony in his charge to the jury. He noted that the elders normally had no medical training or expertise.[31] He instructed the jurors that, since this was a case about caring for the sick, they were obliged to "consider carefully the testimony of the physicians called in this case."[32] Moreover, in regard to the testimony about the book of James, the judge said, "the same inspired writer, whose injunctions the defendant has sought so literally and conscientiously to observe, informs us that 'as the body, without the spirit, is dead, so faith without works is dead also.'"[33]

With the Butler, Pennsylvania decision of 1903, the Church had to abandon the argument that the First Amendment guaranteed the right to practice divine healing. Adults could choose to rely on prayer for healing, but everyone had to submit to medical examinations, and therefore the legally recognized superiority of medical knowledge, in cases involving communicable diseases. The state could even force children to take medicine. After the trial in Butler, the *Trumpet* included only brief notices of trials and arrests.

The change in editorial policy was most striking with the last major divine healing trial mentioned in the *Gospel Trumpet,* which went all the way to the Supreme Court of Oklahoma. On June 20, 1911, *Owens v. State of Oklahoma* upheld Lawrence Owens's conviction for misdemeanor child neglect.[34] This was the highest court a Church of God trial attained, and it presumably would have been a great opportunity to publicize the Church's teachings about healing and its opposition to medicine and coercive health laws. The Oklahoma newspapers covered the case, and it was arguably the most important legal decision related to the Church of God.[35] Further, the child had recovered, so *Owens* was nearly an exact parallel of the Fort Wayne case that received an entire divine healing page in 1897. By this time, however, the Church of God's reaction to divine healing trials had changed markedly, and there were only two brief notices about it in the *Gospel Trumpet.* The first was a "General Notes and News" item that said simply, "The case of Bro. Lawrence Owens is to be decided in the Supreme court [sic] in July."[36] Two years later, and almost an entire year after the final court decision, another note in the *Trumpet* said that Owens had lost both the county court case and the appeal, but that donations had covered all his expenses. Further, Lawrence Owens and his daughter were well and still in the faith.[37] The editors of the *Trumpet* clearly no longer wanted the saints to go to prison for Christ's sake.

Failure and Success

The most important lesson of the divine healing trials was that the experiences of the Church of God were not the same as those of the New Testament church. Peter and John had been persecuted for successful healings, not prosecuted for failures (Acts 4:16). Throngs of people believed and were converted, including Paul's jailer (Acts 4:4; 16:27–33). Moreover, in the time of the apostles, the Holy Spirit shook the prisons and opened the doors (Acts 5:19; 12:17; 16:26). In contrast, the Church of God's trials produced very few converts, and the closest thing to a sign from God was the plague the town of Butler, Pennsylvania, suffered after convicting one of the saints. This divine judgment may have comforted some members of the Church, but it was far from the miraculous unification of the saints for which they had hoped and prayed.[38]

In the first decade of the twentieth century, it was becoming clear that divine healing was not gathering all true Christians into the Church of God. The movement was about thirty years old and was growing quickly, but the worldwide reformation and the imminent return of Christ predicted by the first generation were becoming increasingly unlikely.[39] Church members were realizing that they could not completely separate from the world, and the world was not likely to end anytime soon. Therefore, they had to reevaluate their doctrines of healing. If divine healing was not the key to spreading the gospel—if healing did not have the same function in the evening light dispensation as in the morning light—then perhaps the Church of God had overstated it. Maybe spreading the gospel and living in the world required a selective use of divine healing.[40]

Quarantine and Inoculation

The smallpox epidemic of 1901 to 1903 compelled the *Trumpet* to clarify the Church's position on healing contagious diseases. It is impossible to say how many Church of God members contracted smallpox, but the disease would certainly have been an immediate concern for many of them. Among the areas hardest hit were the state of Ohio and the cities of Detroit and Chicago—centers of Church of God activity.[41] George Cole, the superintendent of the Church's missionary and healing home in Chicago, contracted smallpox in 1901 and was quarantined for five weeks. No announcement of his illness appeared in the *Trumpet*, but his condition must have been well known in the Church. Upon his release, he wrote to the *Trumpet* reporting his healing and thanking the saints for their prayers and letters of encouragement. He could not respond individually because he had burned the letters after reading them.[42]

This epidemic was the first major health crisis in the United States since the Church had begun emphasizing the doctrine of divine healing. A careful study of the trial reports shows that the *Trumpet* had always recommended cooperating with health officials in cases of contagious diseases. However, that message was easily lost under headings trumpeting the virtues of suffering legal persecution for divine healing. The saints were understandably confused about their religious and legal obligations, so this was a precarious situation for the movement. If a few of the saints had prayed the prayer of faith for smallpox and then gone about their normal routines, discounting lingering symptoms as temptations from the devil—standard procedure for non-contagious conditions—the negative publicity could have been devastating.[43] The last thing the leaders of the Church wanted was a reputation for spreading disease.

The May 23, 1901 issue of the *Trumpet* included two articles about quarantines. One explained that there were quarantines in the Bible and that Jesus had submitted to the law. According to the author, separation from the public had nothing to do with the belief in divine healing; so Church members were encouraged to follow secular laws for the benefit of those who did not know the Lord.[44] In the second article, E. E. Byrum told a story from 1896 about the Trumpet Home to show that quarantines were consistent with the historic practices of the Church of God. A member of the Trumpet Family, William Bixler, left the Trumpet Home to pray for his brother and nephew. They died from diphtheria, and Bixler was quarantined for a week longer than the law required, "due to religious prejudice." The day he returned to the Home, he began to show symptoms of diphtheria. Faith healed him but other members of the house became ill. A physician came to investigate on behalf of the county, and E. E. Byrum granted him permission to enter. However, the doctor declined to investigate because his experiences with the saints told him that they were law-abiding citizens who would be healed by prayer. The prayer of faith did heal them all, and this showed God's approval of the entire situation. Thus, Byrum concluded that notifying health officials was "right and proper, as it is for protection against the spread of infectious diseases."[45]

The saints appear to have accepted the argument that quarantines protected the unsaved. Protection of other Church members proved more difficult, because the afflicted wanted to attend divine healing services. In 1906, W. J. Henry exhorted *Trumpet* readers to be mindful of others. They should not expect to be greeted with the holy kiss if they had a disease. Children should not attend meetings where there is sickness, and diseased children should not come to meetings. Henry anticipated the objection that Church members "ought to have faith enough not to get [the disease], or to get healed if they do get it." He replied, "[Y]ou ought to have faith enough to get healed; or, if you do not, you ought to have love enough for your brethren and the cause of Christ not to spread it."[46]

Henry's warning was insufficient. In 1909, E. E. Byrum tried another tack. He said that a few years previous someone with smallpox attended the camp meeting. If God had not softened the heart of the health official, the camp could have been closed. A few more incidents like that one could have jeopardized the entire camp meeting system.[47] The Camp Meeting Committee minutes for 1913 reported that a father had brought two tubercular children and that "Sister Luther's daughter has whooping cough." The Committee decided to isolate the children in a tent and asked Sister Luther to please be careful with her daughter. E. E. Byrum also made an announcement to the entire assembly that contagious diseases were not to be brought to camp meeting. In 1916, the Camp Meeting Committee placed a notice in the *Trumpet* asking everyone with a contagious disease to stay away.[48] For the good of the whole movement, the afflicted needed to stay away from camp meetings, refrain from calling the elders, and write for a handkerchief.[49]

Another development from the smallpox epidemic was compulsory vaccination. By 1906, several school boards required students to be vaccinated before enrolling. The new policies "caused a furor" and much confusion. Parents who wanted to send their children to school feared that vaccines violated the prohibition of medicines. No one *had* to go to school, so what were the saints to do? E. E. Byrum assured them that they could submit to the regulations imposed by school boards. He was certain that inoculations did not do any good and had been foisted on well-meaning school officials by doctors and drug companies, but parents should give them to their children so as not to bring hostility to the child, the family, or the Church of God.[50] Serious damage to the Church's reputation would have resulted if an un-inoculated Church of God child exposed other schoolchildren to disease. Further, immunization was not the same as medicine. It fell under the biblical injunction to be subject to the ruling authorities. It was an imposition on a well person, not a remedy designed to cure a sick one. Thus, Byrum told Church of God members to accept the shot and trust God to protect them from the poison.[51] Technically, vaccines and quarantines did not violate the divine healing doctrine of the Church. In practice, they were significant concessions designed to show that Church members were good neighbors.

Remedies and Medicines

Accepting vaccinations and quarantines was not the same as embracing medicine. E. E. Byrum in particular worked hard to remind the members of the Church of the distinction. The straightforward approach was to reprint articles by physicians and scientists who opposed particular drugs.[52] An important subset consisted of medical doctors who rejected vaccinations. Byrum discovered a Dr. Hodge of New York who said that the smallpox vaccination was toxic, and William Hickman, M.D., said that inoculations stripped youth of its vitality and turned a girl's blood into contagious poison. Medical opinion, in Byrum's estimation, was turning against vaccinations and aligning with the Word of God.[53]

A subtler approach turned a standard argument against faith healing back on the medical establishment. Byrum suggested that unethical doctors played on the credulity and fears of the American people to bilk them of their money. Honest doctors did the same, but they did so from delusions of healing power.[54] Commenting on the American Medical Association's efforts to establish a National Health Bureau and to enforce the examination of all schoolchildren by an allopathic physician, Byrum said they were sly attempts to instill the idea that doctors were "the saviors of the race." The amount of money and effort expended on improbable treatments proved to Byrum that religion was failing and the "medical trust" was succeeding. One example was congressman Robert Gunn Bremner, who died impoverished after spending over $100,000 for a radium treatment for cancer.[55]

A particularly interesting article by Byrum told of a new treatment for tuberculosis that was attracting crowds to a doctor in New York City. According to the newspaper, Friedrich Franz Friedmann, a medical doctor from Berlin, was curing tuberculosis in humans with injections of a strain of the disease found in turtles. As one would expect, Byrum noted that doctors in Germany and the United States opposed this treatment as dangerously experimental. He also asked rhetorically who was trustworthy, God or a man taking tuberculosis out of turtles. Then the article took an important turn. Byrum observed that throngs of people had gone to New York to visit the doctor because he promised to heal them, just as people had done with Jesus. Friedmann had nothing to give them other than an injection, but Byrum believed the doctor's example should have been a model for the Church of God. True "Apostolic healing power" could have brought throngs of people to the healing of soul and body. If a man and a turtle could produce crowds, then the Church should have been ashamed for two reasons. It was not bringing in nearly enough converts, and its message of healing had failed to keep people from listening to doctors like Friedmann. Thus, the *Trumpet* reminded readers that doctors did not deserve their faith, and divine healing was "super scientific: far superior to man's science; so far superior that man's attempts are, comparatively speaking, exceedingly foolish."[56]

If the only challenge to the Church's commitment to divine healing had been medical treatments for cancer and tuberculosis, divine healing might have continued without revision well into the middle of the twentieth century. However, medical healing also included material remedies for less catastrophic conditions, and the Pure Food and Drug Act of 1906 ensured for the first time government oversight of patent medicines. These remedies were the first to attract the saints.[57] In fact, one of the most important players in the transformation of the Church's practice of divine healing was the itch mite. Infestations of these bugs were common and painful, but a solution of carbolic acid and water brought quick relief. Willis M. Brown, a successful healing evangelist, reported on a camp meeting in the late 1890s where everyone got the itch. Most relied on prayer for healing, but Willis's son Charley—who grew up to become the fourth editor of the *Gospel Trumpet*—continued to suffer after his father had prayed for him. He lost his faith in divine healing and left the camp to seek treatment from his uncle who was a doctor. The uncle did not want to contribute to Charley's delinquency, so he suggested they pray together. Charley observed that his father's specialty was praying for healing and that had failed. He wanted the doctor to try medicine.[58]

In 1909, the itch mite returned to the Church. A writer pointedly asked Byrum if it was "more to the glory of God" for him to apply the carbolic acid or "to trust the Lord and be unable to work, suffer untold misery, and endanger others for months." Byrum thought this was a false dichotomy; he and many others had relied on faith and had been healed quickly. Because the statement of the question showed a lack of faith in healing, however, he had to recommend the medicine in this case. Byrum had also heard of saints testifying that they would never use a remedy for the itch. God never required such testimony. As long as they were under the vow, they could not use the remedy. However, if they received "new light" on the subject, they could so testify and then use the carbolic acid with a clear conscience.[59]

Those Not Healed

In a sense, the *Trumpet* was testifying to new light on the limits and requirements of divine healing when it counseled the saints to accept quarantines, inoculations, and some kinds of medicine. Reckless statements from the 1890s led to unexpected consequences when the saints encountered the epidemics and societal pressures of the twentieth century. When a radical reliance on divine healing imperiled the camp meetings, barred Church of God children from schools, and made an itch mite infestation into a crisis of faith, revisions and clarifications became necessary. The changes implied that the Church had over-stated the testimonial function of divine healing.

None of the above-mentioned challenges affected the central idea behind divine healing: if a person met the conditions for physical healing, God would grant it. This idea proved remarkably resilient. The saints managed to explain most cases in which God did not answer the prayers as they had expected. Undisclosed sins or imperfect faith were options. Another was that the person had reached the appointed time for death. The early trials showed that suffering and dying for the promotion of the cause of Christ was yet another explanation. The fact that the Church consisted of individuals and congregations spread out across the country and united by the *Gospel Trumpet* greatly facilitated this kind of argument. The *Trumpet* reported many successes and few failures, giving the impression of a great movement of healing in the Church that overshadowed any local disappointments. Failures from distant congregations would have been sad, but would not shake faith. If the victim were not a personal friend, it would have been easier to attribute suffering and death to one of the above-mentioned reasons than to question the theology of divine healing. Thus, the structure of the Church impeded the collection of convincing examples of unanswered prayers. However, in the early twentieth century, tragedies befell people with wide reputations for holiness. The circumstances of these cases were a difficult test for divine healing and contributed to a revision of the Church's doctrine.

The first happened just a year after seventy Church of God ministers signed an affirmation of the divine healing in the atonement doctrine. At the 1903 camp meeting in Claypool, Indiana, twin infant daughters of Clarence and Nora Hunter became ill and died, despite fasting and fervent prayers by all the ministers. To suggest that this assembly lacked faith for healing was unthinkable. The girls themselves were too young to have sinned or to understand God's reproof, so they could not have caused the sickness. Moreover, the parents were tireless evangelists who had unimpeachable reputations for holiness.[60]

The only explanation in Hunter's report to the *Trumpet* was that "the Lord gave, and the Lord hath taken away." God called the girls to heaven, but had shown mercy by doing so at a camp meeting where he and Nora would have comfort from the saints. Additionally, God had in fact answered their prayers. After they requested healing, God let them know that their prayers "were of no avail as far as restoration to health was concerned." They needed to trust God and pray in accordance with God's will. Nora asked God to relieve the suffering, and "God recognized [her] prayer by letting his glory fill the room and soon our little one was asleep in the arms of Jesus."

Hunter concluded with a quote from a poem: "He gives his very best to those/who leave the choice to him."[61] Soon thereafter he channeled his grief into writing a new hymn, "God's Way is Best." The third verse states the theme well and shows that this hymn was a significant departure from the Church's prevailing theology of divine healing:

He leadeth true; I will not question; Tho' thro' the valley I shall go,
Tho' I should pass thro' clouds of trial, And drink the cup of human woe.
God's way is best, I will not murmur, Although the end I may not see;
Where'er he leads I'll meekly follow—God's way is best, is best for me.[62]

Hunter's hymn acknowledged that God's purposes lay beyond human understanding. Divine healing hymns also said God's way was best, but they meant that divine healing was the best way to obtain physical healing. Hunter meant that following God's will was best, whether God chose to heal or not.

The single most important person in the reinterpretation of the Church's doctrine of divine healing was Charles Wesley Naylor (1874–1950), Hunter's collaborator on "God's Way is Best." Naylor joined the Trumpet Family just before D. S. Warner's death in 1895 and soon began writing and preaching. At least two of his contributions to the *Trumpet* defended divine healing.[63] In 1908, Naylor was critically injured in a tent accident at a camp meeting in Florida. Prayer did nothing to relieve the pain or improve his mobility. Two years later, a car accident left him physically incapacitated, and he was confined to a bed for his remaining forty years.[64]

Naylor's protracted suffering was a significant problem for the Church's advocates of divine healing. Some "insisted that he was the worst thing that ever happened to the movement's theology of healing."[65] A few even suggested that Naylor was responsible for his condition and that God's delay in granting healing indicated sin or lack of faith. An unsigned editorial in the *Trumpet* said, "The Lord doubtless has some lesson for [Brother Naylor]."[66] This was a reasonable conclusion given the previously published explanations for unanswered prayers.

Yet, Naylor rejected all allegations of sin or faithlessness. Unlike previous cases, Naylor would not go away. He lived a long time just off the campgrounds in Anderson, he remained a faithful member of the Church of God and a prolific hymn writer, and he periodically wrote to the *Trumpet* to report that he had not received physical healing. In 1912, for instance, he wrote to remind the saints— especially the ministers, who never wrote to him—that he was still alive and was never free from suffering. He also asked that correspondents "not try to write comforting letters." He was not despairing, so the most comforting letters told of God's work in the Church. Similar reports in 1913 and 1914 said that Naylor saw no improvement but was "enjoying the blessings of the Lord."[67] Thus, readers of the *Trumpet* could not escape the fact that the man who wrote the songs of praise they sang on Sunday mornings was confined to a hospital bed. For most of the saints, Naylor's testimony to sanctification—in the *Trumpet* and especially in his hymns—was too persuasive to ignore. There had to be some reason for Naylor's physical condition. His own explanation was that God did indeed have a lesson for him and the Church. It took a while to develop the full implications, but the lesson was that the Church's entire theology of suffering and pain was wrong.

In 1919, the Gospel Trumpet Co. published *Winning a Crown*, Naylor's first contribution to the Christian Life Series. The subtitle, "A practical treatise on how to find God, what salvation is and does, and how to live a happy and successful Christian life," sounded like another guide to home, health, and success. However, the preface—which Naylor wrote in the third person—indicated differently: "For the past nine years [Naylor] has been a shut-in as the result of a serious injury, but these years upon his bed, with Pain for his constant companion, have taught him many things that might have escaped him the in the busy days of a more active life."[68] Specifically, he learned that winning the crown of salvation required pressing on to the goal despite trials and tribulations. The sanctified life was not a magical deliverance from every problem. Those who believed it was lacked true faith and found every challenge a stumbling block. "As children of God," Naylor wrote, "we are still human. And with others we must bear the things that belong to human life—its cares, its perplexities, its unsolved problems, its frailties, in fact, all those things which fall to the lot of other mortals."[69] Although he did not specifically mention physical pain, his condition implied that a Christian life did not guarantee physical healing.[70]

Irregular Healings

Successful healings were as problematic as failures when people used them to promote doctrines contrary to those of the Church of God. Testimony after testimony in the *Trumpet* had identified healings as proof of sanctification, holy living, renunciation of Babylon, or some other spiritual development. E. E. Byrum and other ministers pointed to healing as proof that God was well pleased with the evening light reformation. When the Church granted healing this much significance, cases of healing occurring outside the movement required careful explanation. To simply deny that the healings had occurred would have cast doubt on all healing testimonies, thereby aiding the Church's critics. The Church of God found itself in the difficult position of having to affirm the healing testimonies of Catholics, Spiritualists, Mormons, and Christian Scientists while rejecting the theological claims of those groups.

In 1901, J. W. Byers wrote an article specifically addressing the problems posed by divine healing. Byers had a long history of interaction with other healing groups. He began his ministry of healing because a Spiritualist in his neighborhood in Los Angeles was performing healings and leading people away from Christianity. Byers believed that the Christian church needed to have similar power to compete for adherents, so he prayed for the gifts of healing. God granted the request in 1895. Byers then moved to Oakland to open a divine healing home near to Carrie Judd Montgomery's Home of Peace. In contrast to his relations with the Spiritualist, Byers appears to have approved of Montgomery's work, at least until she joined the Pentecostal movement. He provided contact information for her and advertised her book *The Prayer of Faith* in his periodical. One testimony from Byers's book suggests that he and Montgomery may have worked together.[72] In any case, from his locations in Los Angeles and Oakland, Byers encountered a variety of groups that performed healings, and he saw firsthand how divine healing could pull people away from the Church of God.[73]

The first problem Byers addressed, however, was the internal challenge divine healing could create. He said it was common to find people who believed their healings proved that they were right and pleasing to God, even though they were "living contrary to the word of God." At a recent Church of God camp meeting, Byers had confronted a man who was "introducing non-scriptural beliefs." The man appealed to a healing of a child he had performed as evidence of God's approval. This clearly was a problem, and Byers offered several explanations. One possibility was that the child himself had faith for healing, so the man's ministrations were irrelevant. Perhaps the healing power coursed through the other ministers who prayed and anointed. A final explanation was simply that man could perform healing because he "believed that much of the truth," but Byers insisted, "the healing was no evidence of the approval of God upon the error." The saints had to reject anything that was not according to the gospel, no matter how plausible or effective. Separating faith for healing from holy living and theological rectitude was an important step in reducing the significance of divine healing.[74]

Byers also cited the case of a friend who had been healed by a Christian Science practitioner. The woman was grateful for the relief and concluded that Mary Baker Eddy was right and Christian. She decided to study Christian Science, so she obtained Eddy's book *Science and Health.* According to Byers, she was perceptive and saw that Christian Science made "Christ's blood to no effect." However, the woman's experience with healing had been so powerful that she concluded that she must have misunderstood the Bible. Byers eventually succeeded in reclaiming her for Christianity, but many were not so lucky. What then explained the healing? Byers said this was an example of an honest and devout soul who did not have enough light but did have a relationship with God. It happened in various religions that, in spite of the preachers and the false doctrines, people grasped and appropriated divine healing. In this specific case, the woman did not learn anything about Christian Science until after her healing. The Christian Science practitioner had only required her to read the Bible, not *Science and Health.* One could therefore obtain divine healing directly from God even when associated with a heretical movement. This created the illusion that Christian Science or Spiritualism had power for healing.[75]

Byers's final example was John Alexander Dowie, the most prominent divine healer in the United States at the turn of the century. Byers believed that Dowie's success was due to his preaching. Whatever else was wrong with his message—and there was a lot from the Church of God's perspective—Dowie was right about divine healing, and God was answering his prayers. Those who were healed by him, however, should have considered themselves on probation. God had touched their lives, so they needed to pursue the truth and conform to God's standards, or else they would have to pay a price.[76] Thus, divine healing could exist on its own, separate from the rest of a ministry. Successful healings showed only that God approved of the message of healing. Byers adopted a similar perspective with respect to the Pentecostal movement, accepting the healings but rejecting the doctrine of tongues.[77]

Institutional Development

The Gospel Trumpet Co. published C. W. Naylor's first book about suffering for the gospel and E. E. Byrum's final book about divine healing in the same year, 1919. Just a few years earlier, publishing antithetical books about healing would have been unthinkable. The editors would have interpreted Naylor's book as a direct challenge to their ministerial authority. However, by 1919 the Church of God movement had begun a radical restructuring. Between 1916 and 1926, the organization of the work of the Church changed from a loose affiliation of charismatic leaders into a managerial bureaucracy, complete with ministerial credentialing committees, a training school, and a General Assembly.[78] The change in polity affected all aspects of the movement's self-perception, but its significance for this study is that spiritual gifts—divine healing in particular—became less important for the day-to-day life of the Church. Ordained ministers who were employed by congregations and were active participants in the General Ministerial Assembly did not need to perform miracles to attract crowds and claim authority. Similarly, people who attended Church of God congregations and camp meetings, contributed to the national and international ministries of the Church, and followed the behavioral strictures of the movement were confident in their membership status, even without divine healing. Therefore, divine healing became one aspect of the ministry of the Church, largely performed by traveling specialists. This separation ensured that successful healings would function as evidence of the return of the apostolic power, but failures would not undermine the movement as a whole.

E. E. Byrum's career is the best illustration of the de-centering of divine healing. In 1916, resentment over Byrum's heavy-handed managerial practices led—for the first time—to a formal separation between the positions of president and editor-in-chief of the Gospel Trumpet Co. Byrum resigned the editorship under pressure but retained the presidency. F. G. Smith became the new editor. One year later, at the June 1917 camp meeting, the entire structure of the Church changed in an attempt to "place the great work [of publishing] in more immediate touch with the ministry, and thereby increase the responsibility for and interest in this important phase of Gospel work."[79] In other words, the company was in debt and hoped to improve relations with the Church members.

The governing board of the Gospel Trumpet Co.—which included E. E. Byrum—met for four days to amend the Articles of Incorporation. Under the old structure, the company legally had no formal ties to the Church of God movement. The board of directors was independent and self-perpetuating. The new plan provided for the election of all board members by the General Ministerial Assembly, which also had the sweeping power to "'expel' any of those members 'for cause'."[80] At the same time, the committee to draft the constitution and by-laws for the General Ministerial Assembly was meeting so that there would be an Assembly to govern the Gospel Trumpet Co.[81] By the end of camp meeting, in addition to all the other changes, J. T. Wilson was elected president, leaving E. E. Byrum without a major office in the Gospel Trumpet Co. for the first time in thirty years.[82] According to the report in the *Trumpet*, "All things of the meeting have been marked by a sweet spirit of unity that is convincing to those who visit these camp grounds that God is truly in our midst."[83]

E. E. Byrum used his new freedom from editorial work to focus exclusively on the ministry of divine healing. He maintained an office and a prayer room at the Gospel Trumpet Co., the latter decorated with crutches, medicine bottles, and braces left behind by those who had been healed.[84] Most of his time, however, was spent traveling. Byrum covered over 41,000 miles in 1920 anointing the sick and holding divine healing services. A biographical note in the *Trumpet* in 1924 said he was "traveling almost constantly in all parts of the United States in answer to calls to instruct or pray for the afflicted."[85]

With Byrum gone from the *Trumpet*, its emphasis on divine healing gradually decreased. It is not clear how intentional this was. The new editor, F. G. Smith, believed in divine healing and affirmed the strongest statements of the doctrine, although he initially expressed some reservations about the atonement doctrine.[86] In *What the Bible Teaches*, he wrote, "the Lord has been pleased to grant divine healing as a sort of forerunner of immortality," and further, "the ministry of healing belongs to all of God's ministers and is part of their regular work."[87] In no sense, however, was divine healing as important to Smith as it was to Byrum. Smith prayed for healing, but he and his wife also called for a doctor and gave medicine to their sick children.[88] He may have used Byrum's absence as an opportunity to change the direction of the *Trumpet*. It is more likely, however, that the greatly increased official activities of the Church—including home and foreign missions, Church Extension, education, Christian education and Sunday school, free literature campaigns, and publishing for the blind—demanded attention and space in the publication. Without Byrum to write and solicit divine healing articles, other topics displaced healing. In any case, under Smith's editorship the divine healing page lost its place of honor in the *Trumpet*. It became a column like those for "The Sunday School" and "The Family Circle," and its placement in the *Trumpet* became unpredictable, no longer occupying the final page of every issue. By 1926, most issues lacked a divine healing page or column.[89]

At the same time, Byrum began to show affinity with divine healing evangelists who were not associated with the Church of God movement. *Miracles and Healing* (1919) was his first book to acknowledge material from outside the Church of God. The "Witnesses of Today" section mentioned Dorothea Trudel, Charles Cullis, and Mrs. Sarah Mix. Byrum included Carrie Judd's entire testimony from *The Prayer of Faith*, and he printed a testimony from Maggie H. Scott, who is notable here only because she received healing not from Byrum but from Cullis, Mix, and Judd.[90] Byrum's recognition of legitimate healing faith outside of the Church of God was a remarkable development that shows that Byrum believed that the message of divine healing could overcome denominational barriers.[91]

More remarkable was an issue of the *National Labor Tribune* entirely devoted to "E. E. Byrum, Mighty Miracle Man of God, Author of Great Works on Divine Healing." The *Tribune*, published in Pittsburgh, Pennsylvania, from its founding in 1872, claimed to be "The Oldest and most Conservative labor paper in America," and its masthead promised to reflect the "opinions, conditions, and demands of 30,000,000 American Toilers." According to Arno C. Gaebelein, it was also the advertising medium of choice for F. F. Bosworth and his divine healing crusade.[92]

F. F. Bosworth (1877–1958) was a Pentecostal pioneer and a healing evangelist. As a young man he was director of John Alexander Dowie's Zion City, Illinois, band. When he received the gift of tongues in 1906 under the guidance of Charles F. Parham, Bosworth left Zion to found an independent charismatic church in Dallas. He was one of the founding members of the Assemblies of God until he left the denomination over a dispute about the "initial evidence" of tongues. He affiliated with the Christian and Missionary Alliance in 1918, and he began holding large healing revivals in 1920. The meeting in Pittsburgh reportedly produced 4,800 conversions, and the one in Detroit saw a woman healed of blindness. Bosworth remained an important figure among divine healers into the mid-century and was one of the few living links between Dowie and the 1950s revivals of William Branham and Oral Roberts.[93]

Bosworth's affiliations made him an unlikely companion for E. E. Byrum; yet, they worked together for at least one revival and planned to work together in Anderson. This connection explains the *Tribune*'s interest in Byrum. A large-type advertisement in the issue said, "America's Greatest Bodily Healing Camp Meeting June 12 to 19. E. E. Byrum and F. F. Bosworth to be present. All roads are leading to Anderson, Indiana, where the great camp meeting opens June 12. Multitudes of sick and afflicted will be dealt with there." The announcement added that Byrum had participated in Bosworth's evangelistic campaign in Detroit, where he personally invited Bosworth to the Anderson camp meeting.[94] Another notice reiterated that Bosworth was coming to camp meeting. This one featured a photograph of a throng of people standing outside the Anderson tabernacle. The text explained:

> Here vast crowds are seen waiting on the outside of the auditorium, while
> E. E. Byrum, author of 'Miracles of [sic] Healing,' the man of mighty
> power, and other workers are conducting Divine healing services on the
> inside and praying for the sick and afflicted, many of whom are in the last
> stages of some dread disease or maimed, crippled, blind, deaf, or racked
> with palsy or writhing with epilepsy.... It is evident the crowds shown in
> the accompanying cut cannot be accommodated in the auditorium and
> many are left to take their turn or await Byrum's presence on the outside.

Byrum may indeed have been preaching in the tabernacle, but the photograph was obviously posed and not an overflow crowd. Moreover, in stark contrast to the description, the people shown on the campground appeared happy and healthy.[95] The implication of the *National Labor Tribune* was that the Church of God camp meeting—the occasion for the General Ministerial Assembly, Mission Board meetings, and every other form of Church business—was a nondenominational divine healing meeting with Byrum as the central attraction.

It is impossible to determine the degree to which Byrum was responsible for this portrait of himself and the Church of God. The *National Labor Tribune* was interested in promoting F. F. Bosworth's healing campaign, not the Church of God camp meeting. Their writers likely created the caption for the photograph. However, the editors must have thought that the meeting would be congenial for Bosworth. This impression could only have come from Byrum and *Miracles and Healing.* By working with F. F. Bosworth and inviting him to Anderson, E. E. Byrum was working as a healing evangelist first and a Church of God minister second. According to the *National Labor Tribune*, Byrum's labors were "nonsectarian, responding to calls wherever duty demands, indifferent to creed or party, seeking only to relieve the suffering who will believe in the Lord Jesus Christ and his teaching."[96]

F. F. Bosworth never came to camp meeting. The *Trumpet* never mentioned that Byrum worked with him or invited him to camp meeting. There was not even a note about the issue of the *Tribune* devoted to Byrum. The silence regarding Byrum's participation in a nationally famous healing campaign combined with the fact that no one other than Byrum extended an invitation to Bosworth illustrates Byrum's decreasing influence in the Church. Byrum was the acknowledged divine healing specialist, but that did not mean that he could invite evangelists from outside the Church of God to transform camp meeting into a healing revival.

Theological Revision

By the time of the Church's reorganization, its functional doctrine of divine healing had changed markedly from the doctrine the Church articulated at the beginning of the twentieth century in *Grace and Healing* and *The Great Physician*. This early doctrine—generally called "the atonement" doctrine—had three main points.[97] First, God's will for healing was perfectly clear to human beings. Jesus' atonement was for sin and sickness, and "the prayer of faith shall save the sick." All Christians who met the conditions for healing would receive the perfect cure; therefore, praying "if it be thy will" completely misunderstood God's self-revelation. At best this form of prayer was ineffectual; at worst it was a crutch used by those who wanted to blame God for their faithlessness. Second, the gospel of healing was the gospel of Jesus Christ. All true ministers had to preach and perform divine healing. The duties of an elder as described in the epistle of James showed that all ministers needed the gifts of healing, so separating healing from Christian ministry crippled the ministry. Third, faith for healing demanded action. People who truly believed that God would heal acted on that belief and abandoned other remedies. All other healing systems were at best temporary fixes for those unacquainted with the Lord, and no true saint would see the use of medicine as anything other than a lack of faith. The sections above have shown that each of these points figuratively received an asterisk in the early twentieth century. All the Church lacked to complete the doctrinal revision were theological statements matching the Church's practices. These first appeared in Gospel Trumpet Co. literature in the 1920s.

God's Will

The text of the Church's strongest refutation of divine healing theology, C. W. Naylor's *God's Will and How to Know It* (1926), never mentioned healing. Naylor chose less controversial examples such as prayers for success or money. However, the book's front matter effectively inserted God's will *for healing* into every discussion of God's will. The first printed page was a photograph of the author in his bed holding an open Bible. The caption directed the reader to the publisher's statement "concerning the author," which reported on Naylor's accidents and explained the apparent contradiction between physical condition and his expertise concerning God's will. According to the notice, he was "peculiarly qualified for his task by a training of the soul in the school of suffering." His joy in the face of lifelong pain testified to a particularly advanced and blessed spiritual state. Physical debility in this case was not evidence of sin or a lack of faith in God's power to heal: In fact, the publisher claimed that

> Though a firm believer in divine healing, and instrumental in the healing
> of those who kneel at his bedside for prayer, yet he has not received per-

manent healing, because, as he believes, this is God's method of developing his heart and making him more useful in helping others.[98]

Naylor knew suffering and also the power of healing. God certainly would
not use a minister to impart healing if he were unsaved or heretical.

The book was an extended discussion of the sanctified life and the divine
will. Its stated purpose was to share Naylor's thoughts on "daily problems" with
those who "have not been able to solve some of them to their own satisfaction."
Many of these people had written Naylor for advice.[99] He explained that many
Christians were burdened with a great misconception about living according to
God's will. Those outside the holiness movement too often thought God's will
was unknowable or impossible to follow. Naylor affirmed the Church of God's
belief that "it is our great privilege to know the will of God, to abide in it, and to
do it." However, he also corrected the misconceptions of holiness people who
frequently mistook their own desires for God's. Knowing and following the divine will required a willingness to be led into God's will and away from one's
own.[100] God was good and willed good for human beings, but—in contrast to the
popular conception of divine healing—Naylor said that that did not imply that
God would grant everything humans thought they wanted. To presume to know
God's will was to close oneself off from God, and the picture at the front of the
book showed that one could not presume that God willed physical healing.
Therefore, every legitimate prayer implicitly or explicitly followed Jesus' example, saying "thy will be done."[101]

The Gifts of Healing

The second part of the Church's divine healing doctrine—all ministers should
have the gifts of healing—logically would have succumbed to *God's Will and
How to Know It*, given enough time. A direct challenge expedited the process. In
1924, the *Trumpet* published Naylor's four-part series on spiritual gifts.[102] He
was responding to the success of the Pentecostal movement, and his primary
goal was to show that Pentecostals had an unscriptural doctrine of the gift of
tongues. However, he chose to reevaluate spiritual gifts in general, showing that
there were no universal gifts. Because glossolalia had never been a significant
focus in the Church of God, these articles implied more for divine healing than
for tongues.

Naylor specifically opposed the "theory that every preacher already has [the
gifts of healing]." This was, it will be remembered, E. E. Byrum's breakthrough
insight that inspired *Divine Healing of Soul and Body* and propelled him into the
ministry of healing. Naylor refrained from mentioning Byrum's name but did
say, "such theology is based upon a misinterpretation or misapplication of certain texts which contain no trace of this idea when rightly interpreted."[103] Further, Naylor claimed that preaching this theory was actually interfering with

healing by crippling the general ministry's ability to pray the prayer of faith. Many ministers "tried to make themselves believe they had the gift when at the same time they were convinced that they did not have it."[104] No healing power could come from such false testimony. Naylor himself experienced this. Once he quit trying to make himself believe that he had the gift of healing, he became able to pray the prayer of faith and follow James 5:14–15 "with a fairly good degree of success."[105] Thus, the prayer of faith—a requirement for every minister and, to a lesser extent every saint—had nothing to do with the gift of healing.[106]

It is important to note that Naylor affirmed all the spiritual gifts, including tongues and healing. In no way did he deny that an individual had a specific spiritual gift. His problem was with any doctrine that limited God's freedom to bestow gifts or that exalted one gift over another. "The prophet prophesies, the minister ministers, the teacher teaches, the exhorters exhort, the rulers rule with diligence, all do their part, and all things work together for the edification of the body."[107] Every gift was important and given for a specific purpose. Only God could know the needs of the body of Christ; therefore, the ministry of healing was a—not the—ministry of the Church.[108]

Healing Divine

The Gospel Trumpet Co. published J. Grant Anderson's *Divine Healing* in 1926, one year after *God's Will and How to Know It*. Anderson edited the "Home Problems" department of the *Trumpet* and wrote *Sex Life and Home Problems*. He was an expert on diet, hygiene, and relationships, not the ministry of divine healing. The introduction by H. M. Riggle, whose prayers led to Anderson's miraculous healing from tuberculosis, detailed Anderson's work as an evangelist and member of the Gospel Trumpet Co. but did not mention a single prayer for healing.[109] Riggle commended the book because Anderson knew divine healing as a recipient: "What minister can better feed the church with food than he who himself has tasted thereof? The writer, in this instance like the husbandman of old, has first been a partaker of the fruit."[110] Anderson's own justification was that he had "combed all available literature on the subject," especially the works of "Gordon, Torrey, Bosworth, La Rose, Byrum, and Lindhahr."[111]

Anderson was more interested in divine healing than in the ministry of divine healing. His object in writing was "that afflicted persons understand and obtain the privileges and blessings made possible through the suffering and death of Jesus Christ, our Lord."[112] To that end, *Divine Healing*'s first section provided the scripture and arguments to prove that it was God's eternal will to grant physical healing, and the second section consisted of testimonies. The only significant difference between these sections and earlier Church of God books about divine healing was that Anderson never mentioned the gifts of healing.

Ministers were of little consequence, as were the prayers of the elders. Healing came through faith and a personal relationship with Jesus.

The truly remarkable feature of *Divine Healing* was its final section, "Vital Facts on Health." The entire chapter explained the six laws of health: right eating, right drinking, right breathing, right thinking, right exercising, and right sleeping.[113] Much of the material had appeared before in other Gospel Trumpet literature, and it is only surprising here because Anderson used it to conclude a book about divine healing. The part about right thinking, however, was a departure that suggested a scientific explanation for faith cure:

> Health conditions must first be established in the mind. The afflicted person should form a mental picture of a person in perfect health, strong, robust, with reservoirs of natural forces overflowing. Dr. Coué was not far from truth when he taught the afflicted to repeat: Every day in every way I'm getting better and better.[114]

This was surprisingly close to saying that prayer was a form of right thinking that automatically and without divine intervention healed the body. In any case, healing derived from harmony with God's laws, not from miraculous power.

Anderson retained the part of the radical doctrine of divine healing that promised that health was part of God's perfect plan and that the prayer of faith always brought a cure. Naylor's criticisms had not affected Anderson. However, Anderson stretched the definition of divine healing, suggesting that all health— be it from faith, observing God's laws, positive thinking, or some other source— was divine. He stopped short of affirming medicine but only because he considered it unreliable.[115] His quotes from doctors who opposed drugs were irenic. For example, he chose to include Dr. W. Hutchinson's opinion that "No drugs, save quinine and mercury, will cure a disease; only rest, food, sunshine, and fresh air can do that miracle." This was hardly a condemnation of medicine, and it was a deflation of the kinds of "miracles" that brought healing. Thus, healing was a benefit from God, but it was not a system in conflict with medicine.

At the 1928 Anderson camp meeting, Herbert McClellan Riggle—noted healing minister, J. Grant Anderson's mentor, and president of the Publication Board of the Gospel Trumpet Co.—exhorted the Church of God to preach and practice divine healing.[116] It was part of the atonement and the commission, so the Church must not neglect divine healing. However, Riggle's sermon continued Anderson's work and subtly redefined divine healing to emphasize "healing" rather than "divine," minimizing the importance of miracles and the opposition to medicine. He insisted that divine healing as taught by the Church of God was not "fanaticism or extremism." It bore no relation to Christian Science, mind healing, or to "so-called 'divine healers' floating all over the country ... trying to assume the appearance of a Messiah."[117] The kind of divine healing practiced by the Church of God was, Riggle believed, a "doctrine that, commonly understood, can be accepted by the medical profession and by all people the world over if only they will understand it."[118]

In essence, divine healing was "healing by divine power administered by the virtues of the Lord Jesus Christ though the instrumentality of the Holy Ghost." The Bible proved that healing was a fact resting on the "same basis as salvation, altho less important." Testimonies also showed that divine healing was working inside and outside the Church of God. None of these—the definition, the Bible, or the testimonies—stated exactly how divine healing worked. Riggle resisted attempts to put a finer point on how God granted healing. Referring to Mark 16—a classic proof text for gifts of healing—he said:

> "They shall lay hands on the sick," folks, and after they inquire for healing, does it say that they shall get a voice in the air somehow that will work a miracle for them? My Book does not read that way. "They shall lay hands on the sick and they shall recover."[119]

The saints were to follow God's plan in the Bible and expect that faith would bring recovery, but they should not expect a spectacular or extraordinary sign. God's regular business was healing. To expect more was fanatical.

Riggle, a "notorious coffee drinker," then discussed proper health care and natural causes of sickness.[120] He said that many of the sins that caused sickness were sins of intemperance. Simply quitting these bad habits would bring recovery. That was the meaning of "Confess your faults one to another, and pray one for another that ye may be healed" (James 5:16). Confessing secret sins would help one to stop committing them, and that would bring healing.[121] The saints could treat other health problems with God-given remedies. Instead of praying for relief from constipation, for example, people should drink more water.[122] Riggle said the benefits of remedies were well attested in the Bible, especially with Paul's advice to Timothy and with Isaiah's application of a "poultice" of figs to Hezekiah's boil. Much of the healing offered by God's plan was "simply a matter of using your own common sense." Thus, Riggle rejected E. E. Byrum's interpretation of remedies and recommended the Church return to D. S. Warner's.

Finally, Riggle openly criticized the saints for the way they presented divine healing. He said that berating the medical world and calling doctors "quacks" did nothing to add power to divine healing and only brought the Church into disrepute. In fact, he said that believers in the biblical doctrine of divine healing (read "revised according to Riggle") were "generally men who respect the medical profession." This would have surprised the saints who remembered *Trumpet* articles in which George Cole, J. W. Byers, and E. E. Byrum accused doctors of being confidence men who used addictive drugs to make money off the weakest and most desperate members of society. However, Riggle did not stop there. He warned the saints that dentistry and remedies were no different from medical care, so virtually everyone in the congregation had sought medical attention of some kind. His point was not that they should stop visiting the dentist, but that they needed to reconsider their opposition to medicine and make their testimonies match their practices.

According to Riggle's camp meeting sermon, the Church of God needed to change its message. Divine healing correctly understood and responsibly practiced healed the body of Christ, attracted converts, and strengthened the Church. It was reasonable and compatible with common sense remedies. It was power for healing from God, not miraculous change imparted by a divine healer. It did not alienate reasonable people or bring opprobrium on the Church. If the saints would stop attacking medicine and abandon their fanatical misconceptions, they could preach true healing as God intended:

> I tell you there are things spoken from this pulpit that do not help us. You had better practice healing and win the respect of the medical profession. Practice divine healing. It is a reasonable thing. It is a necessary thing. Practice healing. The thing you need is healing and healing is the thing you want.[123]

Notes

1. For a fascinating study of the legal aspects of religious healing, see Barry Nobel, "Religious Healing and American Courts in the Twentieth Century: The Liberties and Liabilities of Healers, Patients, and Parents" (Ph.D. diss., University of California, Santa Barbara, 1991). For examples of arrests and prosecution of holiness and Pentecostal people for practicing divine healing, see Paul Chappell, "The Divine Healing Movement in America," 311–20; Mickey Crews, *The Church of God* [Cleveland, Tenn.]: *A Social History* (Knoxville: University of Tennessee Press, 1990), 74–75; Hardesty, *Faith Cure*, 135–36; Shirley Nelson, *Fair, Clear, and Terrible: The Story of Shiloh, Maine* (Latham, N.Y.: British American Publishing, 1989), 239–40; Vinson Synan, "A Healer in the House? A Historical Perspective on Healing in the Pentecostal/Charismatic Tradition," *Asian Journal of Pentecostal Studies* 3:2 (2000): 197–98; Grant Wacker, "Marching to Zion: Religion in a Modern Utopian Community," *Church History* 54 (1985): 500; and Wayne Warner, *The Woman Evangelist Maria B. Woodworth-Etter* (Metuchen, N.J.: Scarecrow Press, 1986). Nobel's dissertation is the only study of divine healing to mention any of the Church of God (Anderson) trials. He discussed *Commonwealth of Pennsylvania v. Hoffman* (1903) but followed the court in misidentifying the defendant as a Christian Scientist (190–92).

2. "Charged With Murder," *GT* 18:23 (June 9, 1898): 4–5. See also Merle D. Strege, *Tell Me Another Tale: Further Reflections on the Church of God* (Anderson, Ind.: Warner Press, 1993), 127–30.

3. "Will Be Arrested," *Fort Wayne Weekly Sentinel*, Nov. 10, 1897, 4; "Faith Cure. That is What a Typhoid Pneumonia Patient is Receiving," *Fort Wayne Weekly Sentinel*, Nov. 10, 1897, 3; "Faith Curist Fined," *Fort Wayne Weekly Gazette*, Nov. 11, 1897, 9;

"The Case of Henry Smith," *Fort Wayne Weekly Sentinel*, Nov. 17, 1897, 2; "Like a Martyr," *Fort Wayne Weekly Sentinel*, Nov. 17, 1897, 5.

4. Henry Smith, "In Prison for Christ's Sake," *GT* 17:47 (Nov. 25, 1897): 4.

5. E. E. Byrum, "The Lord or Doctors, Which?" *GT* 17:47 (Nov. 25, 1897): 4.

6. E. E. Byrum used this passage from Acts in his report on the trial in Fort Wayne. See "The Lord or Doctors, Which?" *GT* 17:47 (Nov. 25, 1897): 4.

7. E. E. Byrum, "Charged with Murder," *GT* 18:23 (June 9, 1898): 5.

8. E. E. Byrum used this phrase in his reports on Fort Wayne (*GT* 17:47 [Nov. 25, 1897]: 4) and Vincennes (*GT* 20:4 [Jan. 25, 1900]: 4).

9. Compare "Prayer," *Western Sun [Vincennes, Indiana]*, Dec. 15, 1899, 1, and *GT* 20:4 (Jan. 25, 1900): 4.

10. See "The Lord or Doctors, Which?" *GT* 17:47 (Nov. 25, 1897): 4, and also the testimony from the Butler, Pennsylvania trial, reprinted in Byrum, *Travels*, 583–84.

11. "Faith Cure," *Fort Wayne Weekly Sentinel*, Nov. 10, 1897, 3.

12. "Involuntary Manslaughter Case," *GT* 18:41 (Oct. 13, 1898): 4.

13. E. E. Byrum, *Travels*, 580.

14. Warren W. Hency, Jr., ed., *Twentieth Century Descendents, Lives & Legacies of Warren Walter Hency Sr. & Effie Lou Burger* (n.p., 1999), 23.

15. "Involuntary Manslaughter Case," *GT* 18:41 (Oct. 13, 1898): 4, 8.

16. E. E. Byrum, "Is There Really a Law in Ohio?" *GT* 22:11 (March 13, 1902): 1–2; E. E. Byrum, "Indiana Health Laws," *GT* 22:12 (March 20, 1902): 1; J. W. Byers, "Death without Medical Attendance in California," *GT* 26:5 (Feb. 1, 1906): 1.

17. The judges threw the Vincennes, Indiana and the Butler, Pennsylvania cases out of court, but no surviving newspapers reported on them. The Ironton, Ohio papers ignored the case in that town entirely.

18. "Gave Bond," *Western Sun [Vincennes, Indiana]*, Dec. 22, 1899, 2; "Divine Healer was Convicted," *The Butler [Pennsylvania] Herald*, Sept. 24, 1903, 2.

19. "Under Bond," *Vincennes [Indiana] Capital*, Dec. 23, 1899, 1.

20. "Relied on Prayer to Cure their Ills," *New York Times*, Sept. 24, 1910, 6.

21. E. E. Byrum, "Charged with Murder," *GT* 18:23 (June 9, 1898): 4–5.

22. "Like a Martyr," *Fort Wayne Weekly Sentinel*, Nov. 17, 1897, 5.

23. See "The Case of Henry Smith," *Fort Wayne Weekly Sentinel*, Nov. 17, 1897, 2.

24. "The Hoffman Case," *The Butler [Pennsylvania] Citizen*, Sept. 24, 1903, 2.

25. In a decision about polygamy, *Reynolds v. United States* (1879), the Supreme Court of the United States declared that the government could regulate religious action. See Anson Phelps Stokes, *Church and State in the United States*, vol. 2 (New York: Harper and Brothers, 1950). See also Nobel, "Religious Healing and American Courts," 189. The articles about the Church of God and religious practice were "The Case of Henry Smith," *Fort Wayne Weekly Sentinel*, Nov. 17, 1897, 2, and "Religious Belief Held no Defense," *Beaver [Oklahoma] Herald*, June 29, 1911, 5.

26. "Faith Curist Fined," *Fort Wayne Weekly Gazette*, Nov. 11, 1897, 9.

27. The cases were in Fort Wayne, Indiana, and Bluefield, West Virginia. "Like a Martyr," *Fort Wayne Weekly Sentinel*, Nov. 17, 1897, 5, reported, "Smith himself was on the witness stand for a long time and gave his story of his conversion to the faith cure, and quoted the Scriptures for his authority." A "General News Notes" entry [*GT* 26:4 (Jan. 25, 1906): 4] said that "a number of witnesses" testified to their faith at the trial in Bluefield, and that "this has awakened interest."

28. Marion, Indiana. See *GT* 18:41 (Oct. 13, 1898): 4, 8.

29. *Commonwealth v. Hoffman* 29 Pa. C.C. 65 (1903), 65.

30. E. E. Byrum, *Travels,* 582.

31. *Commonwealth v. Hoffman,* 69.

32. *Commonwealth v. Hoffman,* 67.

33. *Commonwealth v. Hoffman,* 69.

34. *Lawrence Owens v. State of Oklahoma* 6 Okla. Crim. 110; 116 P. 345; 1911 Okla. Crim. App. LEXIS 302. The *Gospel Trumpet* reported one case after the *Owens,* but it was simply a notice that a grand jury in Pocahontas, Arkansas, had rendered a "true bill" for manslaughter against Bro. L. E. Rogers. The judge dismissed it because of a lack of material witnesses. See "General News Notes," *GT* 32:6 (Feb. 8, 1912): 10, and "General News Notes," *GT* 32:37 (Sept. 19, 1912): 11. The Oran, Missouri case of 1914 did not appear in the *Trumpet.*

35. The other important Church of God case was from Butler, Pennsylvania, *Commonwealth v. Hoffman* (1903). It was a precedent in *Owens v. State of Oklahoma* and in a number of other cases. It established the principle that parents have a duty to provide orthodox medical care to minors. Barry Nobel discusses this case in his dissertation, "Religious Healing and American Courts," 190–92.

36. *GT* 30:17 (April 28, 1910): 8.

37. "General News Notes," *GT* 32:17 (April 25, 1912): 11.

38. According to Byrum, the divine retribution included the following: The doctor who led the persecution died one day before the trial. Soon after the trial, a fire destroyed the business block containing the lawyers' offices. Typhoid fever hit Butler six weeks after the verdict, resulting in 1,277 cases and 111 deaths. Among the casualties were a minister and a doctor who worked for the prosecution. (E. E. Byrum, *Travels,* 590.) The Butler newspaper reported on the typhoid epidemic but attributed it to impure water. See "The Typhoid Scourge," *Butler [Pennsylvania] Citizen,* Dec. 17, 1903, 2, and "Epidemic Conditions," Jan. 28, 1904, 4.

39. C. W. Naylor, *The Teachings of D. S. Warner and His Associates* (Anderson, Ind.: privately published, n.d.), 1–6.

40. See C. E. Hunnex, "Physicians and Remedies," *GT* 29:37 (Sept. 23, 1909): 16; J. D. Ferrill, "Fanaticism," *GT* 32:26 (July 4, 1912): 12. For an opposing view, see R. L. Berry, "Convincing Evidence," *GT* 27:43 (Nov. 7, 1907): 16. Berry said that too many of the saints were calling for doctors. He believed that it would have been better for the cause of Christ for them to die for the truth.

41. "U.S. Smallpox Epidemic of 1901–1903," in George Childs Kohn, ed., *Encyclopedia of Plague and Pestilence from Ancient Times to the Present,* rev. ed. (New York: Facts on File, 2001): 368.

42. George Cole, "Restored to Health," *GT* 21:50 (Dec. 19, 1901): 4. For a full account of Cole's quarantine, see Mary Cole, *Trials and Triumphs of Faith* (Anderson, Ind.: Gospel Trumpet Co., 1914), 249–59. According to Mary Cole, as soon as they were certain George had smallpox, they called "a physician to come and quarantine us so that others would be protected" (252). However, because the doctor resented George's refusal to take medicine, he "created all the resentment he could against us in the neighborhood" (255).

43. On claiming a healing, see chapter three.

44. Emil Kreutz, "Dealing with Contagious Disease," *GT* 21:21 (May 23, 1901): 4–5.

45. E. E. Byrum, "Experience with Diphtheria," *GT* 21:21 (May 23, 1901): 4. It is curious that no one reported this before 1901.

46. W. J. Henry, "Contagious Diseases," *GT* 26:49 (Dec. 13, 1906): 5.

47. "Committee Minutes, Anderson, June 6, 1913," *Minute Book of the Camp-meeting Committee*, Archives of the Church of God, 90.

48. "Camp-meeting Committee Planning Session Minutes, March 1, 1916," *Minute Book of the Camp-meeting Committee*, 177. In 1918, the Spanish influenza pandemic hit the Gospel Trumpet Co. This was not mentioned in the *Trumpet*, but a wing of the Trumpet Home became an influenza ward. See Harold Phillips, *Miracle of Survival*, 161.

49. E. E. Byrum once laid hands on a person with undiagnosed smallpox. Byrum suffered no ill effects but preferred to send handkerchiefs for known cases of contagious diseases. See "Questions Answered," *GT* 29:36 (Sept. 16, 1909): 8–9.

50. E. E. Byrum, "What to Do," *GT* 26:40 (Oct. 11, 1906): 8.

51. E. E. Byrum, "Questions Answered," *GT* 26:8 (Feb. 22, 1906): 4.

52. See D. O. Teasley, "Our Physician—Chapter I," *GT* 21:20 (May 16, 1901): 3; J. W. Byers, "Questions on Divine Healing Answered," *GT* 20 [22]: 12 (March 20, 1902): 8; J. W. Byers, *Two Hundred Genuine Instances of Divine Healing*, 466–74; A. B. Frost, "William Osler's Estimate of Medicine," *GT* 35:13 (April 1, 1915): 9; and E. E. Byrum, *Miracles and Healing*, 148.

53. "Compulsory Vaccination," *GT* 32:16 (April 18, 1912): 2; "Compulsory Medical Treatment," *GT* 32:32 (Aug. 15, 1912): 2.

54. "Too Many Doctors," *GT* 32:12 (March 21, 1912). This article excerpted part of Abraham Flexner's highly critical report on medical education in the United States. The editorial comment charitably noted that not all doctors are charlatans from terrible schools. Another report, this one from the Kentucky Tuberculosis Commission, said, "most of us [doctors] place too much faith in medicine" and do more harm than good (*GT* 33:35 [Sept. 4, 1913]: 10). For the Flexner Report, see Rothstein, *American Physicians*, 289.

55. "Uncertainty of Modern Curatives," *GT* 34:12 (March 19, 1914): 2. See also "A Medico-Political Outrage," *GT* 31:33 (Aug. 31, 1911): 2. The comment about the "medical trust" was from "Something is Radically Wrong," *GT* 32:9 (Feb. 29, 1912): 2. For the development of medicine as a profession, see Gerald E. Markowitz and David Karl Rosner, "Doctors in Crisis: A Study in the Use of Medical Education Reform to Establish Modern Professional Elitism in Medicine," *American Quarterly* 25, no. 1 (March 1973): 83–107; Rothstein, *American Physicians*; Starr, *The Social Transformation of American Medicine*.

56. "New Tuberculosis Cure," *GT* 33:13 (April 10, 1913): 2–3.

57. Henry C. Hawkins, "Earthly Physicians and Divine Physician Contrasted," *GT* 27:32 (Aug. 15, 1907): 16. Hawkins made a case for relying on faith to cure internal diseases and insanity, but he noted that doctors had some effectual drugs for minor diseases and their care was invaluable for wounds. For patent medicines and the Food and Drug Act, see Harvey Young, *Pure Food: Securing the Federal Food and Drugs Act of 1906* (Princeton: Princeton University Press, 1989); Stewart H. Holbrook, *The Golden Age of Quackery* (New York: Macmillan, 1959); and Paul Starr, *The Social Transformation of American Medicine*, 129–38. The act was signed June 1906 and activated January 1, 1907 by Theodore Roosevelt.

58. Brown, *From Infidelity to Christianity*, 282, 289–90.

59. E. E. Byrum, "Questions Answered," *GT* 29:36 (Sept. 16, 1909): 8–9. In another interesting decision, the *Trumpet* said that Church members could be veterinarians. See E. E. Byrum, "Questions," *GT* 14:23 (June 7, 1894): 2; "Questions Answered," *GT* 24:45 (Nov. 10, 1904): 4; and "Questions Answered," *GT* 24:50 (Dec. 15, 1904): 5. The atonement was only for human beings, not animals. However, this conceded that veterinary medicine was effective.

60. John W. V. Smith, *Heralds of a Brighter Day*, 123–44; Merle D. Strege, "Hunter, Nora Siens," in Kostlevy, ed., *Historical Dictionary of the Holiness Movement*.

61. Clarence E. Hunter, "God Called Our Darlings Home," *GT* 23:36 (Sept 3, 1903): 4.

62. C. W. Naylor/C. E. Hunter, "God's Way is Best," no. 63 in *Truth in Song* (Anderson, Ind.: Gospel Trumpet Co., 1907). I owe the connection between the deaths and the hymn to Merle Strege. See *I Saw the Church*, 232.

63. "Who is the Safer?" *GT* 27:45 (Nov. 14, 1907): 16, and "Questions Answered," *GT* 28:42 (Oct. 22, 1908): 9.

64. Merle D. Strege, "Naylor, Charles Wesley," in Kostlevy, ed., *Historical Dictionary of the Holiness Movement*; Smith, *Quest for Holiness and Unity*, 138–39.

65. Strege, *I Saw the Church*, 234. Between the deaths of the Hunter children in 1903 and Naylor's injury in 1908, several Church of God missionaries died in India. According to the news release in the July 25, 1907 issue of the *Trumpet*, James Strong and Sister Maiden died in Aswan, India, June 11 and June 14 respectively. They both "trusted God for healing until the end." Maiden was survived by her husband and one young child, and she was preceded in death by less than a month by her other three children. The *Trumpet* requested prayers for Brother Maiden as he continued his missionary work and cared for his son, who was very sick. (Josephine McCrie, "The Death of the Missionaries," *GT* 27:29 (July 25, 1907): 9.) These deaths likely caused the saints to question divine healing. These were missionaries devoting their lives to spreading the gospel and the message of divine healing. However, this notice is the only available information about Strong and Maiden. Missionary deaths may also have contributed to a change in the teachings about divine healing in the Christian and Missionary Alliance. See William Boyd Bedford, Jr., "A Larger Christian Life: A. B. Simpson and the Early Years of the Christian and Missionary Alliance" (Ph.D. diss., University of Virginia, 1992), 323–35.

66. "General News Notes," *GT* 29:50 (Dec. 23, 1909): 8. E. E. Byrum reportedly said, "Naylor would have been healed but he never *claimed* his healing" (quoted in Reardon, *The Early Morning Light*, 36).

67. "A Message from Brother Naylor," *GT* 32:2 (Jan. 11, 1912): 10–11; "General News Notes," *GT* 33:23 (June 5, 1913): 10; "General News Notes," *GT* 34:44 (Nov. 4, 1914): 10.

68. Naylor, *Winning a Crown* (Anderson, Ind.: Gospel Trumpet Co., 1919), 6.

69. Naylor, *Winning a Crown*, 10.

70. See Naylor, *Winning a Crown*, 343–44, where he does discuss pain.

71. J. W. Byers, *The Grace of Healing* (Moundsville, W.Va.: Gospel Trumpet Co., 1899), 292.

72. *Tidings of Healing* 1:1 (April 1896): 4; J. W. Byers, *Grace of Healing*, 314.

73. In another connection with divine healers, Byers's *The Grace of Healing* (1899) was plagiarized in Maria Woodworth-Etter's *Questions and Answers on Divine Healing* (1919). See Warner, *The Woman Evangelist*, 194–99.

74. J. W. Byers, "Thoughts and Explanations on Divine Healing [pt. 1]," *GT* 21:50 (Dec. 19, 1901): 1–2.

75. Byers was more charitable than most Church of God critics of these movements. A common explanation was that the devil was using them as counterfeits of divine healing. This became complicated because Church members did not want to suggest that the devil could perform miracles of healing; therefore, they said that the devil could create the illusion of healing by imposing a sickness and then removing it. See C. E. Brown, *Christian Science Unmasked* (Anderson, Ind.: Gospel Trumpet Co., 1919); Frances Palmer, "Christian Science," *GT* 18:17 (April 28, 1898): 3; Paul Clifford, "Christian Science—A Dangerous Delusion," *GT* 21:35 (Sept. 5, 1901): 8; V. Y. Tilden, "Saved from Spiritualism," *GT* 21:31 (Aug. 8, 1901): 4; no author, "The Horror of Spiritualism," *GT* 22:17 (April 24, 1902): 4; B. E. Warren, "Health by Divine Means," *GT* 32:15 (April 11, 1912): 9; Pina Winters, "My Experience with Spiritualism," four parts, *GT* 33:1–4 (Jan. 2, 9, 16, and 23, 1913): 4–5. For diabolical counterfeits of divine healing, see A. L. Byers, *Two Hundred Genuine Instances*, 374–80. For the devil's inability to perform "genuine apostolic signs," see J. E. Forrest, editorial remarks, *GT* 28:2 (Jan. 9, 1908): 1.

76. John C. Blaney was more critical of Dowie. He said that Protestantism could no longer hold people, so the devil had to use miracles. One of the most successful diabolical counterfeits was Dowie (John C. Blaney, "Dowie-ism vs. the Bible," *GT* 21:32 [Aug. 15, 1901]: 1–3). Most of the Church of God criticism attacked Dowie but not his healing power. For Dowie's love of money, power, and women other than his wife, see William G. Schell, "Dr. Dowie Against the Bible," *GT* 18:15 (April 14, 1898): 1–2. For an assertion than Dowie had copied Joseph Smith's system, see George L. Cole, "Which is the False Prophet?" *GT* 21:41 (Nov. 7, 1901): 1, 5. For Dowie's rejection of holiness, love of gold, his assertion that Jesus was "joking" about the camel and the eye of a needle, his belief in the perseverance of the saints, and his belief that people could be converted after death, see Lottie Theobold, "Dowieism and the Bible Contrasted," *GT* 24:12 (March 24, 1904): 2–3. For Dowie's declining health due to gluttony, lack of exercise, and general flouting of the dictates of good health, see E. E. Byrum, "Dowie a Physical Failure," *GT* 26:47 (Nov. 29, 1906): 9–10.

77. J. W. Byers, "The Gift of Tongues," *GT* 18:25 (June 23, 1898): 1–2; "The Gift of Tongues," *GT* 26:10 (March 8, 1906): 4.

78. Strege, *I Saw the Church,* 134. The literature about the institutional development of the work of the Church of God is extensive. See Barry L. Callen, "The General Assembly," part three of *Following the Light: A Documentary History of the Church of God Movement* (Anderson, Ind.: Church of God Ministries, 2000); Clear, "The Church of God"; Marvin Hartman, "The Origin and Development of the General Ministerial Assembly of the Church of God, 1917–1950" (B.D. thesis, Butler University, 1958); Forrest, "A Study of the Development of the Basic Doctrines and Institutional Patterns in the Church of God"; Phillips, *Miracle of Survival*, 139–68; Smith, *Quest for Holiness and Unity*, 205–54; and Strege, *I Saw the Church*, 134–64.

79. This quote from the June 28, 1917, issue of the *Gospel Trumpet*. It is reprinted in Callen, *Following the Light*, 162. See also Phillips, *Miracle of Survival*, 136–38.

80. *Miracle of Survival*, 143.

81. *Following the Light*, 160–63.

82. *Miracle of Survival*, 142.

83. *Trumpet* report reprinted in Callen, *Following the Light*, 102.

84. Byrum was in charge of the "Spiritual Service Department." The *Trumpet* published a profile of this work with a picture of Byrum in the prayer room on page nine of the January 14, 1926 issue. This article was the first in a series "Published in the Interests of Your Beneficial Budget" that detailed the non-publishing work of the company. For a later picture of Byrum in his prayer room, see Merle D. Strege, *A Look at the Church of God: The Story for the Children of the Church, Vol. I, 1880–1930* (Anderson, Ind.: Warner Press, 1987), 4. John Alexander Dowie also had a "trophy room." See the photograph on page 16 of *Leaves of Healing* 1:1 (Aug. 31, 1894).

85. *National Labor Tribune*, April 7, 1921, 1; editorial note preceding "How to Get Healed," *GT* 44:6 (Feb. 7, 1924): 2.

86. Smith was one of the six named signatories to the healing in the atonement statement published in the June 19, 1902 issue of the *Trumpet*. The others were H. M Riggle, George L. Cole, S. L. Speck, J. N. Howard, and A. J. Kilpatrick. Later that year Smith wrote that he had initially rejected the position that healing was in the atonement but had come to understand that "our bodies are included in the atonement of Christ *to the same extent* that our souls are" ("Christ's Atonement Includes Soul and Body," *GT* 23:37 [Sept. 10, 1903]: 6–7, italics in original).

87. F. G. Smith, *What the Bible Teaches* (Anderson, Ind.: Gospel Trumpet Co., 1914), 197 and 207.

88. Letter from Mrs. F. G. (Birdie) Smith to Mr. F. G. Smith, April 30, 1920. Archives of the Church of God.

89. In 1925, twelve out of fifty-two issues had a divine healing column. Six others had a healing testimony or a news item about divine healing.

90. Byrum, *Miracles and Healing,* 204–18. For Judd's testimony, see the first chapter of *The Prayer of Faith* in *The Life and Teachings of Carrie Judd Montgomery* (New York: Garland, 1985).

91. In 1908, Byrum and H. M. Riggle attended the "International Divine Healing Convention" at the Pentecostal Mission in Indianapolis. Their experience was mixed. All the participants agreed about the importance of divine healing, but Byrum and Riggle also preached on "feet-washing" and "no-sects." The response was negative. Byrum and Riggle also found that most of the people claiming tongues were deluded, but some "seemed clear in doctrine and experience." These spoke in languages and were able to interpret the same." See H. M Riggle, "International Divine Healing Convention," *GT* 28:4 (Jan. 23, 1908): 8.

92. Arno C. Gaebelein, *The Healing Question: An Examination of the Claims of Faith-Healing and Divine Healing Systems in Light of the Scriptures and History* (New York: Publication Office of "Our Hope," 1925), 86–87.

93. R. M. Riss, "Bosworth, Fred Francis" in Burgess and Van Der Maas, eds., *New International Dictionary of Pentecostal and Charismatic Movements*; Baer, "Perfectly Empowered Bodies," 290–94; David Edwin Harrell, Jr., *All Things Are Possible* (Bloomington: Indiana University Press, 1975), 14–15; Nancy A. Hardesty, *Faith Cure*, 124–25.

94. *National Labor Tribune*, April 7, 1921, 2.

95. *National Labor Tribune*, April 7, 1921, 3. The building looked much smaller than it was. It could hold 5,000 people, far more than were in the picture. See the inside cover of the July 2, 1925 *Trumpet*.

96. *National Labor Tribune*, April 7, 1921, 3.

97. For a full discussion, see chapter four.

98. C. W. Naylor, *God's Will and How to Know It* (Anderson, Ind.: Gospel Trumpet Co., 1926), 3.

99. Naylor, *God's Will*, 5. A biographical note from 1925 said that Naylor had written approximately four hundred articles for the *Trumpet* and answered "something like twenty-five hundred letters each year" for the information department (*GT* 45:41 [Oct. 8, 1925]: 5).

100. Naylor, *God's Will*, 79–80.

101. Naylor, *God's Will*, 185–87.

102. C. W. Naylor, "Differences of Administrations: The Work of the Spirit in the Church," *GT* 44:45 (Nov. 6, 1924): 5–6; "Differences of Administration: More About the Gifts of the Spirit," *GT* 44:46 (Nov. 13, 1924): 3–4; "Differences of Administrations: The Gifts in Operation," *GT* 44:47 (Nov. 20, 1924): 3–4; "Differences of Administrations: Hindrances to Receiving Spiritual Gifts," *GT* 44:48 (Nov. 27, 1924): 5.

103. For Byrum's opinion of the gifts of healing, see E. E. Byrum, *Life Experiences,* 131; "Divine Healing: The Commission," *GT* 15:44 (Nov. 7, 1895): 4; and "Divine Healing: The Will of God to Heal," *GT* 15:45 (Nov. 14, 1895): 4. See also chapter three.

104. Naylor typically referred to the gift of healing, rather than the gifts of healing. The plural is from 1 Cor. 13, and Byrum used Matthew 10:1 to explain that the power included gifts for healing disease, sickness, and casting out demons. Naylor must have been aware of Byrum's theory, but he claimed he had never heard an adequate explanation for the plural (Naylor, "Differences of Administrations," *GT* 44:48 [Nov. 27, 1924]: 5). Naylor's assertion that no gift—not even healing—was possessed by every minister echoed D. S. Warner's initial position. See Warner, "Healing in Christ," *GT* 6:1 (Oct. 1, 1883): 2. See also chapter three.

105. Naylor, "Differences of Administrations," *GT* 44:48 (Nov. 27, 1924): 5.

106. Naylor, "Differences of Administration," *GT* 44:46 (Nov. 13, 1924): 4.

107. Naylor, "Differences of Administrations: The Gifts in Operation," *GT* 44:47 (Nov. 20, 1924): 3. See also J. E. Forrest, "The Gift of Tongues: to whom they are given, the use of them, etc.," *GT* 24:14 (April 7, 1904): 1–2. Forrest's main point was that the gift of tongues was for missions only. The saints who lived only with English speakers should not have expected it. Forrest added that the gift of healing was the same; however, it was more generally useful. For more about the gift of tongues for missions—xenoglossy—see James R. Goff, Jr., *Fields White Unto Harvest: Charles F. Parham and the Missionary Origins of Pentecostalism* (Fayetteville: University of Arkansas Press, 1988).

108. See Russell R. Byrum, "Does the Church Need More Gifts of the Spirit?" *GT* 45:41 (Oct. 8, 1925): 3. According to R. R. Byrum, "Though there will always be a need of miraculous, divine workings to confirm men's faith in Christianity, this need is not in the same degree as was the necessity of miracles at the time of the founding of Christianity." R. R. Byrum was E. E. Byrum's nephew and managing editor of the *Trumpet.* In 1925, the Gospel Trumpet Co. published his *Christian Theology.* In 1927, he resigned from the Gospel Trumpet Co. to become professor of theology at Anderson College. See Strege, *I Saw the Church,* 154–62.

109. H. M. Riggle, introduction to *Divine Healing* by J. Grant Anderson (Anderson, Ind.: Gospel Trumpet Co., 1926). Anderson was hospitalized for tuberculosis in 1903. The ward was quarantined because of smallpox, so Riggle was not able to visit. Anderson and Riggle agreed to a time for prayer, and God answered with a full recovery.

110. Riggle, introduction to *Divine Healing* by Anderson, 7.

111. Anderson, *Divine Healing*, preface. Other than E. E. Byrum, none of the authors listed by Anderson was affiliated with the Church of God. La Rose and Lindlahr did not write about divine healing. Their full names and their most influential publications about health and healing are: Adoniram Judson (A. J.) Gordon, *The Ministry of Healing* (1883); Reuben Torrey, *Divine Healing: Does God Perform Miracles Today?* (1924); Fred Francis (F. F.) Bosworth, *Christ the Healer* (1924); William E. La Rose, *Youth at Seventy* (n.d.); Henry Lindhahr, *Nature Cure: Philosophy and Practice Based on the Unity of Disease and Cure* (1922).

112. Anderson, *Divine Healing*, preface.

113. Anderson, *Divine Healing*, 105.

114. Anderson, *Divine Healing*, 115–16. See Émile Coué, *Self Motivation Through Conscious Autosuggestion* (New York: American Library Service, [1922]). Reuben A. Torrey, one of the authors Anderson cited as an influence in his preface, denounced "Couéism" in *Divine Healing: Does God Perform Miracles Today?* (Grand Rapids, Mich.: Baker Book House, 1924), 13–14.

115. The strong prejudice against medicine must also have been a factor; however, his only stated objection was that medicine was often dangerous and seldom helpful.

116. For more about Riggle, see his autobiography *Pioneer Evangelism* (Anderson, Ind.: Gospel Trumpet Co., 1924). See also William C. Kostlevy, "Riggle, H(erbert) M(cClellan)," in Kostlevy, ed., *Historical Dictionary of the Holiness Movement*; John W. V. Smith, *Heralds of a Brighter Day*, 100–122. Riggle had an overriding interest in eschatology. He wrote several books on the topic, including finishing a manuscript D. S. Warner began, *The Cleansing of the Sanctuary* (1903). For specific information about Riggle's eschatology, see Strege, *I Saw the Church*, 165–81, and John Stanley, "Unity Among Diversity: Interpreting the Book of Revelation in the Church of God (Anderson)," *Wesleyan Theological Journal* 25:2 (Fall, 1990): 64–98. For accounts of divine healing in Riggle's ministry, see "Healings in the Ministry of H. M. Riggle," in J. Grant Anderson, *Divine Healing*, 99–103, and A. L. Byers, *Two Hundred Genuine Instances of Divine Healing*, 270–73.

117. H. M. Riggle, "Divine Healing," in *Select Camp-Meeting Sermons Preached at the International Camp-Meeting of the Church of God, Anderson, Indiana, June 16–24, 1928* (Anderson, Ind.: Gospel Trumpet Co., 1928), 245–46.

118. Riggle, "Divine Healing," in *Select Camp-Meeting Sermons 1928*, 246.

119. Riggle, "Divine Healing," in *Select Camp-Meeting Sermons 1928*, 257.

120. On Riggle's coffee drinking, see Strege, *I Saw the Church*, 180, n. 23.

121. Riggle, "Divine Healing," in *Select Camp-Meeting Sermons 1928*, 259. See D. S. Warner, "Question," *GT* 15:42 (Oct. 24, 1895): 2. This article also appeared as "An Explanation About Divine Healing," in Warren C. Roark, comp., *Divine Healing* (Anderson, Ind.: Gospel Trumpet Co., 1945), 114–19. See also, Strege, *I Saw the Church*, 72–73.

122. This example is an interesting choice. There is no evidence that Riggle knew this, but constipation was the affliction Josephine Courtney had when she took Warner's advice to use remedies. She became worse until she prayed the prayer of faith. Her testimony supported E. E. Byrum's revision of Warner's article and helped to begin the radical, anti-medicine period in the Church of God (Josephine Courtney, "Praise God for Healing," *GT* 16:6 [Feb. 6, 1896]: 6). See chapter three.

123. Riggle, "Divine Healing," in *Select Camp-Meeting Sermons 1928*, 261.

CONCLUSION

JUST THE SAME TODAY

> He is Just the Same Today,
> He is Just the Same Today,
> Yes, He Healed in Galilee,
> Set the Suff'ring Captives Free,
> And He's Just the Same Today.
> (J. W. Byers/A. L. Byers, "He Is Just the Same Today")

Physical healing is a biblical theme and a perennial emphasis in Christian movements. Historians of American Christianity, however, have largely ignored religious healing as a topic for serious study, even though metaphors of healing pervade Christian theology and more mundane issues of health have shaped Christian institutions. Even if we set aside ministries and movements specifically devoted to miraculous healing, we still have the fact that all the major Christian groups have hospitals, chaplains, or religious services for the sick and the dying. The prayers, institutions, and doctrines related to healing reflect, among other things, a group's understanding of the Bible, miracles, spiritual gifts, religious leadership, charity, Christology, and pneumatology. This study of the Church of God, an extreme (but not unique) example of the integration of physical healing into theology and religious life, demonstrates how a study of physical healing can illuminate a religious movement's theology, ecclesiology, and historiography. Religious doctrines and practices of healing show how individuals enact their faith, and healing is often a point of conflict where theology and practices are negotiated and changed. Because of the potential for healing to affect every aspect of the life of a religious movement, healing should at least be

183

considered in any history of a Christian movement. For histories of restorationist holiness and Pentecostal groups like the Church of God, it is absolutely essential.

The most obvious reason for studying physical healing in the Church of God is that it was a core emphasis that performed a variety of functions. This is reflected by the voluminous material on healing, including articles, hymns, tracts, children's literature, books, and testimonies. For historical studies of the Church of God itself, it is impossible to have an accurate picture of the life and theology of the early years without studying divine healing and the physical perfectionism of health reform. For studies of divine healing in America that are not directly related to the Church of God, this study very clearly shows a wide range of religious applications of divine healing, including but not limited to the direct physical benefits felt by believers. Physical healing provided evidence of sanctification and membership in the Church, improved testimonies by bridging the gap between telling about grace and feeling the power of the Holy Spirit, and spread the message of the Church of God by attracting potential converts and by providing a physical parallel to the religious experience of entire sanctification. For organization and leadership, the gifts of healing functioned as validation of ministerial authority and evidence that God was healing the Body of Christ and beginning a new age of Christianity with the Church of God. The members of the Church of God believed that physical healing made the Church visible to anyone who cared to look by identifying members, ministers, and God's work in the world. Thus, the early Church of God experimented with divine healing and eventually integrated it into every aspect of the life and thought of the Church.

A more subtle reason for studying religious healing is to explore the interaction between a religious movement and the wider culture. This is particularly useful for radical healing movements like the Church of God, which were extreme examples of what Sidney Mead identified as "historylessness" in American religion.[1] That is, divine healing collapsed the distance between the present and the apostolic church as well as the distance between human beings and God. Healing was "in the atonement," or it was available because Jesus "is just the same today" as he was in Galilee. This rhetoric built on the assumed definitions of "health" and "healing" to obscure all theological change and to deny any significant influence from extra-biblical doctrine. However, the actual practice of healing belied these claims. Amanda Porterfield has said that healing is always culturally conditioned.[2] In the case of divine healing movements, an even stronger statement is possible: the doctrinal formulations and practices of healing expose the cultural context that the message of divine healing denies.

For example, although the Church of God claimed to be separate from the world, this study has shown that the Church was firmly entrenched in the culture of the nineteenth and early twentieth centuries. It adopted its practical definitions of holy living and healing from contemporary health reform and divine healing movements. The actions of Church members show that the proclaimed rejection of all possible medicine was in fact much more practical and calculated. It was a rejection of the specific medical care of the nineteenth century. Examining healing shows that the entire history of the Church of God has been informed by interaction with other religious groups and the wider culture.

The Church of God changed its theology and practice of healing in an effort to maintain its (continually evolving) message of holiness and unity. In the nineteenth century, when the Church was competing with Seventh-day Adventists and radical holiness groups, it increasingly emphasized healing. When the doctrine of divine healing became a problem in the early twentieth century, Church members gradually changed their practices and beliefs. In one sense, they sacrificed their clear message of separation from the world in favor of respectability and what they hoped would be numerical growth. In another sense, they maintained their commitment to holiness and unity. The vision of the Church—the unity of the saints—became more inclusive and compassionate, but it also became harder to define, demonstrate, and maintain.

This brings the third and final benefit of studying religious healing: it can show theological and ecclesiological change. Healing is multivalent and performs many functions. In a group like the Church of God, which emphasized healing and integrated it into every aspect of the movement, the practice and doctrine of healing had minute, carefully-examined distinctions. Therefore, changes in the understanding of healing can be a sensitive gauge of theological or organizational change. This is especially true when, as in the Church of God, the validity of divine healing itself was never in question; only the details of the doctrine and the practice needed perfecting. Thus, "divine healing" remained a constant emphasis, but the content of that emphasis changed.

D. S. Warner's opinion of divine healing, which accepted some remedies and emphasized sanctification and healthful living, was, for example, different from the gifts and miracles of healing E. E. Byrum preached. This change reflected new leadership and a new organizational style based on a spiritually-gifted ministry. During Byrum's long tenure as editor of the *Gospel Trumpet*, his teaching about healing gradually changed to include inoculations for schoolchildren, quarantines for the contagious, and medicine for children. These transformations showed the Church's growth, maturation, and change from a "flying ministry" of evangelists into a congregation-based church with families, children, and neighbors. Finally, C. W. Naylor rejected the whole foundation of Byrum's radical divine healing doctrine by asserting that God's will for physical healing cannot be known; yet Naylor insisted that he believed in the true doctrine of divine healing, and he continued to anoint people from his hospital bed for healing from God.

Members of the Church of God did not write about the history of divine healing in the movement. They felt the changes but did not examine them. In 1946, the Church commissioned and sent its first medical missionary, David Gaulke, to take the gospel and modern medicine to China and Africa.[3] Five years later, C. E. Brown, the editor of the *Gospel Trumpet*, published *When the Trumpet Sounded: A History of the Church of God Reformation Movement*. By omitting all but a few references to divine healing, Brown's history said that physical healing was not essential to the movement. This theological judgment did not reflect the opinions of many of the early saints, but it proved enormously influential for Church of God historians.[4] In 1954, Brown's *When Souls Awaken* said that refusing to use medicine was, along with the other traditional behaviors of the Church, an ascetic discipline, and not a particularly good one at that.[5] This made divine healing into an option without significant consequences, a position far removed from the doctrine of divine healing in the atonement, which portrayed the choice between prayer and medicine as a choice between heaven and hell. This new vision of the past made more peaceful the coexistence of prayer and medicine, but it avoided the question of how the Church of God of 1895 came to be the Church of God of 1926 and then the Church of God of 1955.

Physical healing, therefore, represented the greatest hopes and beliefs of members of the Church of God. By trusting God to heal their bodies and their children, they testified to their experiences of God's redeeming power and demonstrated their faith that God would perfect physical bodies as well as the spiritual body of Christ. The Church of the late nineteenth century expected divine healing to be an unmistakable and irrefutable sign that the Church was separate from the world. Yet, it was precisely in living out the implications of divine healing that the world intruded most rudely into the life of the Church. Tragic failures of divine healing, epidemics, medical advances, court trials, mandatory inoculations of schoolchildren, and general opprobrium combined to prevent a simplistic equation of the Church of God and the church of the apostles. Church members continued to affirm that Jesus is just the same today, but their changing behavior in the early twentieth century showed that they reinterpreted Jesus' earthly healing ministry: he saved souls and healed the church universal from division; fixing individual bodies was secondary.

Notes

1. Sidney E. Mead, *The Lively Experiment: The Shaping of Christianity in America* (New York: Harper and Row, 1963), 108.

2. Amanda Porterfield, "Healing in the History of Christianity," 227–42. See esp. 227.

3. David W. Gaulke was converted and sanctified in 1928 at the age of fifteen. He graduated with an A.B. from Anderson College in 1934, and he earned an M.D. from Indiana University in 1942. In a letter to the editor of the *Trumpet*, Gaulke said, "From 1938 to 1946 I was in preparation for medical missionary work. Spent three and a half years in China at Peace Memorial Hospital and half a year at Kima Station in Kenya" [Letter dated "Missionary Board. June 22, 1950" from D. W. Gaulke, M.D., to Rev. C. E. Brown, Church of God Archives B650, Box 4, Charles E. Brown Papers, Personal Histories (1949–1950), G].

4. Brown, *When the Trumpet Sounded*. See page xi for Brown's reason for omitting healing from the story.

5. C. E. Brown, *When Souls Awaken: An Interpretation of Radical Christianity* (Anderson, Ind.: Gospel Trumpet Co., 1954), 69–100. Brown did give some historical perspective on healing. He refuted the belief that divine healing was novel or original with the Church of God reformation, and he mentioned many authors and leaders from the divine healing movement (58–62). However, he did not discuss how or why the doctrine changed in the Church of God.

BIBLIOGRAPHY

Newspapers and Periodicals

Beaver [Oklahoma] Herald
Butler [Pennsylvania] Citizen
Butler [Pennsylvania] Herald
Century Magazine
Chicago Tribune
Fairmont [Indiana] News
The Firebrand
Fort Wayne Weekly Gazette
Fort Wayne Weekly Sentinel
Gospel Trumpet/Vital Christianity
Graham Journal of Health and Longevity
Latter Rain Evangel
Leaves of Healing
National Labor Tribune
New York Times
Pentecostal Evangel
Presbyterian Review
The Revivalist
Shining Light
Tidings of Healing
Vincennes [Indiana] Capital
Western Sun [Vincennes, Indiana]

Primary Sources

Account of the Union Meeting for the Promotion of Scriptural Holiness, Oxford, August 29–September 7, 1874. "The Higher Christian Life": Sources for the Study of Holiness, Pentecostal, and Keswick Movements. New York: Garland, 1985.

Alcott, William A. *The Young Husband, or Duties of Man in the Marriage Relation.* 5th ed. Boston: George W. Light, 1840.

———. *Tea and Coffee: Their Physical, Intellectual and Moral Effects on the Human System.* London: Holyoake, 1859.

Anderson, J. Grant. *Divine Healing.* Anderson, Ind.: Gospel Trumpet Co., 1926.

———. *Sex Life and Home Problems.* Anderson, Ind.: Gospel Trumpet Co., 1921.

Arthur, William. *The Tongue of Fire; or the True Power of Christianity.* New York: Harper, 1856.

Austin, E. A. *Christian Science.* Anderson, Ind.: Gospel Trumpet Co., n.d.

Bainbridge, Harriette S. *Life for Soul and Body.* New York: Alliance Press, 1906.

Bartleman, Frank. *Witness to Pentecost: The Life of Frank Bartleman.* "The Higher Christian Life": Sources for the Study of Holiness, Pentecostal, and Keswick Movements. New York: Garland, 1985.

Berry, Robert L. *Adventures in the Land of Canaan.* Anderson, Ind.: Gospel Trumpet Co., 1924.

Boardman, W. E. *Faith-Work; or the Labours of Dr. Cullis, in Boston.* 2d ed. London: Daldy Isbister, 1875.

———. *Faith Work under Dr. Cullis, in Boston.* Beacon Hill Place, Boston: Willard Tract Repository, 1880.

———. *Gladness in Jesus.* New and rev. ed. Boston: Willard Tract Repository, 1870.

———. *The Great Physician (Jehovah Rohpi).* Boston: Willard Tract Repository, 1881.

———. *The Higher Christian Life.* New York: D. Appleton, 1859.

———. *In the Power of the Spirit; or, Christian Experience in the Light of the Bible.* Boston: Willard Tract Repository, 1875.

Booth, William. *In Darkest England and the Way Out.* Chicago: C. H. Sergel & Co., 1890.

Bosworth, F[red] F[rancis]. *Christ, the Healer: Sermons on Divine Healing.* Racine, Wisc.: F. F. Bosworth, 1924.

Brengle, Samuel Logan. *Heart Talks on Holiness*. New York: Salvation Army Publishing House, 1900.

Brooks, John P. *The Divine Church: A Treatise on the Origin, Constitution, Order and Ordinances of the Church; Being a Vindication of the New Testament Ecclesia, and an Exposure of the Anti-Scriptural Character of the Modern Church of Sect*. Columbia, Mo.: Herald Publishing House, 1891.

Brown, Charles Ewing. "Christian Science Unmasked." Anderson, Ind. and Kansas City, Mo.: Gospel Trumpet Co., 1919.

———. *The Church Beyond Division*. Anderson, Ind.: Gospel Trumpet Co., 1939.

———. *The Meaning of Sanctification*. Anderson, Ind.: Gospel Trumpet Co., 1945.

———. *When Souls Awaken: An Interpretation of Radical Christianity*. Anderson, Ind.: Gospel Trumpet Co., 1954.

———. *When the Trumpet Sounded: A History of the Church of God Reformation Movement*. Anderson, Ind.: Gospel Trumpet Co., 1951.

Brown, Willis M. *From Infidelity to Christianity: Life Sketches of Willis M. Brown*. Moundsville, W.Va.: Gospel Trumpet Co., 1904.

Buckley, James Monroe. "Faith-Healing and Kindred Phenomena." *Century Magazine*, June 1886, 221–36.

———. "Faith-Healing and Kindred Phenomena (Supplementary Article)." *Century Magazine*, March 1887, 781–87.

———. *Faith-Healing, Christian Science, and Kindred Phenomena*. New York: The Century Co., 1898.

Byers, Andrew L. *Birth of a Reformation*. Anderson, Ind.: Gospel Trumpet Co., 1921.

———. *The Gospel Trumpet Publishing Work, Described and Illustrated*. Anderson, Ind.: Gospel Trumpet Co., 1907.

———, ed. *His Praise Anew: A Treasury of New Sacred Song Including Many Old Favorites*. Anderson, Ind.: Gospel Trumpet Co., 1936.

———. *Two Hundred Genuine Instances of Divine Healing: The Doctrine Explained*. Anderson, Ind.: Gospel Trumpet Co., 1911.

Byers, Andrew L., and Barney E. Warren, eds. *Melodies of Zion: A Compilation of Hymns and Songs, Old and New, Intended for All Kinds of Religious Services*. Anderson, Ind.: Gospel Trumpet Co., 1926.

———, eds. *Reformation Glory: A New and Inspiring Collection of Gospel Hymns for Evangelistic Services*. Anderson, Ind.: Gospel Trumpet Co., 1923.

Byers, Jacob Whistler. *The Grace of Healing; or Christ Our Physician*. Moundsville, W.Va.: Gospel Trumpet Co., 1899.

———. "Questions and Answers on Divine Healing." Anderson, Ind.: Gospel Trumpet Co., n.d.

Byrum, Enoch Edwin. *The Boy's Companion, or a Warning against the Secret Vice and Other Bad Habits*. Grand Junction, Mich.: Gospel Trumpet Co., 1893.

———. *Divine Healing of Soul and Body; Also How God Heals the Sick, and the Conditions Upon Which They Are Restored; Giving Wonderful Testimonies of His Miraculous Power in These Last Days*. Grand Junction, Mich., 1892.

———. "The Doctrine of Healing." Anderson, Ind.: Gospel Trumpet Co., n.d.

———. *The Great Physician and His Power to Heal*. Moundsville, W.Va.: Gospel Trumpet Co., 1899.

———. *Life Experiences: Containing Narratives, Incidents, and Experiences in the Life of the Author*. Anderson, Ind.: Gospel Trumpet Co., 1928.

———. *Little Things*. Moundsville, W.Va.: Gospel Trumpet Co., 1895.

———. *The Man of Galilee*. Anderson, Ind.: Gospel Trumpet Co., 1907.

———. *Miracles and Healing: Scriptural Incidents and Evidences of the Miraculous Manifestation of the Power of God, and of the Healing of Sicknesses and Diseases*. Anderson, Ind.: Gospel Trumpet Co., 1919.

———. "The Power of Healing." Anderson, Ind.: Gospel Trumpet Co., n.d.

———. *The Secret of Salvation, How to Get It and How to Keep It; Showing the Way of Salvation, Giving the Reader the Key with Which to Unlock Its Great Storehouse of Peace and Happiness*. Anderson, Ind.: Gospel Trumpet Co., 1896.

———. *Startling Incidents and Experiences in the Christian Life; Narratives of the Wonderful Dealings of the Lord with Those Who Put Their Trust in Him and of Their Deliverance in Time of Adversity, Trial, and Temptation*. Anderson, Ind.: Gospel Trumpet Co., 1915.

———. *Travels and Experiences in Other Lands*. Moundsville, W.Va.: Gospel Trumpet Co., 1905.

———. *What Shall I Do to Be Saved? Words of Advice, Warning, and Encouragement to the Unsaved, Pointing out the Way of Salvation, and the Requirements Necessary to Obtain It*. Moundsville, W.Va.: Gospel Trumpet Co., 1903.

———. *Why Some Are Not Healed: 35 Reasons or Excuses with Answers Given*. Anderson, Ind., and Kansas City, Mo.: Gospel Trumpet Co., n.d.

Byrum, Isabel. *The Pilot's Voice; Words of Warning to the Youth and Enlightenment for Parents*. Anderson, Ind.: Gospel Trumpet Co., 1916.

———. *The Value of a Praying Mother*. Anderson, Ind.: Gospel Trumpet Co., 1911.

Byrum, Noah H. *Familiar Names and Faces; a Collection of Cuts from Photo-graphs of Ministers, Gospel Workers, Writers, and Others, Whose Names Are Mostly Familiar to the Readers of the Gospel Trumpet...Also a History of the Gospel Trumpet Publishing Work, with Cuts Representing the Same and Other Things of Interest.* Moundsville, W.Va.: Gospel Trumpet Co., 1902.

———. "Diary, Noah H. Byrum." Archives of the Church of God, Anderson, Ind., 1888–1898.

Byrum, Russell R. *Christian Theology: A Systematic Statement of Christian Doctrine for the Use of Theological Students.* Anderson, Ind.: Gospel Trumpet Co., 1925.

———. *Holy Spirit Baptism and the Second Cleansing.* Anderson, Ind.: Gospel Trumpet Co., 1923.

Camp-Meeting Sermons: Sermons Preached at the General Annual Camp-Meeting of the Church of God, Held at Anderson, Indiana, June 6–15, 1913. Anderson, Ind.: Gospel Trumpet Co., 1913.

Carter, Russell Kelso. *The Atonement for Sin and Sickness; or, a Full Salvation for the Soul and Body.* Boston: Willard Tract Repository, 1884.

———. *Divine Healing, or, the Atonement for Sin and Sickness.* New York: J. B. Allen, 1888.

———. "Divine Healing; or, 'Faith Cure.'" *Century Magazine*, March 1887, 777–80.

———. *"Faith Healing" Reviewed after Twenty Years.* Boston: Christian Witness Co., 1897.

Causes of Disease and Sickness. Anderson, Ind.: Gospel Trumpet Co., n.d.

Cole, Mary. *Trials and Triumphs of Faith.* Anderson, Ind.: Gospel Trumpet Co., 1914.

Counsel to Young Saints. Moundsville, W.Va.: Gospel Trumpet Co., n.d.

Cullis, Charles. *Faith Cures; or, Answers to Prayer in the Healing of the Sick.* Boston: Willard Tract Repository, 1879.

———. *More Faith Cures; or, Answers to Prayer in the Healing of the Sick.* Boston: Willard Tract Repository, 1881.

———. *Other Faith Cures; or, Answers to Prayer in the Healing of the Sick.* Boston: Willard Tract Repository, 1885.

Davis, Henry Turner. *Modern Miracles.* Cincinnati: Martin Wells Knapp, 1901.

Doctrine and Discipline of the Free Methodist Church. Chicago: Free Methodist Publishing House, 1905.

Dowie, John Alexander. *Our Second Year's Harvest Being a Brief Record of a Year of Divine Healing Missions on the Pacific Coast of America, in California, Oregon, Washington and British Columbia Conducted by the Rev. John Alex. Dowie and Mrs. Dowie, from Melbourne, Australia: With an*

Appendix Containing Farewell Addresses, and a Full Report of the First General Convention of the Divine Healing Association. Chicago: International Divine Healing Association, 1891.

Eddy, Mary Baker. *Science and Health, with Key to the Scriptures.* 16th, rev. ed. Boston: the author, 1886.

Egermeier, Elsie E. *Bible Story Book.* 5th ed. Anderson, Ind.: Gospel Trumpet Co., 1922.

Flory, J. S. *Mind Mysteries Phenomena of Spiritism, Christian Science, and Faith Healing: Gospel Healing from a Bible Standpoint Completely Vindicated.* Mount Morris, Ill.: J. S. Flory, 1897.

Forney, Christian Henry. *The Bible Doctrine of Sanctification.* Harrisburg, Penn.: Central Printing and Publishing House, Churches of God, 1906.

Fowler, Harriet P. *Vegetarianism: The Radical Cure for Intemperance.* New York: Fowlers & Wells, 1886.

Fowler, Orson Squire. *Creative and Sexual Science: Or Manhood, Womanhood, and Their Mutual Interrelations; Love, Its Laws, Power, Etc.; Selection or Mutual Adaptation.* New York: Fowlers & Wells, 1875.

———. *Physiology, Animal and Mental: Applied to the Preservation and Restoration of Health of Body, and Power of Mind.* 6th ed. New York: Fowlers and Wells, 1851.

———. *Religion; Natural and Revealed: Or, the Natural Theology and Moral Bearings of Phrenology and Physiology.* 10th ed. New York: Fowlers and Wells, 1847.

———. *Self-Culture, and Perfection of Character; Including the Management of Youth.* New York: Fowlers & Wells, n.d.

"Friend, A." *Startling News to Mothers.* Grand Junction, Mich.: Gospel Trumpet Co., 1895.

Gaebelein, Arno C. *The Healing Question: An Examination of the Claims of Faith-Healing and Divine Healing Systems in Light of the Scriptures and History.* New York: Publications Office of "Our Hope," 1925.

Godbey, William B. *Divine Healing.* Greensboro, N.C.: Apostolic Messenger Office, 1909.

———. *Six Tracts.* "The Higher Christian Life": Sources for the Study of Holiness, Pentecostal, and Keswick Movements. New York: Garland, 1985.

Gordon, Adoniram Judson. *In Christ, or, the Believer's Union with His Lord.* Boston: Gould and Lincoln, 1872.

———. *The Ministry of Healing, or, Miracles of Cure in All Ages.* Rev. ed. Boston: Howard Gannett, 1883.

———. *The Ministry of the Spirit.* New York: Fleming H. Revell, 1894.

———. *The Twofold Life, or, Christ's Work for Us and Christ's Work in Us.* New York: Fleming H. Revell, 1883.

Graham, Sylvester. *A Lecture to Young Men*. 1834. Reprint, New York: Arno Press, 1974.

Gray, Albert F. *Christian Theology*. Anderson, Ind.: Warner Press, 1946.

Gunn, John C., and Johnson H. Jordan. *Gunn's New Domestic Physician: Or, Home Book of Health*. Cincinnati: Moore Wilstach Keys and Co., 1859.

Hahn, Fred L. *Hints on Healing*. Grand Junction, Mich.: Gospel Trumpet Co., 1894.

Haynes, W. A. *Save the Girls*. Grand Junction, Mich.: Gospel Trumpet Co., 1898.

———. *Social and Sexual Purity*. Grand Junction, Mich.: Gospel Trumpet Co., n.d.

Henry, William J. *The Evil Effects of Tight Lacing*. Moundsville, W.Va.: Gospel Trumpet Co., 1898.

Holiness Tracts Defending the Ministry of Women. "The Higher Christian Life": Sources for the Study of Holiness, Pentecostal, and Keswick Movements. New York: Garland, 1985.

Howe, Joseph W., M.D. *Excessive Venery Masturbation and Continence: the etiology, pathology, and treatment of the diseases resulting from venereal excess, masturbation, and continence*. New York: E. B. Treat, 1887. Reprint, New York: Arno Press, 1975.

Hussey, A. H. *Divine Healing in Mission Work*. Nyack, N.Y.: Christian Alliance Publishing Co., 1902.

Hypnotism. Anderson, Ind.: Gospel Trumpet Co., 1904.

Johnson, Anna Jane Sample. *The Healing Voice: On the Power of Prayer, Faith Literature and the Science of Healing: Proving to the World That a Living Faith Gives Us a Practical Christianity*. New York: Press of James N. Johnston, 1885.

Judd, Carrie F. *The Prayer of Faith*. Chicago: F. H. Revell, 1880.

Kiergan, A. M. *Washing Feet: Historical and Scriptural View*. Chillicothe, Mo.: The Good Way Publishing House, 1891.

Lewis, Dio. *Chastity; or, Our Secret Sins*. Philadelphia, New York, Boston, Cincinnati and Chicago: George Maclean & Co., 1874.

———. *Our Digestion; or, My Jolly Friend's Secret*. Philadelphia: G. Maclean, 1872.

———. *Our Girls*. New York: Harper and Brothers, 1871.

McPherson, Aimee Semple. *This Is That*. "The Higher Christian Life": Sources for the Study of Holiness, Pentecostal, and Keswick Movements. New York: Garland, 1985.

Miller, Frankie. "Diary, Miss Frankie Miller, Battle Creek, Michigan." Archives of the Church of God. Anderson, Ind., 1886.

Minute Book of the Camp-meeting Committee. Archives of the Church of God. Anderson, Ind.

Mix, Mrs. Edward. *Faith Cures, and Answers to Prayer.* Syracuse, N.Y.: Syracuse University Press, 2002.

Montgomery, Carrie Judd. *The Life and Teaching of Carrie Judd Montgomery.* "The Higher Christian Life": Sources for the Study of Holiness, Pentecostal, and Keswick Movements. New York: Garland, 1985.

———. *"Under His Wings": The Story of My Life.* "The Higher Christian Life": Sources for the Study of Holiness, Pentecostal, and Keswick Movements. New York: Garland, 1985.

Murray, Andrew. *Divine Healing: A Series of Addresses and a Personal Testimony.* Fort Washington, Penn.: Christian Literature Crusade, n.d.

Myland, D. Wesley, George Floyd Taylor, and Bennett Freeman Lawrence. *Three Early Pentecostal Tracts.* "The Higher Christian Life": Sources for the Study of Holiness, Pentecostal, and Keswick Movements. New York: Garland, 1985.

Naylor, Charles Wesley. *God's Will and How to Know It.* 2d ed. Anderson, Ind.: Gospel Trumpet Co., 1925.

———. *The Teaching of D. S. Warner and His Associates.* Anderson, Ind: n.p., [1940s].

———. *Winning a Crown: A Practical Treatise on How to Find God, What Salvation Is and Does, and How to Live a Happy and Successful Christian Life.* Anderson, Ind.: Gospel Trumpet Co., 1919.

Nelson, Thomas. *Home, Health, and Success; or a Guide to a Happy Home and a Successful Life.* Anderson, Ind.: Gospel Trumpet Co., 1908.

Noble, Louis A. "Diary of Louis A. Noble." [1893] Church of God in Michigan: General Assembly: Louis Noble Folder, 9. Bentley Historical Library, University of Michigan. Ann Arbor, Mich.

Oerter, J. H. *Divine Healing in the Light of Scripture.* Brooklyn, N.Y.: Christian Alliance Publishing Co., 1900.

Orr, Charles Ebert. *Food for the Lambs; or, Helps for Young Christians.* Anderson, Ind.: Gospel Trumpet Co., 1904.

———. *The Gospel Day; or, the Light of Christianity.* Moundsville, W.Va.: Gospel Trumpet Co., 1904.

———. *The Hidden Life; or, Walks with God.* Anderson, Ind.: Gospel Trumpet Co., 1908.

———. *A Religious Controversy.* Anderson, Ind.: Gospel Trumpet Co., n.d.

Palmer, Phoebe. *Full Salvation; Its Doctrine and Duties.* Salem, Ohio: Schmul, 1979.

————. *Pioneer Experiences, or, the Gift of Power Received by Faith: Illustrated and Confirmed by the Testimony of Eighty Living Ministers, of Various Denominations.* New York: W. C. Palmer, 1869.

————. *Promise of the Father: Or, a Neglected Specialty of the Last Days. Addressed to the Clergy and Laity of All Christian Communities.* New York: W. C. Palmer, 1872.

————. *The Way of Holiness, with Notes by the Way; Being a Narrative of Religious Experience Resulting from a Determination to Be a Bible Christian.* 2d ed. New York: Lane & Scott, 1849. Reprint, Holiness Data Ministries, Digital Edition 09/30/98.

Pardington, G. P. *Twenty-Five Wonderful Years 1889–1914: A Popular Sketch of the Christian and Missionary Alliance.* "The Higher Christian Life": Sources for the Study of Holiness, Pentecostal, and Keswick Movements. New York: Garland, 1985.

Parham, Sarah E. *The Life of Charles F. Parham, Founder of the Apostolic Faith Movement.* "The Higher Christian Life": Sources for the Study of Holiness, Pentecostal, and Keswick Movements. New York: Garland, 1985.

Pierson, Arthur Tappan. *Forward Movements of the Last Half Century.* "The Higher Christian Life": Sources for the Study of Holiness, Pentecostal, and Keswick Movements. New York: Garland, 1985.

Proceedings of Holiness Conferences. "The Higher Christian Life": Sources for the Study of Holiness, Pentecostal, and Keswick Movements. New York: Garland, 1985.

Proceedings of the Western Union Holiness Convention Held at Jacksonville, Ill., Dec. 15th–19th, 1880. Bloomington, Ill.: Western Holiness Association, L. Hawkins, agent, 1881.

Rees, Seth Cook. *Miracles in the Slums.* "The Higher Christian Life": Sources for the Study of Holiness, Pentecostal, and Keswick Movements. New York: Garland, 1985.

Riggle, Herbert McClellan. *Christ's Kingdom and Reign.* Anderson, Ind.: Gospel Trumpet Co., 1918.

————. *Christ's Second Coming and What Will Follow.* Anderson, Ind.: Gospel Trumpet Co., 1918.

————. *The Christian Church, Its Rise and Progress.* Anderson, Ind.: Gospel Trumpet Co., 1912.

————. *The Kingdom of God and the One Thousand Years' Reign.* Moundsville, W.Va.: Gospel Trumpet Co., 1899.

————. *Pioneer Evangelism, or Experiences and Observations at Home and Abroad.* Anderson, Ind.: Gospel Trumpet Co., 1924.

Roberts, John E. *Spiritualism or, Bible Salvation vs. Modern Spiritualism, the Doctrine of the Bible Arrayed against the Doctrine of Devils.* Grand Junction, Mich.: Gospel Trumpet Co., n.d.

Rutty, Jennie C. *The Faith of Hannah.* Grand Junction, Mich.: Gospel Trumpet Co., n.d.

———. *Letters of Love and Counsel for "Our Girls."* Moundsville, W.Va.: Gospel Trumpet Co., 1898.

———. *Mothers' Counsel to Their Sons.* Moundsville, W.Va.: Gospel Trumpet Co., 1899.

———. *Words of Love to Girls.* Moundsville, W.Va.: Gospel Trumpet Co., 1904.

Schauffler, A. F. "Faith-Cures." *Century Magazine,* Dec. 1885, 274–78.

Schell, William G. *The Better Testament; or, the Two Testaments Compared: Demonstrating the Superiority of the Gospel over Moses' Law According to the Epistles of Paul, Especially That Addressed to the Hebrews.* Moundsville, W.Va.: Gospel Trumpet Co., 1899.

Select Camp-Meeting Sermons, Anderson, Ind., 1928. Anderson, Ind.: Gospel Trumpet Co., 1928.

Shaw, S. B. *Echoes of the General Holiness Assembly, Chicago, May 3–13, 1901.* "The Higher Christian Life": Sources for the Study of Holiness, Pentecostal, and Keswick Movements. New York: Garland, 1984.

Simpson, A. B. *Discovery of Divine Healing.* New York: Alliance Press Co., 1903.

———. *Divine Healing Pamphlets.* New York, N.Y.: Christian Alliance Publishing Co., 1885.

———. *The Four-Fold Gospel.* Harrisburg, Penn.: Christian Publications, Inc., 1925.

———. *Friday Meeting Talks, or, Divine Prescriptions for the Sick and Suffering.* New York: Christian Alliance Publishing Co., 1894.

———. *The Gospel of Healing.* Rev. ed. New York: Christian Alliance Publishing Co., 1915.

———. *Inquiries and Answers Concerning Divine Healing.* New York: Christian Alliance Publishing Co., n.d.

———. *The Lord for the Body with Questions and Answers on Divine Healing.* New York: Christian Alliance Publishing Co., 1925.

———. *My Medicine Chest; or, Helps to Divine Healing.* New York: Christian Alliance Publishing Co., n.d.

Smith, Frederick George. *Evolution of Christianity; or, Origin, Nature, and Development of the Religion of the Bible.* Anderson, Ind.: Gospel Trumpet Co., 1911.

———. *Is Man Immortal?* Anderson, Ind.: Gospel Trumpet Co., n.d.

———. *The Last Reformation*. Anderson, Ind.: Gospel Trumpet Co., 1919.

———. *The Revelation Explained*. Anderson, Ind.: Gospel Trumpet Co., 1907.

———. *Sanctification and the Baptism of the Holy Spirit*. Anderson, Ind.: Gospel Trumpet Co., n.d.

———. *What the Bible Teaches; A Systematic Presentation of the Fundamental Principles of Truth Contained in the Holy Scriptures*. Anderson, Ind.: Gospel Trumpet Co., 1914.

Smith, Sarah. *Life Sketches of Mother Sarah Smith: "A Mother in Israel."* Moundsville, W.Va.: Gospel Trumpet Co., 1902.

Smith, Uriah. *The Sanctuary and its Cleansing*. Battle Creek, Mich.: Steam Press, 1877.

Stanton, R. L. *Gospel Parallelisms: Illustrated in the Healing of Body and Soul*. Buffalo, N.Y.: Offices of Triumphs of Faith, 1883.

———. "Healing through Faith." *Presbyterian Review* 5, no. 17 (1884): 49–79.

Steele, Daniel. *Half-Hours with St. Paul and Other Bible Readings*. Boston: Christian Witness Co., 1895.

———. *Love Enthroned; Essays on Evangelical Perfection*. New York: Nelson and Phillips, 1875. Reprint, Holiness Data Ministries, Digital Edition 07/24/2001.

———. *Milestone Papers*. Kaifeng, Honan, China: Kaifeng Bible School, n.d. Reprint, Holiness Data Ministries, Digital Edition 07/14/95.

———. *A Substitute for Holiness, or, Antinomianism Revived; or, the Theology of the So-Called Plymouth Brethren Examined and Refuted*. "The Higher Christian Life": Sources for the Study of Holiness, Pentecostal, and Keswick Movements. New York: Garland, 1984.

Stockmayer, Otto. *Sickness and the Gospel*. New York: A. C. Gaebelein, [ca. 1878].

Teasley, D. Otis. *Private Lectures to Men and Boys*. Moundsville, W.Va.: Gospel Trumpet Co., 1905.

———. *Private Lectures to Mothers and Daughters on Sexual Purity*. Moundsville, W.Va.: Gospel Trumpet Co., 1904.

Torrey, Reuben A. *Divine Healing: Does God Perform Miracles Today?* Grand Rapids, Mich.: Baker Book House, 1924.

Trall, R. T. *The Hydropathic Encyclopedia: A System of Hydropathy and Hygiene, in Eight Parts, Designed as a Guide to Families and Students, and a Text-Book for Physicians*. New York: Fowlers and Wells, 1854.

———. *Sexual Physiology: A Scientific and Popular Exposition of the Fundamental Problems of Sociology*. New York: M. L. Holbrook, 1881. Reprint, New York: Arno Press, 1974.

Vincent, Marvin R. "Dr. Stanton on 'Healing through Faith.'" *Presbyterian Review* 5, no. 18 (1884): 305–29.

——. "Modern Miracles." *Presbyterian Review* 4, no. 15 (1883): 473–502.

Warfield, Benjamin Breckinridge. *Miracles: Yesterday and Today: True and False*. 1918. Reprint (original title *Counterfeit Miracles*), Grand Rapids, Mich.: Eerdmans, 1965.

Warner, Daniel Sidney. *The Altar and the Mercy-Seat*. Grand Junction, Mich.: Gospel Trumpet Co., n.d.

——. *Bible Proofs of the Second Work of Grace, or, Entire Sanctification as a Distinct Experience, Subsequent to Justification, Established by the United Testimony of Several Hundred Texts, Including a Description of the Great Holiness Crisis of the Present Age, by the Prophets*. Goshen, Ind.: Evangelical United Mennonite Publishing Society, 1880.

——. *The Church of God; or, What Is the Church and What Is It Not*. Moundsville, W.Va.: Gospel Trumpet Co., n.d.

——. *The Evening Light*. Grand Junction, Mich.: Gospel Trumpet Co., 1895.

——. "An Explanation About Divine Healing." Pages 114–19 in *Divine Healing*. Edited by Warren C. Roark. Anderson, Ind.: Warner Press, 1945.

——. *The Great Tobacco Sin*. Grand Junction, Mich.: Gospel Trumpet Co., n.d.

——. *Innocence*. Grand Junction, Mich.: Gospel Trumpet Co., 1896.

——. Journal. Archives of the Church of God. Anderson, Ind., 1872–1879.

——. *Marriage and Divorce*. Grand Junction, Mich.: Gospel Trumpet Co., 1895.

——. *Poems of Grace and Truth*. Grand Junction, Mich.: Gospel Trumpet Co., 1890.

——. *The Sabbath; or, Which Day to Keep*. Grand Junction, Mich.: Gospel Trumpet Co., 1884.

——. *Salvation: Present, Perfect, Now or Never*. Grand Junction, Mich.: Gospel Trumpet Co., n.d.

——. *Train Your Children for Heaven*. Grand Junction, Mich.: Gospel Trumpet Co., n.d.

——. *What Is the Soul? or, 100 Scriptures Proving That Man Possesses a Spiritual and Immortal Element Called the Soul, the Spirit, and the Inner Man, Which Goes to God and the Death of the Body*. Grand Junction, Mich.: Gospel Trumpet Co., n.d.

Warner, Daniel Sidney, and Herbert McClellan Riggle. *The Cleansing of the Sanctuary; or, the Church of God in Type and Antitype, and in Prophecy and Revelation*. Moundsville, W.Va.: Gospel Trumpet Co., 1903.

Warner, Daniel Sidney, and Barney E. Warren, eds. *Anthems from the Throne*. 2d ed. Grand Junction, Mich.: Gospel Trumpet Co., 1888.

Warren, Barney E., and Andrew L. Byers, eds. *Junior Hymns; Prepared for the Sunday School and for Religious Meetings of Children and Young People Generally.* Anderson, Ind.: Gospel Trumpet Co., 1914.

———. *Songs of the Evening Light; for Sunday-Schools, Missionary and Revival Meetings, and Gospel Work in General.* Moundsville, W.Va.: Gospel Trumpet Co., 1897.

Warren, Barney E., Andrew L. Byers, D. Otis Teasley, and C. E. Hunter, eds. *Salvation Echoes; a New Collection of Spiritual Songs Hymning the Tidings of Full Salvation, Suitable for Evangelistic Work and Gospel Services in General.* Moundsville, W.Va.: Gospel Trumpet Co., 1900.

Warren, Barney E., and Daniel Sidney Warner, eds. *Echoes from Glory; for Sunday-School and for Prayer, Praise and Gospel Meetings, with Primary Instruction in Music.* Grand Junction, Mich.: Gospel Trumpet Co., 1893.

Washburn, Josephine M. *History and Reminiscences of the Holiness Church Work in Southern California and Arizona.* "The Higher Christian Life": Sources for the Study of Holiness, Pentecostal, and Keswick Movements. New York: Garland, 1985.

Weaver, Edward E. *Mind and Health: With an Examination of Some Systems of Divine Healing.* New York: Macmillan, 1913.

Weaver, George S. *Lectures on Mental Science According to the Philosophy of Phrenology: Delivered to the Anthropological Society of the Western Liberal Institute of Marietta, Ohio, in the Autumn of 1851.* New York: Fowlers and Wells, 1852.

Wells, Samuel R. *How to Read Character: A New Illustrated Hand-Book of Phrenology and Physiognomy: For Students and Examiners: With a Descriptive Chart.* New York: Samuel R. Wells Publisher, 1869.

Wesley, John. *A Plain Account of Christian Perfection.* London: Epworth Press, 1952.

White, Ellen G. *The Ministry of Healing.* Mountain View, Calif.: Pacific Press Publishing Association, 1942.

———. *Spiritual Gifts: Important Facts of Faith: Laws of Health, and Testimonies Nos. 1–10.* Washington, D.C.: Review and Herald Publishing Association, 1945. Reprint, facsimile reproduction.

———. *Steps to Christ.* Washington, D.C.: Review and Herald Publishing Association, 1921.

White, Ronald C., Jr. *Liberty and Justice for All: Racial Reform and the Social Gospel, 1877–1925.* San Francisco: Harper & Row, 1990.

Wickersham, Henry C. *A History of the Church: From the Birth of Christ to the Present Time: Embracing an Account of the Lives of the Apostles, and Many Eminent Christians and Reformers That Have Lived since Christ; Also a Biographical Notice of the Principal Martyrs and Promoters of*

Christianity, Illustrating Their Constancy and Zeal, Suffering and Fortitude. Moundsville, W.Va.: Gospel Trumpet Co., 1900.

———. *Holiness Bible Subjects.* Grand Junction, Mich.: Gospel Trumpet Co., 1890.

Winebrenner, John. *A Brief Scriptural View of the Church of God.* Rev. ed. Harrisburg, Penn.: Board of Publication of the Church of God, 1878.

Wood, J. A. *Perfect Love.* Rev. and enl. ed. Noblesville, Ind.: J. Edwin Newby, 1967.

———. *Purity and Maturity.* North Attleboro, Mass.: J. A. Wood, 1882. Reprint, Holiness Data Ministries, Digital Edition 07/26/95.

Worship the Lord: Hymnal of the Church of God. Anderson, Ind.: Warner Press, 1989.

Secondary Sources

Abzug, Robert H. *Cosmos Crumbling: American Reform and the Religious Imagination.* New York: Oxford University Press, 1994.

Adams, Robert H. "The Hymnody of the Church of God (1885–1980) as a Reflection of That Church's Theological and Cultural Changes." D.M.A. diss., Southwestern Baptist Theological Seminary, 1980.

Albanese, Catherine L. *Nature Religion in America.* Chicago History of American Religion. Chicago: University of Chicago Press, 1990.

———. "Physic and Metaphysic in Nineteenth-Century America: Medical Sectarians and Religious Healing." *Church History* 55, no. 4 (1986): 489–502.

———. "The Poetics of Healing: Root Metaphors and Rituals in Nineteenth-Century America." *Soundings* 63, no. 4 (1980): 381–406.

Albrecht, Daniel. *Rites in the Spirit: A Ritual Approach to Pentecostal/Charismatic Spirituality.* Edited by John Christopher Thomas, Rickie D. Moore, and Steven J. Land. Journal of Pentecostal Theology Supplement Series 17. Sheffield: Sheffield Academic Press, 1999.

Arnett, William M. "The Role of the Holy Spirit in Entire Sanctification in the Writings of John Wesley." *Wesleyan Theological Journal* 14, no. 2 (1979): 15–30.

Baer, Jonathan R. "Perfectly Empowered Bodies: Divine Healing in Modernizing America." Ph.D. diss., Yale University, 2002.

———. "Redeemed Bodies: The Functions of Divine Healing in Incipient Pentecostalism." *Church History* 70, no. 4 (2001): 735–71.

Bassett, Paul M. "The Interplay of Christology and Ecclesiology in the Theology of the Holiness Movement." *Wesleyan Theological Journal* 16, no. 2 (1981): 79–94.

———. "Study in the Theology of the Early Holiness Movement." *Methodist History* 13 (1975): 61–84.

Bassett, Paul M., and William M. Greathouse. *Exploring Christian Holiness: The Historical Development.* 3 vols. Vol. 2. Kansas City, Mo.: Beacon Hill Press, 1985.

Bederman, Gail. "'The Women Have Had Charge of the Church Work Long Enough': The Men and Religion Forward Movement of 1911–1912 and the Masculinization of Middle-Class Protestantism." Pages 107–40 in *A Mighty Baptism: Race, Gender, and the Creation of American Protestantism.* Edited by Susan Juster and Lisa MacFarlane. Ithaca, N.Y.: Cornell University Press, 1996.

Bedford, William Boyd, Jr. "'A Larger Christian Life': A. B. Simpson and the Early Years of the Christian and Missionary Alliance." Ph.D. diss., University of Virginia, 1992.

Bellah, Robert N. *Beyond Belief: Essays on Religion in a Post-Traditionalist World.* Berkeley, Calif.: University of California Press, 1991.

Bendroth, Margaret L. "Children of Adam Children of God: Christian Nurture in Early Nineteenth-Century America." *Theology Today* 56, no. 4 (2000): 495–505.

Berg, Daniel N. "The Theological Context of American Wesleyanism." *Wesleyan Theological Journal* 20, no. 1 (1985): 45–60.

Bittlinger, Arnold, ed. *The Church Is Charismatic: The World Council of Churches and the Charismatic Renewal.* Geneva: Renewal and Congregational Life, World Council of Churches, 1982.

Bloom, Lynn Z. "'It's all for Your Own Good:' Parent-Child Relationships in Popular American Child Rearing Literature, 1820–1970." *Journal of Popular Culture* 10, no. 1 (1976): 191–98.

Blumhofer, Edith. *Aimee Semple McPherson: Everybody's Sister.* Edited by Mark A. Noll and Nathan O. Hatch, *Library of Religious Biography.* Grand Rapids, Mich.: William B. Eerdmans Publishing Co., 1993.

———. *The Assemblies of God: A Chapter in the Story of American Pentecostalism.* Vol. 1. Springfield, Mo.: Gospel Publishing House, 1989.

———. *Restoring the Faith: The Assemblies of God, Pentecostalism, and American Culture.* Urbana: University of Illinois Press, 1993.

Blumhofer, Edith L., Russell P. Spitler, and Grant A. Wacker. *Pentecostal Currents in American Protestantism.* Urbana: University of Illinois Press, 1999.

Braude, Ann. *Radical Spirits: Spiritualism and Women's Rights in Nineteenth-Century America.* Boston: Beacon Press, 1989.

Brereton, Virginia Lieson. *From Sin to Salvation: Stories of Women's Conversions, 1800 to the Present.* Bloomington: Indiana University Press, 1991.

Brockwell, Charles W. "John Wesley's Doctrine of Justification." *Wesleyan Theological Journal* 18, no. 2 (1983): 18–32.

Brooke, John H. *Science and Religion: Some Historical Perspectives.* Cambridge: Cambridge University Press, 1991.

Brown, Delwin, ed. *Converging on Culture: Theologians in Dialogue with Cultural Analysis and Criticism.* New York: Oxford University Press, 2001.

Brown, Kenneth O. *Inskip, McDonald, Fowler: "Wholly and Forever Thine": Early Leadership in the National Camp Meeting Association for the Promotion of Holiness.* Hazelton, Pa.: Holiness Archives, 1999.

Bundy, David D. "The Historiography of the Wesleyan-Holiness Tradition." *Wesleyan Theological Journal* 30, no. 1 (1995): 55–77.

———. "Spiritual Advice to a Seeker: Letters to T. B. Barratt from Azusa Street, 1906." *Pneuma* 14 (1992): 159–170.

Burgess, Stanley M., and Gary B. McGee, eds. *Dictionary of Pentecostal and Charismatic Movements.* Grand Rapids, Mich.: Zondervan, 1988.

Burgess, Stanley M., and Eduard M. Van Der Maas, eds. *New International Dictionary of Pentecostal and Charismatic Movements, Revised and Expanded Edition.* Grand Rapids, Mich.: Zondervan, 2002.

Burnham, John C. *Bad Habits: Drinking, Smoking, Taking Drugs, Gambling, Sexual Misbehavior, and Swearing in American History.* New York: New York University Press, 1993.

———. *Paths into American Culture: Psychology, Medicine, and Morals.* Philadelphia, Pa.: Temple University Press, 1988.

Bushman, Richard L., and Claudia L. Bushman. "The Early History of Cleanliness in America." *Journal of American History* 74, no. 4 (1988): 1213–38.

Butler, Jon. *Awash in a Sea of Faith: Christianizing the American People.* Cambridge: Harvard University Press, 1992.

Calhoun, Charles, ed. *The Gilded Age: Essays on the Origins of Modern America.* Wilmington, Del.: Scholarly Resources, 1996.

Callen, Barry L. *Confessing and Celebrating: A Tract for Transitional Times.* Anderson, Ind.: Anderson University Press, 2001.

———. "Daniel Warner: Joining Holiness and All Truth." *Wesleyan Theological Journal* 30, no. 1 (1995): 92–110.

———, ed. *Following the Light: Teachings, Testimonies, Trials and Triumphs of the Church of God Movement, Anderson.* Anderson, Ind.: Warner Press, 2000.

———. *Guide of Soul and Mind: The Story of Anderson University*. Anderson, Ind.: Anderson University and Warner Press, 1992.

———. *It's God's Church: The Life & Legacy of Daniel Sidney Warner*. Anderson, Ind.: Warner Press, 1995.

———. *Radical Christianity: The Believers Church Tradition in Christianity's History and Future*. Nappanee, Ind.: Evangel Publishing House, 1999.

———. "Wesleyan and Pentecostal Dialogue." *Pneuma* 21, no. 2 (1999): 181–287.

———. *The Wisdom of the Saints*. Anderson, Ind.: Anderson University Press, 2003.

Carson, Gerald. *Cornflake Crusade*. New York: Rinehart and Co., 1957.

Carter, Paul A. *The Spiritual Crisis of the Gilded Age*. DeKalb: Northern Illinois University Press, 1972.

Carver, Frank G. "Biblical Foundations for the 'Secondness' of Entire Sanctification." *Wesleyan Theological Journal* 22, no. 2 (1987): 7–23.

Cayleff, Susan E. *"Wash and Be Healed": The Water-Cure Movement and Women's Health*. Philadelphia: Temple University Press, 1987.

Cerillo, Augustus. "The Beginnings of American Pentecostalism: A Historiographical Overview." In *Pentecostal Currents in American Protestantism*. Edited by Edith Blumhofer, Russell P. Spittler, and Grant A. Wacker. Urbana: University of Illinois Press, 1999.

Chappell, Paul Gale. "The Divine Healing Movement in America." Ph.D. diss., Drew University, 1983.

Clear, Valorous B. "The Church of God: A Study in Social Adaptation." Ph.D. diss., University of Chicago, 1953.

———. *Where the Saints Have Trod: A Social History of the Church of God Reformation Movement*. Chesterfield, Ind.: Midwest Publications, 1977.

Cochrane, Sharlene Voogd. "Letters from Mudlavia: '...It Is Just Very Hard to Get Well.'" *Indiana Magazine of History* 97, no. 4 (2001): 296–314.

Conkin, Paul K. *American Originals: Homemade Varieties of Christianity*. Chapel Hill: University of North Carolina Press, 1997.

Cook, Philip L. *Zion City, Illinois: Twentieth-Century Utopia*. Syracuse, N.Y.: Syracuse University Press, 1996.

Coppedge, Allan. "Entire Sanctification in Early American Methodism, 1812–1835." *Wesleyan Theological Journal* 13, no. 1 (1978): 34–50.

Corbin, J. Wesley. "Christian Perfection and the Evangelical Association through 1875." *Methodist History* 7 (1969): 28–44.

Courtwright, David T. *Forces of Habit: Drugs and the Making of the Modern World*. Cambridge: Harvard University Press, 2001.

Cox, Harvey G. *Fire from Heaven: The Rise of Pentecostal Spirituality and the Reshaping of Religion in the Twenty-First Century.* Reading, Mass.: Addison-Wesley, 1995.

Creech, Joe. "Visions of Glory: The Place of the Azusa Street Revival in Pentecostal History." *Church History* 65, no. 3 (1996): 405–24.

Crews, Mickey. *The Church of God: A Social History.* Knoxville, Tenn.: University of Tennessee Press, 1990.

Crose, Lester. *Passport for a Reformation.* Anderson, Ind.: Warner Press, 1981.

Csordas, Thomas J. *Body/Meaning/Healing.* New York: Palgrave Macmillan, 2002.

Cunningham, Raymond J. "From Holiness to Healing: The Faith Cure in America, 1872–1892." *Church History* 43, no. 4 (1974): 499–513.

Danforth, Loring. *Firewalking and Religious Healing: The Anastenaria of Greece and the American Firewalking Movement.* Princeton: Princeton University Press, 1989.

Darnton, Robert. *Mesmerism and the End of the Enlightenment in France.* Cambridge: Harvard University Press, 1968.

Davies, John D. *Phrenology Fad and Science: A 19th-Century American Crusade.* New Haven: Yale University Press, 1955.

Dayton, Donald. "Asa Mahan and the Development of American Holiness Theology." *Wesleyan Theological Journal* 9, no. 1 (1974): 60–69.

———. *Discovering an Evangelical Heritage.* New York: Harper and Row, 1976.

———. "The Doctrine of the Baptism of the Holy Spirit: Its Emergence and Significance." *Wesleyan Theological Journal* 13, no. 1 (1978): 114–26.

———. "Pneumatological Issues in the Holiness Movement." *Greek Orthodox Theological Review* 31, no. 3–4 (1986): 361–87.

———. "The Rise of the Evangelical Healing Movement in Nineteenth-Century America." *Pneuma* 4, no. 1 (1982): 1–18.

———. *Theological Roots of Pentecostalism.* Metuchen, N.J.: Scarecrow Press, 1987.

———. "Yet Another Layer of the Onion; or Opening the Ecumenical Door to Let the Riffraff In." *Ecumenical Review* 40, no. 1 (1988): 87–110.

Dayton, Donald W., D. William Faupel, and David D. Bundy, eds. *"The Higher Christian Life": A Bibliographical Overview.* New York: Garland, 1985.

Dayton, Lucille Sider, and Donald Dayton. "'Your Daughters Shall Prophesy': Feminism in the Holiness Movement." *Methodist History* 14 (1976): 67–92.

Degler, Carl. "What Ought to Be and What Was: Women's Sexuality in the Nineteenth Century." *American Historical Review* 79, no. 5 (1974): 1467–90.

Delp, Robert W. "Andrew Jackson Davis: Prophet of American Spiritualism." *The Journal of American History* 54, no. 1 (1967): 43–56.

Dieter, Melvin E. "The Development of Nineteenth Century Holiness Theology." *Wesleyan Theological Journal* 20, no. 1 (1985): 61–77.

———. *The Holiness Revival of the Nineteenth Century*. Lanham, Md.: Scarecrow Press, 1996.

———. "Primitivism in the American Holiness Tradition." *Wesleyan Theological Journal* 30, no. 1 (1995): 78–91.

———. "The Wesleyan/Holiness and Pentecostal Movements: Commonalities, Confrontation, and Dialogue." *Pneuma* 12, no. 1 (1990): 4–13.

Diner, Steven J. *A Very Different Age: Americans of the Progressive Era*. New York: Hill and Wang, 1998.

Duffy, John. *From Humors to Medical Science: A History of American Medicine*. 2d ed. Urbana: University of Illinois Press, 1993.

———. *The Sanitarians: A History of American Public Health*. Chicago: University of Illinois Press, 1990.

Dunlap, E. Dale. "Tuesday Meetings, Camp Meetings, and Cabinet Meetings: A Perspective on the Holiness Movement in the Methodist Church in the U.S. in the 19th Century." *Methodist History* 13 (1975): 85–106.

DuPree, Sherry Sherrod. *African-American Holiness Pentecostal Movement: An Annotated Bibliography*. Garland Reference Library of Social Science 526. New York: Garland, 1996.

Dye, Dwight L. "The Asceticism in the Church of God Reformation Movement from 1880 to 1913." Master of Religious Education thesis, University of Tulsa, 1963.

Engs, Ruth Clifford. *Clean Living Movements in America: Cycles of Health Reform*. Westport, Conn.: Praeger, 2000.

Epstein, Barbara Leslie. *The Politics of Domesticity: Women, Evangelism, and Temperance in Nineteenth-Century America*. Middletown, Conn.: Wesleyan University Press, 1981.

Faupel, D. William. *The Everlasting Gospel: The Significance of Eschatology in the Development of Pentecostal Thought*. Journal of Pentecostal Theology Supplement Series 10. Sheffield: Sheffield Academic Press, 1996.

Fellman, Michael, and Anita Fellman. *Making Sense of Self: Medical Advice Literature in Late Nineteenth-Century America*. Philadelphia: University of Pennsylvania Press, 1981.

Fischer, Gayle Veronica. "Who Wears the Pants? Women, Dress Reform, and Power in the Mid-Nineteenth-Century United States." Ph.D. diss., Indiana University, 1995.

Fleming, James Rodger. "Science and Technology in the Second Half of the Nineteenth Century." Pages 19–37 in *The Gilded Age: Essays on the Ori-*

gins of Modern America. Edited by Charles W. Calhoun. Wilmington, Del.: Scholarly Resources, 1996.

Fletcher, Robert Samuel. *A History of Oberlin College: From Its Foundation through the Civil War*. Vol. I. Chicago: R. R. Donnelley & Sons, 1943.

Flexner, Abraham. *Medical Education in the United States and Canada: A Report to the Carnegie Foundation for the Advancement of Teaching*. New York: n.p., 1910.

Forney, Christian Henry. *History of the Churches of God in the United States*. Harrisburg, Penn.: Board of Directors of the Publishing House and Book Rooms of the Churches of God, 1914.

Forrest, Aubrey Leland. "A Study of the Development of the Basic Doctrines and Institutional Patterns in the Church of God (Anderson, Indiana)." Ph.D. diss., University of Southern California, 1948.

Foucault, Michel. *The Birth of the Clinic: An Archaeology of Medical Perception*. Translated by A. M. Sheridan Smith. New York: Vintage Books, 1975.

Frankhauser, Craig Charles. "The Heritage of Faith: An Historical Evaluation of the Holiness Movement in America." M.A. thesis, Pittsburg State University, 1983.

Fudge, Thomas A. *Daniel Warner and the Paradox of Religious Democracy in Nineteenth-Century America*. Lewiston, N.Y.: Edwin Mellen Press, 1998.

Fuller, Robert C. *Alternative Medicine and American Religious Life*. New York: Oxford University Press, 1989.

———. *Stairways to Heaven: Drugs in American Religious History*. Boulder, Colo.: Westview Press, 2000.

Garroutte, Eva Marie. "When Scientists Saw Ghosts and Why They Stopped: American Spiritualism in History." Pages 57–74 in *Vocabularies of Public Life: Empirical Essays in Symbolic Structure*. Edited by Robert Wuthnow. London: Routledge, 1992.

Geiger, Kenneth, ed. *Insights into Holiness: Discussions of Holiness by Fifteen Leading Scholars of the Wesleyan Persuasion*. Kansas City, Mo.: Beacon Hill Press, 1962.

Gevitz, Norman, ed. *Other Healers: Unorthodox Medicine in America*. Baltimore: Johns Hopkins University Press, 1988.

Ginzberg, Lori D. *Women and the Work of Benevolence: Morality, Politics, and Class in the Nineteenth-Century United States*. New Haven: Yale University Press, 1990.

Goff, James R., Jr. *Fields White Unto Harvest: Charles F. Parham and the Missionary Origins of Pentecostalism*. Fayetteville: University of Arkansas Press, 1988.

Goff, James R., Jr., and Grant Wacker, eds. *Portraits of a Generation: Early Pentecostal Leaders*. Fayetteville: University of Arkansas Press, 2002.

Grob, Gerald. "The Social History of Medicine and Disease in America: Problems and Possibilities." *Journal of Social History* 10, no. 4 (1977): 391–409.

Hall, David D., ed. *Lived Religion in America: Toward a History of Practice.* Princeton: Princeton University Press, 1997.

———. "The Victorian Connection." *American Quarterly* 27, no. 5 (1975): 561–74.

Hall, Donald E. *Muscular Christianity: Embodying the Victorian Age.* Cambridge: Cambridge University Press, 1994.

Haller, John S., Jr. *American Medicine in Transition, 1840–1910.* Urbana: University of Illinois Press, 1981.

Handy, Robert T. *A Christian America: Protestant Hopes and Historical Realities.* London: Oxford University Press, 1971.

———. *Undermined Establishment: Church-State Relations in America, 1880–1920.* Princeton: Princeton University Press, 1991.

Hardesty, Nancy A. *Faith Cure: Divine Healing in the Holiness and Pentecostal Movements.* Peabody, Mass.: Hendrickson, 2003.

Harrell, David Edwin, Jr. *All Things Are Possible: The Healing and Charismatic Revivals in Modern America.* Bloomington: Indiana University Press, 1975.

———. *Oral Roberts: An American Life.* Bloomington: Indiana University Press, 1985.

Hartman, Marvin. "The Origin and Development of the General Ministerial Assembly of the Church of God, 1917–1950." B.D. thesis, Butler University, 1958.

Hatch, Nathan O. *The Democratization of American Christianity.* New Haven: Yale University Press, 1989.

Hazen, Craig James. *The Village Enlightenment in America: Popular Religion and Science in the Nineteenth Century.* Urbana: University of Illinois Press, 2000.

Heitzenrater, Richard P. *Wesley and the People Called Methodists.* Nashville, Tenn.: Abingdon, 1995.

Hetrick, Gale. *Laughter among the Trumpets: A History of the Church of God in Michigan.* n.p.: General Assembly of the Church of God in Michigan, 1980.

Holbrook, Stewart H. *The Golden Age of Quackery.* New York: Macmillan, 1959.

Howe, Daniel Walker. "American Victorianism as a Culture." *American Quarterly* 27, no. 5 (1975): 507–32.

Hughes, Richard T., ed. *The American Quest for the Primitive Church.* Urbana: University of Illinois Press, 1988.

Hughes, Richard T., and C. Leonard Allen, eds. *Illusions of Innocence: Protestant Primitivism in America, 1630–1875*. Chicago: University of Chicago Press, 1988.

Hynson, Leon O. "Original Sin as Privation: An Inquiry into a Theology of Sin and Sanctification." *Wesleyan Theological Journal* 22, no. 2 (1987): 65–83.

Ivey, Paul Eli. *Prayers in Stone: Christian Science Architecture in the United States, 1894–1930*. Urbana: University of Illinois Press, 1999.

Jacobsen, Douglas. *Thinking in the Spirit: Theologies of the Early Pentecostal Movement*. Bloomington: Indiana University Press, 2003.

Jones, Charles Edwin. "Beulah Land and the Upper Room: Reclaiming the Text in Turn-of-the-Century Holiness and Pentecostal Spirituality." *Methodist History* 32, no. 4 (1994): 250–59.

———. *A Guide to the Study of the Holiness Movement*. ATLA Bibliography Series 1. Metuchen, N.J.: Scarecrow Press, 1974.

———. "The Inverted Shadow of Phoebe Palmer." *Wesleyan Theological Journal* 31, no. 2 (1996): 120–31.

———. *Perfectionist Persuasion: The Holiness Movement and American Methodism, 1867–1936*. Metuchen, N.J.: Scarecrow Press, 1974.

———. "Tongues-Speaking and the Wesleyan-Holiness Quest for Assurance of Salvation." *Wesleyan Theological Journal* 22, no. 2 (1987): 117–24.

Kaufman, Martin. *American Medical Education: The Formative Years, 1765–1910*. Westport, Conn.: Greenwood Press, 1976.

Kelsey, Morton T. *Healing and Christianity in Ancient Thought and Modern Times*. New York: Harper and Row, 1973.

Kerber, Linda K. "Separate Spheres, Female Worlds, Woman's Place: The Rhetoric of Women's History." *Journal of American History* 75, no. 1 (1988): 9–39.

Kern, Richard. *John Winebrenner: Nineteenth Century Reformer*. Harrisburg, Penn.: Central Publishing House, 1974.

Kern, Richard, Jack Parthemore, and Richard E. Wilkin. *Time for Review: Facts about the Founding of the Churches of God, General Conference*. Harrisburg, Penn.: Central Publishing House, 1975.

Koenig, Harold G., Michael McCullough, and David B. Larson, eds. *Handbook of Religion and Health*. New York: Oxford University Press, 2001.

Kohn, George Childs, ed. *Encyclopedia of Plague and Pestilence from Ancient Times to the Present*. Rev. ed. New York: Facts on File, 2001.

Kostlevy, William C. "Culture, Class and Gender in the Progressive Era: The Social Thought of the Free Methodist Church During the Age of Gladden, Strong and Rauschenbusch." Pages 157–82 in *Perspectives on the Social Gospel: Papers from the Inaugural Social Gospel Conference at Colgate*

Rochester Divinity School. Edited by Christopher H. Evans. Lewiston, N.Y.: Edwin Mellen Press, 1999.

———, ed. *Historical Dictionary of the Holiness Movement*. Lanham, Md.: Scarecrow Press, 2001.

———. *Holiness Manuscripts: A Guide to Sources Documenting the Wesleyan Holiness Movement in the United States and Canada*. ATLA Bibliography Series, no. 34. Metuchen, N.J.: Scarecrow Press, 1994.

Lambert, Bryon Cecil. "'Experience' in Two Church Traditions: Differing Semantic Worlds." *Wesleyan Theological Journal* 30, no. 1 (1995): 134–53.

Lindberg, David C., and Ronald L. Numbers, eds. *When Science and Christianity Meet*. Chicago: University of Chicago Press, 2003.

Lindstrom, Harald. *Wesley and Sanctification: A Study in the Doctrine of Salvation*. Grand Rapids, Mich.: Francis Asbury Press, 1980.

Lowery, Kevin T. "A Fork in the Wesleyan Road: Phoebe Palmer and the Appropriation of Christian Perfection." *Wesleyan Theological Journal* 36, no. 2 (2001): 187–222.

MacDonald, Robert H. "The Frightful Consequences of Onanism: Notes on the History of a Delusion." *Journal of the History of Ideas* 28, no. 3 (1967): 423–31.

McLoughlin, William G. "Pietism and the American Character." *American Quarterly* 17, no. 2 (1965): 163–86.

———. *Revivals, Awakenings, and Reform: An Essay on Religion and Social Change in America, 1607–1977*. Chicago: University of Chicago Press, 1978.

Maddocks, Morris. "Health and Healing in the Ministry of John Wesley." Pages 138–49 in *John Wesley: Contemporary Perspectives*. Edited by John Stacey. London: Epworth Press, 1988.

Magnuson, Norris A. *Salvation in the Slums: Evangelical Social Work, 1865–1920*. Metuchen, N.J.: Scarecrow Press, 1977.

Markowitz, Gerald E., and David Karl Rosner. "Doctors in Crisis: A Study in the Use of Medical Education Reform to Establish Modern Professional Elitism in Medicine." *American Quarterly* 25, no. 1 (1973): 83–107.

Marsden, George M. *Fundamentalism and American Culture: The Shaping of Twentieth Century Evangelicalism, 1870–1925*. New York: Oxford University Press, 1982.

Mead, Sidney E. *The Lively Experiment: The Shaping of Christianity in America*. New York: Harper and Row, 1963.

Mechling, Jay E. "Advice to Historians on Advice to Mothers." *Journal of Social History* 9, no. 1 (1975): 44–63.

Meyer, Donald. *The Positive Thinkers: Religion as Pop Psychology from Mary Baker Eddy to Oral Roberts*. New York: Pantheon Books, 1980.

Mix, Mrs. Edward. *Faith Cures and Answers to Prayer*. With a critical introduction by Rosemary D. Gooden. Syracuse, N.Y.: Syracuse University Press, 2002.

Money, John. *The Destroying Angel: Sex, Fitness & Food in the Legacy of Degeneracy Theory, Graham Crackers, Kellogg's Corn Flakes & American Health History*. Buffalo, N.Y.: Prometheus Books, 1985.

Moore, D. Marselle. "Development in Wesley's Thought on Sanctification and Perfection." *Wesleyan Theological Journal* 20, no. 2 (1985): 29–53.

Moore, R. Laurence. *In Search of White Crows: Spiritualism, Parapsychology, and American Culture*. New York: Oxford University Press, 1977.

Morantz, Regina Markell. "Feminism, Professionalism, and Germs: The Thought of Mary Putnam Jacobi and Elizabeth Blackwell." *American Quarterly* 34, no. 5 (1982): 459–78.

Morgan, H. Wayne, ed. *The Gilded Age*. Syracuse, N.Y.: Syracuse University Press, 1970.

Mullin, Robert Bruce. *Miracles and the Modern Religious Imagination*. New Haven: Yale University Press, 1996.

Mullins, Jeffrey Alan. "Making the Moral Mind: Contestations over Self-Government, Personal Responsibility, and the Body in American Culture, 1780–1860." Ph.D. diss., Johns Hopkins University, 1997.

Nelson, Shirley. *Fair, Clear, and Terrible: The Story of Shiloh, Maine*. Latham, N.Y.: British American Publishing, 1989.

Neumann, R. P. "Masturbation, Madness, and the Modern Concepts of Childhood and Adolescence." *Journal of Social History* 8, no. 3 (1975): 1–27.

Nissenbaum, Stephen. *Sex, Diet, and Debility in Jacksonian America: Sylvester Graham and Health Reform*. Westport, Conn.: Greenwood Press, 1980.

Nobel, Barry. "Religious Healing and American Courts in the Twentieth Century: The Liberties and Liabilities of Healers, Patients, and Parents." Ph.D. diss., University of California, Santa Barbara, 1991.

Numbers, Ronald L. *Prophetess of Health: Ellen G. White and the Origins of Seventh-Day Adventist Health Reform*. Knoxville: University of Tennessee Press, 1992.

Numbers, Ronald L., and Darrel W. Amundsen, eds. *Caring and Curing: Health and Medicine in the Western Religious Traditions*. Baltimore: Johns Hopkins University Press, 1998.

Numbers, Ronald L., and Jonathan M. Butler, eds. *The Disappointed: Millerism and Millenarianism in the Nineteenth Century*. Knoxville: University of Tennessee Press, 1993.

Opp, James William. "Religion, Medicine, and the Body: Protestant Faith Healing in Canada, 1880–1930." Ph.D. diss., Carleton University, Ottawa, Canada, 2000.

Ownby, Ted. *Subduing Satan: Religion, Recreation, and Manhood in the Rural South, 1865–1920.* Chapel Hill: University of North Carolina Press, 1990.

Painter, Nell Irvin. *Standing at Armageddon: The United States, 1877–1919.* New York: W. W. Norton and Co., 1987.

Peters, John Leland. *Christian Perfection and American Methodism.* Nashville, Tenn.: Abingdon, 1956.

Phillips, Harold. *Miracle of Survival.* Anderson, Ind.: Warner Press, 1979.

———. "Warner and Charles Finney" *Vital Christianity* (Oct. 6, 1974): 7–8.

Porterfield, Amanda. "Healing in the History of Christianity." *Church History* 71, no. 2 (2002): 227–41.

Purkiser, W. T. *Exploring Christian Holiness.* Vol. 1, *The Biblical Foundations.* Kansas City, Mo.: Beacon Hill Press, 1985.

Putney, Clifford. *Muscular Christianity: Manhood and Sports in Protestant America, 1880–1920.* Cambridge: Harvard University Press, 2001.

Reardon, Robert H. *The Early Morning Light.* Anderson, Ind.: Warner Press, 1979.

Reinhardt, Douglas Edward. "Faith Healing: Where Science Meets Religion in the Body of Believers." Ph.D. diss., University of North Carolina, 1982.

Ricour, Paul. "The Hermeneutics of Testimony." In *Essays on Biblical Interpretation.* Edited by Lewis S. Mudge. Philadelphia: Fortress, 1980.

Riegel, Robert E. "The Introduction of Phrenology to the United States." *American Historical Review* 39, no. 1 (1933): 73–78.

Risse, Guenter, Ronald L. Numbers, and Judith Walzer Leavitt, eds. *Medicine Without Doctors: Home Health Care in American History.* New York: Science History Publications, 1977.

Roark, Warren C., ed. *Divine Healing.* Anderson, Ind.: Warner Press, 1945.

Robins, Roger Glenn. "Plainfolk Modernist: The Radical Holiness World of A. J. Tomlinson." Ph.D. diss., Duke University, 1999.

Rosenberg, Charles. "And Heal the Sick: The Hospital and the Patient in the 19th Century America." *Journal of Social History* 10, no. 4 (1977): 428–47.

———. "The Therapeutic Revolution: Medicine, Meaning, and Social Change in Nineteenth Century America." *Perspectives in Biology and Medicine* 20 (1977).

Rothstein, William G. *American Physicians in the Nineteenth Century: From Sects to Science.* Baltimore: Johns Hopkins University Press, 1972.

Royce, J. E. "Sin or Solace? Religious Views of Alcohol and Alcoholism." *Journal of Drug Issues* 14, no. 1 (1985): 51–62.

Russell, C. Allyn. "Adoniram Judson Gordon: 19th-Century Fundamentalist." *American Baptist Quarterly* 4, no. 1 (1985): 61–89.

Sanders, Cheryl J. *Saints in Exile: The Holiness-Pentecostal Experience in African American Religion and Culture*. New York: Oxford University Press, 1996.

Schlesinger, Arthur M., Sr. "A Critical Period in American Religion, 1875–1900." In *Religion in American History*. Edited by John Mulder and John Wilson. Englewood Cliffs, N.J.: Prentice-Hall, 1978.

Shyrock, Richard H. "Sylvester Graham and the Popular Health Movement, 1830–1870." *Mississippi Valley Historical Review* 18, no. 2 (1931): 172–83.

Sizer, Sandra S. "New Spirit, New Flesh: The Poetics of Nineteenth-Century Mind-Cures." *Soundings* 63, no. 4 (1980): 407–22.

Sloan, R. P., E. Bagiella, and T. Powell. "Religion, Spirituality, and Medicine." *Lancet* 353 (1999): 664–67.

Smith, John W. V. *A Brief History of the Church of God Reformation Movement*. Anderson, Ind.: Warner Press, 1976.

———. *Heralds of a Brighter Day: Biographical Sketches of Early Leaders in the Church of God Reformation Movement*. Anderson, Ind.: Gospel Trumpet Co., 1955.

———. "Holiness and Unity." *Wesleyan Theological Journal* 10 (1975): 24–37.

———. *The Quest for Holiness and Unity: A Centennial History of the Church of God (Anderson, Indiana)*. Anderson, Ind.: Warner Press, 1980.

Smith, Timothy L. *Called Unto Holiness: The Story of the Nazarenes: The Formative Years*. Kansas City, Mo.: Nazarene Publishing House, 1962.

———. "How John Fletcher Became the Theologian of Wesleyan Perfectionism, 1770–1776." *Wesleyan Theological Journal* 15, no. 1 (1980): 68–87.

———. "John Wesley and the Second Blessing." *Wesleyan Theological Journal* 21, nos. 1 and 2 (1986): 137–58.

———. *Revivalism and Social Reform: American Protestantism on the Eve of the Civil War*. Baltimore: Johns Hopkins University Press, 1980.

———. "Righteousness and Hope: Christian Holiness and the Millennial Vision in America, 1800–1900." *American Quarterly* 31, no. 1 (1979): 21–45.

Smith-Rosenberg, Carroll, and Charles Rosenberg. "The Female Animal: Medical and Biological Views of Woman and Her Role in Nineteenth-Century America." *The Journal of American History* 60, no. 2 (1973): 332–56.

Stage, Sarah. *Female Complaints: Lydia Pinkham and the Business of Women's Medicine*. New York: Norton, 1979.

Stanley, John E. "Unity Among Diversity: Interpreting the Book of Revelation in the Church of God (Anderson)." *Wesleyan Theological Journal* 25, no. 2 (1990): 64–98.

Stanley, Susie C. *Holy Boldness: Women Preachers' Autobiographies and the Sanctified Self.* Knoxville: University of Tennessee Press, 2002.

Starr, Paul. *The Social Transformation of American Medicine: The Rise of a Sovereign Profession and the Making of a Vast Industry.* New York: Basic Books, 1982.

Stern, Madeleine B. *Heads and Headlines: The Phrenological Fowlers.* Norman: University of Oklahoma Press, 1971.

Stokes, Anson Phelps. *Church and State in the United States,* Vol. 2. New York: Harper and Brothers, 1950.

Strege, Merle D. *I Saw the Church: The Life of the Church of God Told Theologically.* Anderson, Ind.: Warner Press, 2002.

———. *A Look at the Church of God for Children, Vol. I, 1880–1930.* Anderson, Ind.: Warner Press, 1987.

———. *Tell Me Another Tale: Further Reflections on the Church of God.* Anderson, Ind.: Warner Press, 1993.

———. *Tell Me the Tale: Historical Reflections on the Church of God.* Anderson, Ind.: Warner Press, 1991.

Sweet, Leonard I., ed. *The Evangelical Tradition in America.* Macon, Ga.: Mercer University Press, 1997.

Synan, Vinson. "A Healer in the House? A Historical Perspective on Healing in the Pentecostal/Charismatic Tradition." *Asian Journal of Pentecostal Studies* 3, no. 2 (2000): 189–201.

———. *The Holiness-Pentecostal Tradition: Charismatic Movements in the Twentieth Century.* 2d ed. Grand Rapids, Mich.: Eerdmans, 1997.

———, ed. *Aspects of Pentecostal-Charismatic Origins.* Plainfield, N.J.: Logos International, 1975.

———, ed. *The Century of the Holy Spirit: 100 Years of Pentecostal and Charismatic Renewal, 1901–2001.* Nashville, Tenn.: Thomas Nelson, 2001.

Taves, Ann. *Fits, Trances, & Visions: Experiencing Religion and Explaining Experience from Wesley to James.* Princeton: Princeton University Press, 1999.

Taylor, Mark C., ed. *Critical Terms for Religious Studies.* Chicago: University of Chicago Press, 1998.

Taylor, Richard S. *Exploring Christian Holiness.* 3 vols. Vol. 3. Kansas City, Mo.: Beacon Hill Press, 1985.

Thornton, Wallace. *Radical Righteousness: Personal Ethics and the Development of the Holiness Movement.* Salem, Ohio: Schmul Publishing Co., 1998.

Tomes, Nancy. *The Gospel of Germs*. Cambridge: Harvard University Press, 1998.

Turley, Briane K. *A Wheel within a Wheel: Southern Methodism and the Georgia Holiness Association*. Macon, Ga.: Mercer University Press, 1999.

Van Dussen, D. Gregory. "The Bergen Camp Meeting in the American Holiness Movement." *Methodist History* 21 (1983): 69–89.

Wacker, Grant. *Heaven Below: Early Pentecostals and American Culture*. Cambridge: Harvard University Press, 2001.

———. "The Holy Spirit and the Spirit of the Age in American Protestantism, 1880–1910." *The Journal of American History* 72, no. 1 (1985): 45–62.

———. "Marching to Zion: Religion in a Modern Utopian Community." *Church History* 54 (1985): 496–511.

Wall, Robert Walter. "The Embourgeoisement of the Free Methodist Ethos." *Wesleyan Theological Journal* 25, no. 1 (1990): 117–29.

Walters, Ronald G. *American Reformers 1815–1860*. New York: Hill and Wang, 1978.

———. *Primers for Prudery: Sexual Advice to Victorian America*. Baltimore: Johns Hopkins University Press, 2000.

Ware, Steven L. "Restoring the New Testament Church: Varieties of Restorationism in the Radical Holiness Movement of the Late Nineteenth and Early Twentieth Centuries." *Pneuma* 21, no. 2 (1999): 233–50.

Warner, Wayne E. *The Woman Evangelist: The Life and Times of Charismatic Evangelist Maria B. Woodworth-Etter*. Metuchen, N.J.: Scarecrow Press, 1986.

Warner, Wayne M. *Saint Sebastian: The Long Shadow*. Battle Creek, Mich.: n.p., 2000.

Welch, Douglas E. *Ahead of His Times: A Life of George P. Tasker*. Anderson, Ind.: Anderson University Press, 2001.

Wessinger, Catherine, ed. *Women's Leadership in Marginal Religions: Explorations Outside the Mainstream*. Urbana: University of Illinois Press, 1993.

Wharton, James C. *Crusaders for Fitness: The History of American Health Reformers*. Princeton: Princeton University Press, 1982.

White, Charles E. "Phoebe Palmer and the Development of Pentecostal Pneumatology." *Wesleyan Theological Journal* 23, nos. 1 and 2 (1988): 198–212.

———. "What the Holy Spirit Can and Cannot Do: The Ambiguities of Phoebe Palmer's Theology of Experience." *Wesleyan Theological Journal* 20, no. 1 (1985): 108–21.

White, Ronald C., Jr. *Liberty and Justice for All: Racial Reform and the Social Gospel, 1877–1925*. San Francisco: Harper & Row, 1990.

Wiebe, Robert H. *The Search for Order, 1877–1920*. New York: Hill and Wang, 1967.

Wigger, John H. *Taking Heaven by Storm: Methodism and the Rise of Popular Christianity in America*. Urbana: University of Illinois Press, 1998.

Wilcox, Leslie D. *Be Ye Holy: A Study of the Teaching of Scripture Relative to Entire Sanctification with a Sketch of History and the Literature of the Holiness Movement*. Rev. ed. Salem, Ohio: Schmul Publishing Co., 1994.

Wilhoit, Mel R. "American Holiness Hymnody: Some Questions: A Methodology." *Wesleyan Theological Journal* 25, no. 2 (1990): 39–63.

Wilkinson, John. "Physical Healing and the Atonement." *Evangelical Quarterly* 63, no. 2 (1991): 149–67.

Wood, Laurence W. "Pentecostal Sanctification in Wesley and Early Methodism." *Pneuma* 21, no. 2 (1999): 251–87.

Wrobel, Arthur, ed. *Pseudo-Science and Society in Nineteenth-Century America*. Lexington: The University Press of Kentucky, 1987.

Yearbook of the Church of God: United States and Canada. Anderson, Ind.: Church of God Ministries, 2004.

Young, James Harvey. "American Medical Quackery in the Age of the Common Man." *Mississippi Valley Historical Review* 47, no. 4 (1961): 579–93.

———. *Pure Food: Securing the Federal Food and Drugs Act of 1906*. Princeton: Princeton University Press, 1989.

Zimdars-Swartz, Sandra L. *Encountering Mary: Visions of Mary from La Salette to Medjugorje*. New York: Avon Books, 1992.

INDEX

medicine, 104; on physicians,
106
Byers, Jennie M., 68
Byrum, Enoch E.: *The Boy's
Companion,* 128–29;
decreasing influence of, 165–
68; forward move (1895), 79–
80; on Good Samaritan parable,
103; on healing power, 77–79,
82–83, 97–98, 170, 185; on
health/diet, 105–6, 126, 157–
59; on "if it be thy will," 110–
11; managerial style, 76–77;
marriages, 73–74; on medicinal
remedies, 80–81; on trials, 151–
52
Byrum, Noah H., 53n48, 142n33

Calomel, 5
camp meetings: in Anderson (IN), 167–
68; in Bangor (MI), 71–75;
Byrum's gift of miracles at, 79–
80; contagious diseases at, 158;
early gatherings, 12–13;
importance of, 45–46
Carson City Resolutions, 42–44
Carter, R. Kelso, 113n2
chain of healing testimony, 72
children, 74, 127–31
cholera, 6–7, 17n33
Christian Science, 11, 164
Church of God: forward move (1895),
79–80; histories of, xiv–xv,
186; institutional development,
165–68; name, xixn1; organs,
44–48; origins, 23, 34–36;
splits, 136; theology, xiv, 37–
44, 164–65, 169–74, 185–86
Church of God School of Theology, 47
clay, 103–5
Cole, George, 106–7, 112
Cole, Mary, xxin21, 61n126, 176n42
Coles, Langdon B., 123
Colossians, Epistle to, 107–9
Combe, George, 8–9
congregational ministries, 45
contagious diseases, 157–59
conversions, 72, 82

1 Corinthians, 78
corset wearing, 130
Courtney, Josephine (Miller), 72–74,
81, 182n122
creeds, 43
criminal trials: *Gospel Trumpet* reports,
151–53; lessons learned, 156–
57; outcomes, 150–51, 155–56;
outsider reports, 154–55
Cullis, Charles, 13–14, 93–94, 113n9
cultural context, 184–85

denominations: holiness cleansing of,
42; organs of church as, 47–48;
as sect Babylon, 37, 43–44;
Warner's rejection of, 26–27,
35–36
devil, 179n75
diet: for children, 128; Graham on, 6–8;
Warner on, 26, 29–30, 33–34,
125
diseases. *See* illness
divine healing: benefits, 2–3, 75; Bible
proofs of, 91–95, 97–100; in
Christianity, xvi–xviii; defining
Church of God, xiv, xv, xvii,
112; early theology, 13–14; as
essential for ministry, 78–79,
96–98, 169; importance to
historians, xvi; reinterpretation
of, 161–63, 170–74; as subject
for study, 183–85; trials, *see*
criminal trials. *See also* failures
of divine healing
Divine Healing, 171–72
doctors. *See* medicinal remedies;
physicians
doctrines. *See* atonement doctrine of
divine healing; holiness
doctrine; justification doctrine
domesticity ideals, 127–28
Dowie, John Alexander, 114n16, 164–
65, 179

ecclesiology, 41–44
education, 47

ABOUT THE AUTHOR

Michael S. Stephens lives in Nashville, Tennessee with his wife Heather Harriss and their children, Daniel and Emma Anne. He grew up in Anderson, Indiana, in the Church of God. He has an M.Div. from Princeton Theological Seminary and a Ph.D. in church history from Vanderbilt University. He is an acquisitions editor in the Bible and Reference department at Thomas Nelson Publishers, and he is an adjunct professor of church history in the Distributed and Extended Learning program of Asbury Theological Seminary. Michael and Heather and their children are active members of Belmont United Methodist Church in Nashville.